Extra-Cranial Applications of Diffusion-Weighted MRI

Edited by

Bachir Taouli
Mount Sinai School of Medicine, Department of Radiology, New York, USA

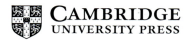

CAMBRIDGE UNIVERSITY PRESS
Cambridge, New York, Melbourne, Madrid, Cape Town, Singapore,
São Paulo, Delhi, Dubai, Tokyo, Mexico City

Cambridge University Press
The Edinburgh Building, Cambridge CB2 8RU, UK

Published in the United States of America by
Cambridge University Press, New York

www.cambridge.org
Information on this title: www.cambridge.org/9780521518697

First published 2011

Printed in the United Kingdom at the University Press, Cambridge

A catalogue record for this publication is available from the British Library

Library of Congress Cataloging-in-Publication data

Extra-cranial applications of diffusion-weighted MRI / edited by Bachir
Taouli.
     p. ; cm.
  Includes bibliographical references and index.
  ISBN 978-0-521-51869-7 (Hardback)
  1. Diffusion magnetic resonance imaging.   I. Taouli, Bachir.
  [DNLM: 1. Diffusion Magnetic Resonance Imaging–methods.
WN 185 E96 2011]
  RC78.7.N83.E98 2011
  616.07'548–dc22
                                                                2010022747

ISBN 978-0-521-51869-7 Hardback

Contents

Contributors

Andriy M. Babsky, PhD
Department of Radiology, Indiana University,
Indianapolis, Indiana, USA

Navin Bansal, PhD
Department of Radiology, Indiana University,
Indianapolis, Indiana, USA

Andrea Baur-Melnyk, MD
Department of Clinical Radiology,
University Hospitals – Grosshadern, LMU
Ludwig Maximilian University of Munich,
Munich, Germany

David J. Collins, PhD
The Royal Marsden NHS Foundation Trust,
Department of Radiology, Sutton, UK

Frederik De Keyzer, MSc
University Hospitals Leuven,
Department of Radiology, Leuven, Belgium

Nandita M. deSouza, MD, FRCR
MRI Unit, Cancer Imaging Centre at the Institute
of Cancer Research and Royal Marsden Hospital,
Sutton, UK

Olaf Dietrich, PhD
Josef Lissner Laboratory for Biomedical Imaging,
Department of Clinical Radiology, University
Hospitals – Grosshadern,
LMU Ludwig Maximilian University of Munich,
Munich, Germany

Yong Guo, MD
Radiology Department, Navy General Hospital of the
PLA, Beijing, China

Tomoaki Ichikawa, MD, PhD
Department of Radiology, University of Yamanashi,
Shimokato, Japan

Jens Jensen, PhD
Department of Radiology, Physiology, and
Neuroscience, New York University Langone Medical
Center, New York, USA

Shenghong Ju
Department of Radiology, Indiana University,
Indianapolis, Indiana, USA

Sooah Kim, MD
Department of Radiology, New York University
Langone Medical Center, Department of Radiology,
New York, USA

Dow-Mu Koh, MD
The Royal Marsden NHS Foundation Trust,
Department of Radiology, Sutton, UK

Thomas C. Kwee, MD, PhD
University Medical Center Utrecht,
Department of Radiology, Utrecht, The Netherlands

Masayuki Maeda, MD
Department of Radiology, Mie University School
of Medicine, Tsu, Japan

Utaroh Motosugi, MD, PhD
Department of Radiology, University of Yamanashi,
Shimokato, Japan

Ali Muhi, MD
Department of Radiology, University of Yamanashi,
Shimokato, Japan

Anwar R. Padhani, FRCP, FRCR
Paul Strickland Scanner Centre, Mount Vernon
Hospital, Northwood, UK

Sophie F. Riches, MPhys, MSc
Cancer Imaging Centre at the Institute of Cancer
Research and Royal Marsden Hospital,
Sutton, UK

Katsuhiro Sano, MD, PhD
Assistant Professor, Department of Radiology,
University of Yamanashi, Shimokato, Japan

Hela Sbano, MRCP, FRCR
Imperial College NHS Trust, Hammersmith Hospital,
London, UK

Eric E. Sigmund, PhD
University Langone Medical Center,
New York, USA

Taro Takahara, MD, PhD
Tokai University School of Engineering,
Department of Biomedical Engineering,

Japan and University Medical Center Utrecht,
Department of Radiology,
Utrecht, The Netherlands

Bachir Taouli, MD
Mount Sinai School of Medicine,
Department of Radiology,
New York, USA

Harriet C. Thoeny, MD
Department of Diagnostic, Interventional, and
Pediatric Radiology, University of Bern, Bern,
Switzerland

Preface

Powered by the tremendous advances in technology over the last few years, MR imaging has the potential to go beyond morphology and provide functional information on organs and tumors. One of the most promising techniques is diffusion-weighted MRI (DWI), which has been routine in brain imaging since the early nineties, and is now applied more and more often in body imaging. I developed an interest in DWI when I was a resident; I thought it was fascinating to provide a different "dimension" to morphology. In the last few years, diffusion image quality outside the brain has improved tremendously, as major vendors and many research groups have focused their interest on this technique. While certain clinical applications of DWI – such as tumor detection and characterization – are more or less established and adopted by many academic and non-academic centers, DWI is still in its infancy, and other applications such as diffuse liver and renal disease and tumor treatment response have to be established in larger confirmatory studies. I am pleased to serve as the editor of this book, compiling the most recent information on DWI applied to the body by world-renowned experts in the field. The text is divided by organ, thus making it more easily searchable, and will serve beginners as well as more advanced diffusion users. With this book, we hope to attract more researchers into body diffusion imaging, which has enormous potential particularly in oncology.

Bachir Taouli, MD
Department of Radiology,
Mount Sinai Medical School,
New York, USA

Chapter

1

Basic physical principles of body diffusion-weighted MRI

Eric E. Sigmund and Jens Jensen

1.1 Introduction

The possibility of sensitizing nuclear magnetic resonance (NMR) signals to molecular diffusion was recognized in the early, pioneering days of NMR by Hahn[1], Carr and Purcell[2]. In the 1960s, the Stejskal–Tanner pulse sequence for measuring diffusion properties was introduced and has been a mainstay of diffusion NMR every since[3–4]. The Stejskal–Tanner sequence is also the prototypical pulse sequence for diffusion-weighted imaging (DWI), although for human imaging there are a number of variants and alternative sequences that help manage the practical challenges of clinical scanning.

Until recently, DWI in humans has been dominated by brain applications, to a large degree because the relatively long transverse relaxation times (T2) in the brain help maintain a sufficient signal-to-noise ratio (SNR) and the good field homogeneity helps minimize imaging artifacts. However, recent improvements in scanning hardware and pulse sequence design have now made feasible good quality DWI for the body, and body applications are becoming increasingly common[5–6].

In this chapter, we review the basic physical principals of DWI, emphasizing issues particularly pertinent to body applications. We begin with diffusion NMR physics, covering both the relevant concepts of molecular diffusion and the essential theory for the Stejskal–Tanner pulse sequence. We will consider practical aspects of image acquisition, such as sequence selection and artifact reduction. The analysis of DWI data and an overview of selected important body applications will be discussed.

1.2 Diffusion NMR physics

Molecules within a liquid move in a complicated pattern that can be regarded as a random process. This process may be quantified by various types of probability distributions – the most commonly used being the probability $P(\mathbf{r}, t)$ of a molecule moving a displacement vector $\mathbf{r}$ in a time t. For DWI, the molecule of interest is generally water.

Since the total probability of moving some amount is always unity, we have the normalization condition

$$\int d^3 r P(\mathbf{r}, t) = 1. \tag{1.1}$$

The mean or average value of an arbitrary function $F(\mathbf{r})$ is simply given by

$$\langle F(\mathbf{r}) \rangle \equiv \int d^3 r P(\mathbf{r}, t) F(\mathbf{r}), \tag{1.2}$$

with the angle brackets being a shorthand for the average.

The molecular motion in a particular direction $\mathbf{n}$ ($|\mathbf{n}| = 1$) is conveniently characterized by the "moments":

$$M_i(\mathbf{n}) \equiv \langle (\mathbf{r} \cdot \mathbf{n})^i \rangle, \tag{1.3}$$

where i is a positive integer. In equilibrium, we have the symmetry property $P(\mathbf{r}, t) = P(-\mathbf{r}, t)$, which implies that M_i vanishes for odd values of i. Note that $M_1 = 0$ is the condition for no net flow of molecules.

The diffusion coefficient in the direction $\mathbf{n}$ is defined by

$$D(\mathbf{n}) \equiv \frac{1}{2t} M_2(\mathbf{n}). \tag{1.4}$$

Extra-Cranial Applications of Diffusion-Weighted MRI, ed. Bachir Taouli. Published by Cambridge University Press.
© Cambridge University Press 2011.

This is the most basic diffusion metric for DWI. For normal, unrestricted diffusion $D(\mathbf{n})$ is time independent and Eq. (1.4) reduces to the well-known Einstein or Fickian relation in which position dispersion grows linearly with time, with a slope given by the diffusion coefficient[7]. Fick's law holds exactly for all regimes for an ideal liquid.

Another metric that has recently been introduced is the diffusional kurtosis defined by[8]

$$K(\mathbf{n}) \equiv \frac{M_4(\mathbf{n})}{[M_2(\mathbf{n})]^2} - 3. \tag{1.5}$$

The average of $D(\mathbf{n})$ over all directions is the mean diffusivity (MD), while the average of $K(\mathbf{n})$ over all directions is the mean kurtosis (MK).

If the diffusion moments are independent of the direction $\mathbf{n}$, the diffusion is referred to as "isotropic." Otherwise, the diffusion is referred to as "anisotropic." Some biological tissues, such as healthy liver, are isotropic to an excellent approximation, while others, such as muscle, cerebral white matter, and renal medulla, are distinctly anisotropic.

For anisotropic tissues (cerebral white matter, renal medulla, skeletal muscle), it is useful to define a diffusion tensor by[9–10]

$$D_{ij} \equiv \frac{1}{2t} \langle r_i r_j \rangle, \tag{1.6}$$

where r_i ($i = 1$, 2, or 3) is a component of the displacement vector $\mathbf{r}$. In terms of the diffusion tensor, the diffusion coefficient can be written as

$$D(\mathbf{n}) = \sum_{i=1}^{3} \sum_{j=1}^{3} D_{ij} n_i n_j, \tag{1.7}$$

where n_i is a component of the direction vector $\mathbf{n}$. Therefore, knowledge of the diffusion tensor allows one to calculate the diffusion coefficient in an arbitrary direction. The diffusion tensor can be written as a 3×3 matrix:

$$D_{ij} \equiv \begin{pmatrix} D_{11} & D_{12} & D_{13} \\ D_{21} & D_{22} & D_{23} \\ D_{31} & D_{32} & D_{33} \end{pmatrix}. \tag{1.8}$$

From the definition of the diffusion tensor, one can show that $D_{21} = D_{12}$, $D_{31} = D_{13}$, and $D_{32} = D_{23}$. The diffusion tensor is thus a symmetric matrix with 6 adjustable degrees of freedom. A spatially resolved technique that measures the full diffusion tensor in each voxel of an image is called diffusion tensor imaging (DTI).

An important property of symmetric matrices is that they can be diagonalized. This means that it is possible to rotate to a coordinate system in which the off-diagonal matrix elements vanish. In such a special or "principal" coordinate system, the diffusion tensor takes the form

$$D_{ij} = \begin{pmatrix} \lambda_1 & 0 & 0 \\ 0 & \lambda_2 & 0 \\ 0 & 0 & \lambda_3 \end{pmatrix}. \tag{1.9}$$

The three elements along the diagonal are the diffusion tensor eigenvalues and correspond to the diffusion coefficients along the coordinate axes of the principal coordinate system.

These eigenvalues play a central role in the analysis of DWI data for anisotropic tissues. The MD can be calculated from

$$\mathrm{MD} \equiv \bar{D} = \frac{1}{3}(\lambda_1 + \lambda_2 + \lambda_3). \tag{1.10}$$

The notation $\bar{D}$ for the MD is sometimes preferred for mathematical equations, since MD could be mistaken for the product of two quantities. Similarly, the "fractional anisotropy" (FA) can be calculated from

$$\mathrm{FA} = \sqrt{\frac{(\lambda_1 - \lambda_2)^2 + (\lambda_1 - \lambda_3)^2 + (\lambda_2 - \lambda_3)^2}{2(\lambda_1^2 + \lambda_2^2 + \lambda_3^2)}}. \tag{1.11}$$

The FA varies from 0 to 1 and quantifies the degree to which a tissue is anisotropic[10].

Unit vectors aligned with the principal coordinate axes are called eigenvectors. The direction that corresponds to the largest eigenvalue (usually chosen to be λ_1) is called the axial or parallel direction, while the other two directions are called the radial or perpendicular directions. This is because the source of anisotropy is often the presence of fibrous structures, as in muscle or renal tubules, which restricts diffusion more strongly in directions perpendicular to the fibers. The axial diffusivity is given by

$$D_{\parallel} \equiv \lambda_1, \tag{1.12}$$

and the radial diffusivity is given by

$$D_{\perp} \equiv \frac{1}{2}(\lambda_2 + \lambda_3). \tag{1.13}$$

By construction, $D_\parallel \geq D_\perp$. Also note that from Eqs. (1.10), (1.12), and (1.13), we find the identity $\bar{D} = (D_\parallel + 2D_\perp)/3$.

For simple aqueous solutions, the diffusion process is well described by the isotropic, Gaussian distribution:

$$P(\mathbf{r}, t) = \frac{1}{(4\pi D t)^{3/2}} \exp\left(-\frac{|\mathbf{r}|^2}{4Dt}\right). \qquad (1.14)$$

For this distribution, one can show that FA = MK = 0. However, in biological tissues, diffusion restrictions, such as cell membranes, may cause $P(\mathbf{r}, t)$ to deviate significantly from this canonical form. For isotropic tissues, we still have FA = 0, but MK will typically have a positive value. In fact, the MK is constructed precisely to be an index for the degree to which the diffusion process is non-Gaussian, and as such, it may be regarded as an indicator of tissue microarchitectural complexity (i.e., the diffusion restrictions). An MK value of around 1 or higher implies a significant degree of diffusional non-Gaussianity. For anisotropic tissues, the FA will be positive, as well. We emphasize that there is no simple connection between the FA and the MK, so that these two metrics provide complementary information about water diffusion in tissues. In analogy with DTI, an imaging protocol that produces maps of diffusional kurtosis metrics (e.g., MK) is termed diffusion kurtosis imaging (DKI).

In principle, diffusion metrics, such as $D(\mathbf{n})$ and $K(\mathbf{n})$, have a time dependence in complex media such as biological tissues. This time dependence is typically strongest when the diffusion length is comparable to characteristic length scales of the media. The diffusion length is defined as

$$l_D \equiv \sqrt{6\bar{D}t} \qquad (1.15)$$

and corresponds to the root-mean-square distance that a molecule moves during an observation time t (often called the diffusion time). For biological tissues, the MD for water is typically about $1\ \mu m^2/ms$, and for DWI, the diffusion times are typically about 50 ms. This gives a diffusion length of about $17\ \mu m$, which is indeed comparable to cell sizes. Thus some dependence of diffusion metrics on the diffusion time may be expected and care should be taken when comparing diffusion measurements obtained with different diffusion times. In most cases studied in the brain[11-12], diffusion time dependence has been found to be relatively modest over the normal range of diffusion

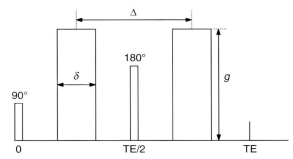

Figure 1.1 The Stejskal–Tanner sequence has been commonly used for DWI. It consists of a conventional spin echo sequence with one diffusion sensitizing gradient lobe inserted between the initial 90° excitation pulse and 180° refocusing pulse and with another inserted between the 180° pulse and the signal readout at the echo time (TE). The interval between the centers of the diffusion gradient lobes corresponds to the diffusion time (Δ). The strength of the diffusion weighting (i.e., the b-value) depends on the magnitude (g) and duration (δ) of the diffusion gradients, as well as the diffusion time, according to Eq. 1.17 (See text).

times (20 to 80 ms), although it is more pronounced over longer diffusion times[13].

So far, we have considered molecular diffusion without reference to how it is measured with NMR or MRI. To illustrate the concepts underlying diffusion measurement, let us consider the famous Stejskal–Tanner sequence[3-4]. The key element of this sequence is the pair of strong gradient lobes that sensitize the signal to molecular diffusion. These "diffusion gradients" are balanced and so have no effect on the signal magnitude if the molecular spins (i.e., water protons) are stationary. But the diffusion gradients cause measurable signal loss for even the small amount of motion associated with molecular diffusion. The diffusion direction corresponds to the orientation of the diffusion gradients. A pulse diagram for the Stejskal–Tanner sequence is shown in Fig. 1.1.

If one applies this sequence to a media with Gaussian diffusion, the signal intensity is given by

$$S(b) = S_0 e^{-bD}, \qquad (1.16)$$

where S_0 is the signal intensity in the absence of diffusion gradients, D is the diffusion coefficient in the direction of the diffusion gradients, and

$$b \equiv (\gamma \delta g)^2 \left(\Delta - \frac{\delta}{3}\right). \qquad (1.17)$$

This defines the so-called b-value. Here γ is the gyromagnetic ratio (equal to $2.675 \times 10^8\ s^{-1}$/Tesla for water protons), g is the magnitude of the diffusion gradients, Δ is the diffusion time, and δ is the pulse duration. For arbitrary pulse sequences the b-value can be calculated from the effective gradient waveform G_{eff} according to the more general formula[14]

$$b = \gamma^2 \int_0^{TE} \left[\int_0^t g_{eff}(t') dt' \right]^2 dt \qquad (1.18)$$

Here g_{eff} reflects the effective diffusion-weighting gradient including the phase reversal effects of radio-frequency pulses in the sequence. Furthermore, in some cases the diffusion-weighting effect of the imaging gradients must also be taken into account for maximal accuracy[15]. For clinical DWI of the brain, b-values typically range from zero to several thousand s/mm^2. For body imaging, b-values usually are not much more than 1000 s/mm^2 due to shorter T2 times limiting signal-to-noise ratio.

Since Eq. (1.16) has two unknown parameters, the diffusion-weighted signal must be measured for at least two different diffusion weightings (i.e., b-values) in order to determine D. If exactly two b-values are used, then one has the simple formula

$$D = \frac{1}{b_2 - b_1} \ln \left[\frac{S(b_1)}{S(b_2)} \right]. \qquad (1.19)$$

Although Eq. (1.16) is the basis of most analyses of DWI data, one should be aware that it is only exact for Gaussian diffusion, while diffusion in biological tissues may be significantly non-Gaussian. Indeed, departures from the monoexponential form of Eq. (1.16) can be used to estimate the MK[8].

Even when Eq. (1.16) appears to be a good fit to experimental data, measured values for D may still depend to some extent on Δ and δ, as well as the echo time, due both to the effect of diffusion restrictions and intravoxel variations in T2 values[12]. Therefore, it is best practice to be consistent with the selection of these parameters.

Strictly speaking, diffusion refers to random molecular motion. However, in biological tissues, blood flow through the capillary network can mimic diffusion and will affect measured diffusion metrics obtained with DWI. This effect is referred to as intravoxel incoherent motion (IVIM). The essential idea is that the capillary network can have a quasi-random arrangement so that flow through the capillaries (and other small blood vessels) leads to random movement of blood referred to as pseudo-diffusion[16–17].

When IVIM is significant, then the diffusion signal is more accurately modeled by the biexponential form

$$S(b) = S(0) \left[f_p e^{-bD^*} + (1 - f_p) e^{-bD_t} \right], \qquad (1.20)$$

where D_t is the tissue diffusion coefficient, D^* is the pseudo-diffusion coefficient for blood, and f_p is the blood volume fraction (a.k.a. "perfusion fraction"). In practice, f_p more precisely refers to the relative water fractions of the blood compartment, since DWI is normally measuring water diffusion.

As Eq. (1.20) suggests, the IVIM effect tends to be large in organs with a high blood volume, such as liver and kidney[17–18]. Pseudo-diffusion coefficients are typically many times larger than tissue diffusion coefficients[17], and the second term of Eq. (1.20) is often negligible for b-values above 300 s/mm^2. If the IVIM effect is substantial, but DWI data are fit to Eq. (1.16) rather than Eq. (1.20), then diffusion coefficient estimates may depend significantly on the choice of b-values.

In part due to IVIM, a diffusion coefficient estimate obtained with DWI became known as an apparent diffusion coefficient (ADC) to remind us that it may be influenced to some degree by effects other than true molecular diffusion. Logically, one may also include the aforementioned dependences of D on pulse duration, intravoxel T2 variations, and non-Gaussian diffusion response as justifications for the moniker "apparent." ADC is used to refer both to D in a given direction and to the MD, although mean diffusivity is preferred for the latter.

In fact, modifications to "apparent" water diffusion due to structural restriction have proven to be a more pervasive MRI contrast mechanism than active flow-induced IVIM. Water embedded in biological media (cells, axons, tubules, blood vessels) undergoes more complex hindered, restricted, or driven motion. However, the average diffusion moments of the whole spin ensemble are still useful descriptors and serve as biomarkers of the tissue structure. To first approximation, diffusion in tissue (and more generally in porous media[19]) obeys Fick's law with a reduced ADC. For isotropic tissues, it suffices to measure diffusion in a single direction, and one often may be primarily interested in determining the ADC. For anisotropic tissues, multiple diffusion directions are

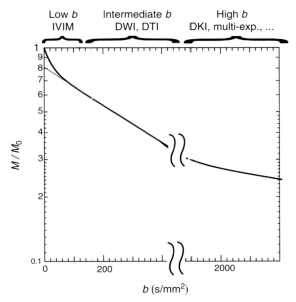

Figure 1.2 Sketch of diffusion-weighted signal decay behavior in several regimes of diffusion-weighting for in vivo tissue response.

required to fully characterize the diffusion process. In particular, in order to estimate the diffusion tensor, at least six directions are needed since the diffusion tensor has six adjustable parameters. However, if only the MD is required, then it can be found from the average of ADCs measured for any three orthogonal directions.

Experimentally, the various effects just described can be organized according to the regimes of diffusion weighting in which they are observed to occur (Figure 1.2). The low b-value regime ($0 < b < 200$ s/mm^2) is where pseudo-diffusion from microcirculation effects are found (i.e., the IVIM regime), since pseudo-diffusivities are typically quite high ($D^* \sim 10 - 50$ mm^2/ms). Studies wishing to avoid vascular contamination typically exclude this range; conversely, those aiming to quantify vascularity with DWI may sample both this regime and the normal diffusion regime heavily. The mostly commonly used regime is the intermediate regime ($200 < b < 1000$ s/mm^2), where diffusion appears Gaussian and DWI signal decays appear monoexponential. In this regime, standard DWI metrics (e.g., ADC) or DTI metrics (MD, FA, eigenvalues) are typically derived. Finally, the high b-value regime ($b > 1000$ s/mm^2) also often shows non-monoexponential signal decay due to microscopic parenchymal structure, which can be

quantified for example with diffusional kurtosis. In clinical scanners, the b-value is typically incremented by adjusting diffusion gradient magnitude g, or equivalently the diffusion wave vector $q = \gamma g \delta$, the inverse of one of the probing length scales of DWI. At high b-values, q^{-1} is comparable to or shorter than parenchymal length scales of a few microns (cell size, axon radius, membrane thickness) and their geometry begins to manifest in a non-monoexponential signal decay[20–21]. Depending on the organ, pathology, data sampling, and precision, one can model this behavior in different ways (either with physical models or empirical descriptions) to extract microstructural markers. Example models include multiexponential functions reflecting tissue compartments[21–23] (similar to the IVIM vascular/parenchymal decomposition), the cumulant expansion model which extracts higher-order displacement moments[8,24–25], or other models of tissue complexity[26–27]. In all cases, the model and interpretation must be chosen with regard to the data precision and tissue prior knowledge; compartmental models for example can be overinterpreted since multiexponentiality does not necessarily equate to compartmentalization[28–29]. These issues will be further discussed below.

1.3 DWI techniques
Pulse sequences (Figures 1.3 and 1.4)
The desired contrast in DWI is an attenuation of the *magnitude* of the spin magnetization following the diffusion-weighting gradient waveform due to microscopic incoherent motion, as described in Sections 1.1 and 1.2. However, macroscopic motion such as respiration, pulsation, or bulk translation/rotation can induce *phase shifts* in the spin magnetization which can be temporally and spatially heterogeneous. In MRI sequences with segmented k-space trajectories, these motional phases can induce phase inconsistency across k-space and therefore image ghosting. For this reason, particularly for body applications, the most common modalities for DWI are single-shot sequences. Also, the magnitude channel is retained and the phase channel is typically discarded. Two examples are echo-planar imaging (EPI)[30] and turbo spin echo (TSE)[31] imaging (see Figure 1.3 for pulse sequence diagrams).

Echo-planar imaging (EPI)
Echo-planar imaging (EPI)[30] is one of the mainstay techniques for fast MRI, and is the key to such

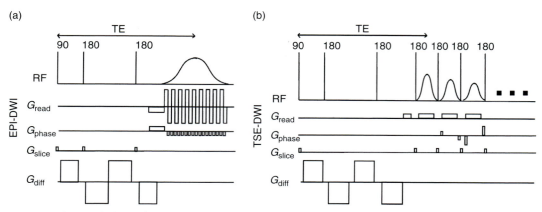

Figure 1.3 DWI single-shot pulse sequence diagrams. (a) Echo-planar imaging (EPI). (b) Turbo spin echo (TSE).

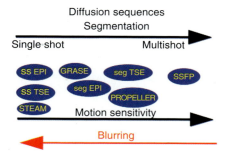

Figure 1.4 Diffusion imaging strategies as a function of k-space segmentation. In general, more segmentation reduces image blurring but requires motion correction, and vice versa.

powerful applications as functional imaging (fMRI), diffusion tensor imaging (DTI), and perfusion-weighted imaging (PWI). For DWI, it is most often run in 2D single-shot mode, where all the required lines of acquisition (k-space) for a 2D spatial slice are all collected in an echo train following a single excitation and diffusion weighting preparation. For full-body human clinical MRI scanners, the standard implementation of the diffusion-weighting preparation is a twice-refocused spin echo with bipolar gradients, as depicted in Figure 1.3a, which has the advantage of eddy-current compensation for improved image quality[32]. A disadvantage of this approach is a longer required echo time (TE) for the same diffusion weighting factor (b) in comparison with a simpler Stejskal–Tanner sequence. While some aspects of this technique carry over smoothly from cerebral to abdominal imaging, other challenges are unique to the abdominal setting and require modifications of the imaging paradigm.

The EPI echo train is collected within the envelope of a single spin echo MR transient, and so suffers attenuation due to intravoxel static magnetic field inhomogeneity (characterized by a spatially dependent time constant T_2^*) as well as phase shifts from the average local field deviations. The former effect induces blurring in the image, while the latter induces distortions, and both are generally referred to under the category magnetic susceptibility artifact. Both can be particularly problematic in abdominal DWI, given the heterogeneous adjacent organs (liver, kidney, spleen), some of which contain air (bowel, stomach, lung). Therefore, measures are taken to reduce the echo train length (ETL) as much as possible. One example is partial Fourier, where as little as half the full k-space is collected and combined with assumptions of phase symmetry is sufficient to generate an image[33]. Another solution, which is very common for body MRI[34–36], is the use of parallel imaging undersampling, where spatially varying receiver coil sensitivity information is used in lieu of full k-space sampling for image reconstruction. Each of these solutions reduces ETL and thus blurring and distortions, but in exchange for lower SNR due to fewer-acquired data and/or the processing cost of coil-based reconstruction.

For further image quality improvement, segmented k-space trajectories where far fewer lines (5–10) are acquired in a single excitation have been used with EPI-DWI[37–38]. Since motional phase errors can induce inconsistency among segments, navigator echoes (with 1D, 2D, or even 3D phase mapping) are required to prevent ghosting in these segmented EPI-DWI sequences[39–40]. For single-shot sequences, even if individual image quality is uncorrupted, the entire image set must be positionally consistent prior to diffusion processing, particularly for the diffusion tensor. During acquisition, physiological triggering (respiratory gating[41–42] or pulse triggering[43]) is employed to minimize bulk motion. Physiological triggering can use signals from either patient devices (finger pulse sensor, abdominal pad/belt transducer) or from simultaneous MR navigation (e.g., of diaphragm motion). When possible, breath-hold acquisitions are performed to minimize patient motion during the acquisition, though usually at the expense of some SNR due to suboptimal repetition times TR. Finally, even in gated or breath-hold acquisitions, post-acquisition registration is often needed to completely align the dataset prior to diffusion processing.

Most clinical abdominal EPI-DWI has been performed at 1.5 T, but 3-T applications are becoming more common[44–47]. The advantage of higher raw SNR at higher field must be considered in balance with the larger susceptibility artifact, and shorter transverse relaxation time T2[48]. Parallel imaging, which generally becomes more favorable at higher field, is one potential solution to these issues.

Turbo spin echo (TSE)

The second most common single-shot diffusion-weighted imaging sequence uses a turbo spin echo (TSE) readout, also known as fast spin echo (FSE) or rapid acquisition with relaxation enhancement (RARE). This sequence, depicted in Figure 1.3b, employs a train of spin echoes generated by a series of 180° refocusing pulses, each of which provides one line of k-space, similar to the EPI gradient echo train. Importantly, however, the spin echo-based TSE signals are insensitive to susceptibility-induced blurring and distortions. Accordingly, the limiting signal envelope is determined not by the total transverse relaxation time T_2^* but by the usually longer irreversible transverse relaxation time T_2; thus TSE images can show "T2-blurring." The temporal advantage is somewhat mitigated by the time required for slice-selective inversion pulses between each echo, but TSE images are in general more morphologically accurate than EPI counterparts.

Other artifacts are unique to the DW-TSE protocol. The most important one arises due to the essentially random phase imparted to the magnetization following diffusion-weighting, but before TSE readout,

due to bulk motion. This phase causes the (Carr–Purcell–Meiboom–Gill) CPMG condition[2,49], which usually provides for echo pathway isolation and also RF pulse error compensation, to be violated. This effect, especially when combined with RF pulse errors generating unwanted stimulated echo pathways, causes interference between the desired signal parity and spurious signals of opposite parity[31,50]. This "non-CPMG" artifact manifests as streaking or banding roughly perpendicular to the frequency-encoding axis, and is regionally pronounced in areas of RF or B0 inhomogeneity. Various solutions have been implemented, including spoilers to isolate desired parity[50], split-echo techniques to separately acquire both parities and combine them offline[51–52], and phase modulations to stabilize both signals' phase histories[53].

Like EPI, the TSE echo train can include complete k-space coverage (single-shot mode) or only portions in each excitation (segmented mode); with diffusion-weighting preparation, the segmented protocol must be accompanied by navigator echo collection to correct intershot motional phase errors[54]. Some strategies solve this problem by using self-navigated radial trajectories that pass through the center of k-space often, allowing measurement and correction of motional phases. Segmented radial TSE sequences such as PROPELLER[55] (a.k.a. BLADE) have had great success in DWI in both the brain and body[52,56–57].

Regarding field strength, TSE-DWI is also progressively migrating to the higher field platform (e.g., 3 T) for body imaging[58]. Unlike EPI, TSE does not suffer increased distortion at higher field and therefore may be preferred in regions of high susceptibility contrast (lung, breast, etc.). However, the refocusing RF pulse train will give rise to higher specific absorption rate (SAR) due to the higher Larmor frequency at higher field, so RF heating restrictions may extend scan time.

Other pulse sequences
GRASE and STEAM

We have seen that EPI generates gradient echo trains with rapid gradient reversals, and TSE generates spin echo trains with rapid refocusing RF pulses. In some cases hybrid methods employing both gradient and spin echo (GRASE) signals to accelerate k-space have also been used for diffusion imaging[57]. Another approach is a stimulated echo acquisition mode (STEAM), in which a series of stimulated echoes

(STE) are generated by two 90° pulses followed by a train ("burst") of low-flip angle pulses, each one "stimulating" a portion of the stored magnetization from the first pulse pair[59–60]. Since each STE is "fresh" from storage mode there is no blurring due to susceptibility or transverse relaxation. However, the STEAM–BURST pulse train progressively depletes the stored magnetization as k-space is acquired, which dictates lower SNR signals and in some cases RF demodulation corrections. STEAM preparation can also be used followed by another readout (EPI or SSFP)[61–62], which has advantages for more specific quantification of tissue microstructure when the diffusion time is a control variable.

Steady-state free precession (SSFP)

The limit of a fully segmented acquisition, i.e., one k-space line per excitation, induces minimum blurring, but maximum motion artifacts and, if full recovery were allowed between lines, maximum acquisition time. One solution to this problem is to use steady-state-free-precession (SSFP) sequences that include diffusion weighting[63–66]. These sequences employ a rapid train of excitations that do not allow full magnetization recovery but instead arrive at a lower driven equilibrium "steady state" value. The reduced magnitude is more than compensated by acquisition speed in overall scan efficiency. Though slower than single-shot modes (inter-signal spacing is TR ~ 30–50 ms), SSFP allows in principle very high quality diffusion imaging in acceptable time-frames. However, there are two complications to this technique which have thus far mostly confined its successful use to the brain. First, as mentioned above, segmentation requires motion correction. In this case, every line must be accompanied by a navigator signal, ideally a multidimensional one to capture non-uniform motion[66–68]. Second, the diffusion-weighting of the SSFP signal is "entangled" in a complicated way with effects of relaxation weighting and RF flip angle excitation[63,69]; thus, successful quantitation requires not only multiple diffusion weightings for good-quality curve fitting, but also prior knowledge or separate maps of relaxation times T1, T2, and RF field B1. Thus, SSFP diffusion imaging potentially provides maximum quality and resolution, but at a high price in navigation and peripheral acquisitions. For abdominal applications it may only apply to relatively immobile organs like the prostate. Alternatively, SSFP can be used as a pure readout modality following a more standard diffusion preparation[70].

1.4 Data analysis

Once a set of DWI images has been obtained, one would then normally like to use them to generate parametric maps of various diffusion metrics. This requires a certain amount of post-processing, the details of which can be fairly complicated. Here, we give a general overview of some of the key considerations, while trying to minimize mathematical formalities. A more in-depth description for one particular image analysis program for DWI is given by Jiang and co-workers[71].

Raw diffusion-weighted images themselves are sometimes considered clinically informative, but it should always be remembered that the observed contrast depends strongly on additional, non-diffusion-related factors such as relaxation rates and proton density. The so-called "T2 shine-through" effect is perhaps the best-known example of this problem[72].

In order to obtain pure diffusion maps, the first step is often to co-register the DWI images to correct for any relative displacements or rotations due to patient motion. This is important, because the images are processed as a set and misregistration between images can lead to significant artifacts and alter estimates of the ADC and other quantities. A variety of image analysis programs are available that can perform the necessary co-registration. However, image co-registration may not always be necessary for certain organs, such as prostate, where motion can be minimal. Alternatively, if gating strategies have been used in the acquisition process as discussed earlier, then some physiological motion will have been minimized.

Once co-registered, the images can be used to calculate the desired diffusion metrics on a voxel-by-voxel basis, yielding parametric maps. The most widely employed diffusion maps are for the MD and FA, although the axial and radial diffusivities are gaining popularity[73].

A useful extension of the FA map is called the FA color or directivity map[74]. Here each pixel of an FA map is converted to red–green–blue (RGB) color by using the eigenvector corresponding to the highest eigenvalue, which in many cases may be reasonably assumed to be oriented parallel to any fiber-like structures. The intensity of the red is determined by the FA multiplied by the x-component of the eigenvector in a specified reference frame, while the green and blue intensities are determined by products of the FA with the y- and z-components. In this way, a directivity map displays both the degree of anisotropy as well as the orientation of the fibers.

An alternative approach for displaying diffusional anisotropy is to perform fiber tracking (FT), which is again based on an assumption that fibers are the source of anisotropy. An FT algorithm generates trajectories, originated from a set of selected starting points (seeds) and guided by using the primary eigenvector field to trace streamlines that are intended to show the fiber paths within a tissue. This method has been used extensively for mapping white matter tracts within the brain and has also been applied to study muscle[75] and kidney[76].

In the brain, the IVIM effect is small and usually ignored in the analysis of DWI data. In body, however, the IVIM effect can be much more significant and may have to be taken into account[17–18]. As previously mentioned, a typical indication of an IVIM effect is finding ADC values that depend on the choice b-value, when a conventional monoexponential model is used to fit the signal data.

In such cases with a large IVIM effect, it can be useful to fit to the biexponential model of Eq. (1.20), provided DWI data is available for a sufficient range of b-values. Since Eq. (1.20) has four unknown parameters, one needs data for at least four different b-values. Ideally, two of these would be for $b < 200$ s/mm^2, as the IVIM effect is mainly important for low b-values. Great care should be taken when performing the fit due to the sensitivity of the fit parameters to noise[77–78]. Sometimes more robust results can be obtained by a "segmented" procedure of first fitting the high b-value (i.e., $b > 300$ s/mm^2) data to a monoexponential to determine f_p and D_t, and then fitting to Eq. (1.20) with D_t fixed to this predetermined value.

As an example, consider a set of DWI measurements for the four b-values: 0, $b_1 = 150$ s/mm^2, $b_2 = 500$ s/mm^2, $b_3 = 1000$ s/mm^2. If it is assumed that the IVIM effect is negligible for $b > 300$ s/mm^2, one can then estimate

$$D_t = \frac{1}{b_3 - b_2} \ln \left[\frac{S(b_2)}{S(b_3)} \right]. \qquad (1.21)$$

From this result, one can in turn determine the other parameters for the biexponential model by using the formulae

$$f_p = 1 - \frac{S(b_3)}{S(0)} e^{b_3 D_t}, \qquad (1.22)$$

$$D^* = -\frac{1}{b_1} \ln \left[\frac{S(b_1)}{f_p S(0)} - \frac{(1 - f_p)}{f_p} e^{-b_1 D_t} \right]. \qquad (1.23)$$

Since the signal intensity of diffusion-weighted images drops sharply with increasing b-value, noise is often an important source of error in the analysis of DWI data. Unless noise is explicitly modeled in the data fits, then the maximum b-value that can be used without causing significant errors in estimated diffusion metrics depends both on the intrinsic SNR (i.e., without diffusion weighting) and the ADC. This maximum b-value is approximately given by[79]

$$b_{max} \approx \frac{1}{D} \ln \left(\text{SNR} \cdot \sqrt{\frac{2}{\pi}} \right). \qquad (1.24)$$

After maps of diffusion metrics have been obtained, then mean values for different regions of interest are usually compared. For large regions of interest, containing many voxels, histogram approaches, such as principal component analysis, may be useful[80–81].

1.5 Body applications

The biophysical mechanisms affecting diffusion weighted imaging in the body, reviewed in previous sections, have a wide range of applications in abdominal imaging. Many pathological mechanisms involve alterations in the parenchymal structure that affect the natural scale or shape of restrictions/hindrances to water motion (cell membranes, sheaths, fibers, tubules, etc.). Others are sensitive to changes in fluid content, such as in cysts, edema, or glandular compartments, as well as desiccation. Finally, the IVIM methodology can reveal changes in the abundance or flow speed (or both) of tissue vascularity. The impacts of these sensitivities are itemized below in several abdominal organ categories, following a few brief comments about common tissue states or pathologies.

Common entities (Table 1.1)

Certain entities are common to multiple organs and/ or pathologies. Edema, or abnormal fluid release surrounding pathological insults to tissue such as carcinoma or injury, tends to increase apparent diffusion coefficients (i.e., ADC, MD, or D$_t$). Simple cysts are isolated pockets of free fluid that show normal

Table 1.1 Typical changes in diffusion MR metrics with common tissue entities

	ADC/MD/D_t	FA	MK	f_p	D_p
Edema	↑	↓	↓	0	NA
Cyst	↑	0	0	0	NA
Fibrosis	↓	↓	↑	0	NA
Tumor	↓	↓	?	↑	↓

Notes: ADC: apparent diffusion coefficient; MD: mean diffusivity; D_t: tissue diffusivity; FA: fractional anisotropy; MK: mean kurtosis; f_p: perfusion fraction; D_p: pseudo-diffusivity.

unrestricted diffusion (high ADC), while complex cysts may show a mixture of free fluid and hemorrhagic fluid, the latter of which shows slower diffusion due in part to higher viscosity. Fibrosis, or an abnormal growth of fibrous parenchymal tissue, increases the prevalence of barriers to diffusion and thus reduces ADC values and would be expected to increase diffusional kurtosis.

Finally, tumors possess several properties for which diffusion imaging can provide biomarkers. First and foremost, the proliferation of cancer cells generally reduces the extracellular space and thus the ADC by an amount depending on aggressiveness. Thus, the ADC is considered a marker of the "cellularity" of malignant tumors throughout the body. While diffusion in the aggressive tumor core is usually isotropic (FA ~ 0), high resolution DTI of brain tumors has revealed significant diffusion anisotropy in the infiltration rim zone, corresponding to either radial or azimuthally oriented cell patterns[82–83]. Diffusional kurtosis can be either higher or lower in tumors than normal tissue. Most tumors (with a few notable exceptions) are hypervascular due to unregulated angiogenesis. This effect generally promotes the IVIM pseudo-diffusion effect in DWI; indeed, a monoexponential model can potentially confuse effects of vascularity and cellularity since they have opposite influences on apparent diffusion. When analyzed properly with an IVIM compartment model, tumors usually display higher perfusion fraction (f_p) than background tissue, and sometimes abnormal pseudo-diffusivity (D_p) for sluggish blood flow. These effects are common to many tumor types but differences exist in the diffusion measurement and interpretation of each organ separately.

Liver

Hepatic tissue possesses several properties in health and disease that diffusion imaging can probe[84]. First, hepatic tissue is highly vascular, which translates to a high IVIM perfusion fraction (f_p ~ 30%)[17–18,85]; accordingly, studies have observed dependencies of ADC results on selected b-values[86]. Compared to other organs, the liver has a short transverse relaxation time T2[48] (and significantly more so in the case of iron overload[87–88]) and thus reduces available SNR for diffusion imaging. Secondarily, sufficient iron deposition can generate local magnetic field inhomogeneities that can interfere with applied gradients and thus alter prescribed b-values. Liver fibrosis and cirrhosis is a prominent pathology in which DWI has been shown to have significant diagnostic potential[17,85,89], since cirrhosis is thought to involve both vascular (reduced flow) and parenchymal (fibrotic growth) abnormalities. Figure 1.5a shows example images of total apparent diffusion coefficient (ADC$_{tot}$), tissue diffusivity (D_t), and perfusion fraction (f_p) in a healthy and cirrhotic patient from IVIM MRI performed at 1.5 T (taken from[89]). All three parametric maps show differences between the two subjects, consistent with multifactorial pathophysiology of cirrhosis. Such information updates previously held convention that diffusion contrast in cirrhosis reflected only fibrotic restriction. Finally, hepatocellular carcinoma (HCC) is a significant health threat in which MRI plays a key role in detection and diagnosis. High cellularity in the tumor zone reduces ADC values, and high vascularity has also been shown to demonstrate high perfusion fractions in IVIM studies[18].

Kidney

The two tissue types in renal parenchyma, cortex and medulla, can be tracked by DWI via several physiological properties: vascular flow, tubular flow, and parenchymal structure. As the kidney is one of the most highly vascularized bodily organs, blood volume and blood flow are significant contributors to overall water transport in the cortex and medulla, and thus a strong pseudo-diffusion component is present in IVIM imaging. Additionally, active tubular flow in both compartments is another source of pseudo-diffusion in the DWI signal. Figure 1.6 shows DWI signal decay data from cortex, medulla, and benign cyst regions of a normal healthy volunteer[90–91]. In comparison with the nearly monoexponential

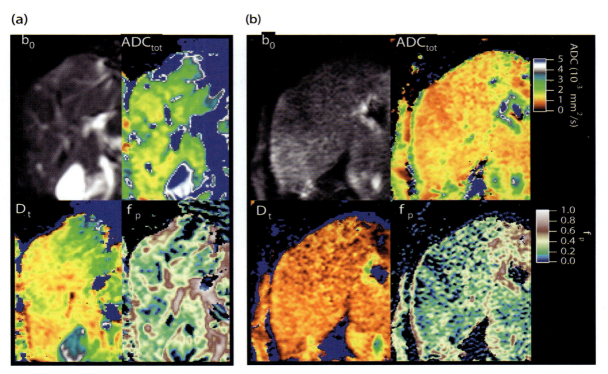

Figure 1.5 Liver DWI image results for (a) normal subject and (b) cirrhosis patient. See text for parameter definitions. $b0$, unweighted image; ADC, apparent diffusion coefficient; D_t, tissue diffusion coefficient; f_p, perfusion fraction. [Reproduced with permission from Patel J *et al.* Diagnosis of cirrhosis with intravoxel incoherent motion diffusion MRI and dynamic contrast-enhanced MRI alone and in combination: preliminary experience. *J Magn Reson Imag* 2010; **31**:589–600.]

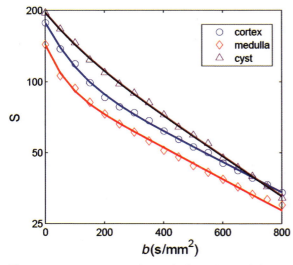

Figure 1.6 IVIM imaging results in a healthy volunteer kidney at 3 T. ROI diffusion-weighted signal decays taken from cortex, medulla, and cyst regions of the same volunteer are shown.

response of the unrestricted cyst fluid, the parenchymal tissues both show a fast pseudo-diffusion component. As a result, use of a monoexponential model (Eq. (1.16)) to produce ADC maps will depend strongly on the choice of diffusion weighting values[91].

As with other cancer types, renal cell carcinomas (RCC) have strong signatures in diffusion-weighted imaging. Numerous reports have found ADC reductions arising from aggressive cellularity[46,92–93]. Renal mass vascularity, however, has also been probed with detailed IVIM analysis and found to correlate with vascular measures from standard contrast-enhanced MRI. IVIM presents opportunities for biomarkers of ischemia, filtration malfunction, or transplant rejection, if those etiologies induce reduced flow in renal tissue. These possibilities have been explored in several studies[94–95], but represent a relatively uncharted area of medical research.

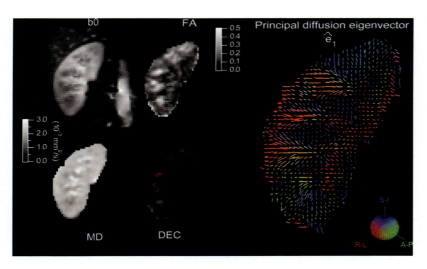

Figure 1.7 Diffusion tensor imaging (DTI) in a healthy volunteer kidney at 3 T. *b*0, T2-weighted reference image; MD, mean diffusivity; FA, fractional anisotropy; DEC, direction encoded color map; e1, principal diffusion eigenvector (length weighted by FA). DEC and e1 maps are color-coded according to standard RGB directional reference (lower right). [Reproduced with permission from Kim S *et al.* Diffusion-weighted MR imaging of the kidneys and the urinary tract. *Magn Reson Imag Clin N Am* 2008; **16**:585–596.]

Parenchymal structure also plays a role in kidney diffusion contrast. While both cortex and medulla show restricted diffusion, in the cortex it is isotropic, while in medulla the apparent diffusion is markedly anisotropic, with the largest diffusivities occurring along the radial direction of the medullary tubules. Figure 1.7 shows example DTI data in a healthy volunteer kidney at 3 T[96–97] illustrating this anisotropy, which a number of reports have demonstrated[76,98]. Medullary compartments show lower MD and higher FA than the cortex, and the primary diffusion eigenvector is radially oriented relative to the central collection system of the kidney. The source of this anisotropy may have contributions both from tubular flow (which is highly oriented in the medullary loops of Henle) as well as from structural restrictions to passive diffusion. Future work employing a combined IVIM and DTI scheme may tease apart these effects. The DTI indices (MD, FA) will likely be useful biomarkers of tubular integrity; they have been shown in pilot studies to be sensitive to hydration level[99] and to transplant rejection status[100].

Prostate

Prostate imaging is another important area of abdominal radiology in which diffusion contrast is playing a significant role, particularly in the assessment of prostate cancer (PCa)[47,101–104]. PCa in the peripheral zone is a complex mixture of intermingled stromal cells, fluid-filled glandular ducts, and infiltrating/malignant tumor cells. The characteristic branching structure of the glandular ducts, and its disruption and replacement by aggressive tumor cellularity, forms the basis for the standard histological PCa grading system, the Gleason score. The sensitivity of DWI to tissue microarchitecture therefore makes it a valuable non-invasive tool for identification and assessment of PCa in vivo. The most common DWI application to PCa to date has been conventional ADC mapping to differentiate and score tumors, primarily in the peripheral zone. As discussed for other carcinomas, the tumor cellularity adds more restrictive barriers and thus lowers the apparent diffusion by an amount determined by the cell density[105]. Diffusion tensor imaging has also been applied[106–109] to attempt to characterize local anisotropy in stroma, glands, tumor cells, prostatic hyperplasia, or fibromuscular tissue, though the results and their biophysical underpinnings are still controversial. Finally, a select few studies[110–111] have performed prostate DWI in the high *b*-value regime and found non-monoexponential behavior, which may be sensitive to higher-order structural features in the stromal, glandular, and tumor compartments. Example DWI results of this type acquired at 3 T are shown in Figure 1.8, where the peripheral zone DWI signal decay shows non-monoexponential (i.e., non-Gaussian) character in the range $0 < b < 2000$ s/mm^2, which gives a non-zero diffusional kurtosis ($K = 0.86$). Modifications of such non-Gaussian diffusion biomarkers in PCa may shed more light on the manifestation of tumors' microstructure in clinical MRI and aid in its use for non-invasive diagnosis, grading, and treatment monitoring.

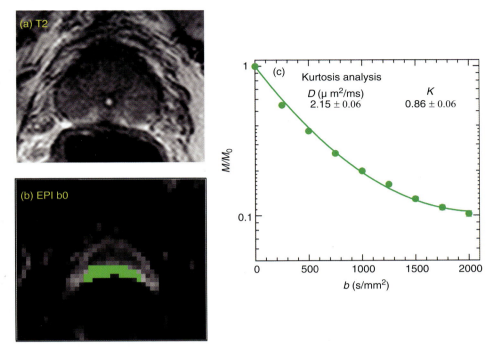

Figure 1.8 Diffusion-weighted imaging in the peripheral zone of the prostate in a normal control healthy volunteer at 3 T. (a) Anatomical T2-weighted image. (b) EPI unweighted ($b0$) image with region-of-interest (ROI) definition in the peripheral zone. (c) DWI signal decay for the ROI shown in (b). Non-monoexponential behavior is evident at high b-values, which can be quantified with the kurtosis model.

1.6   Summary

Diffusion-weighted imaging has been a mainstay of the neuroimaging toolbox for quite some time, but is migrating more and more to other anatomical areas in need of its unique structural and functional specificity. This migration is enabled in part by a vast array of pulse sequence tools, acquisition techniques, and analysis algorithms that have made MRI of fairly mobile abdominal organs feasible. Both standard DWI and advanced techniques like IVIM, DTI, and DKI are opening new avenues of research in abdominal radiology that are expected in turn to lead to new diagnostic tools for pathology detection, monitoring, and treatment guidance in areas as disparate as cirrhosis, transplant malfunction, and cancer. The addition of DWI tools to an abdominal imaging session makes it a much more complete and diagnostically powerful imaging modality.

References

1. Hahn EL. Spin echoes. *Phys Rev* 1950;**80**:580–94.

2. Carr HY, Purcell EM. Effects of diffusion on free precession in NMR experiments. *Phys Rev* 1954; **94**:630.

3. Stejskal EO, Tanner JE. Spin diffusion measurements: spin echoes in the presence of a time-dependent field gradient. *J Chem Phys* 1965;**42**:288–92.

4. Tanner JE, Stejskal EO. Restricted self-diffusion of protons in colloidal systems by the pulsed-gradient, spin-echo method. *J Chem Phys* 1968;**49**:1768–77.

5. Thoeny HC, De Keyzer F. Extracranial applications of diffusion-weighted magnetic resonance imaging. *Eur Radiol* 2007;**17** (6):1385–93.

6. Colagrande S, Carbone SF, Carusi LM, Cova M, Villari N. Magnetic resonance diffusion-weighted imaging: extraneurological applications. *Radiologia Med* 2006;**111** (3):392–419.

7. Einstein A. Diffusion. *Ann Phys* 1905;**17**:549.

8. Jensen JH, Helpern JA, Ramani A, Lu HZ, Kaczynski K. Diffusional kurtosis imaging: the quantification of non-Gaussian water diffusion by means of magnetic resonance imaging. *Magn Reson Med* 2005;**53** (6):1432–40.

9. Basser PJ, Mattiello J, Lebihan D. MR diffusion tensor spectroscopy and imaging. *Biophys J* 1994; **66** (1):259–67.

10. Basser PJ, Pierpaoli C. Microstructural and physiological features of tissues elucidated by quantitative-diffusion-tensor MRI. *J Magn Reson B* 1996;**111** (3):209–19.

11. Clark CA, Hedehus M, Moseley ME. Diffusion time dependence of the apparent diffusion tensor in healthy human brain and white matter disease. *Magn Reson Med* 2001;**45** (6):1126–9.

12. Qin W, Yu CS, Zhang F, *et al*. Effects of echo time on diffusion quantification of brain white matter at 1.5T and 3.0T. *Magn Reson Med* 2009;**61** (4):755–60.

13. Kim S, Chi-Fishman G, Barnett AS, Pierpaoli C. Dependence on diffusion time of apparent diffusion tensor of ex vivo calf tongue and heart. *Magn Reson Med* 2005;**54** (6):1387–96.

14. Callaghan PT. *Principles of Nuclear Magnetic Resonance Microscopy*. Oxford: Oxford University Press; 1993.

15. Basser PJ, Mattiello J, Lebihan D. Estimation of the effective self-diffusion tensor from the NMR spin-echo. *J Magn Reson B* 1994;**103** (3):247–54.

16. LeBihan D, Breton E, Lallemand D, *et al*. Separation of diffusion and perfusion in intravoxel incoherent motion MR imaging. *Radiology* 1988;**168** (2):497–505.

17. Luciani A, Vignaud A, Cavet M, *et al*. Liver cirrhosis: intravoxel incoherent motion MR imaging: pilot study. *Radiology* 2008;**249** (3):891–9.

18. Yamada I, Aung W, Himeno Y, Nakagawa T, Shibuya H. Diffusion coefficients in abdominal organs and hepatic lesions: Evaluation with intravoxel incoherent motion echo-planar MR imaging. *Radiology* 1999;**210** (3):617–23.

19. Mitra PP, Sen PN, Schwartz LM. Short-time behavior of the diffusion coefficient as a geometrical probe of porous media. *Phys Rev B* 1993;**47**:8565.

20. Mulkern RV, Gudbjartsson H, Westin CF, *et al*. Multi-component apparent diffusion coefficients in human brain. *NMR Biomed* 1999;**12** (1):51–62.

21. Clark CA, Le Bihan D. Water diffusion compartmentation and anisotropy at high *b* values in the human brain. *Magn Reson Med* 2000;**44** (6):852–9.

22. Mulkern RV, Zengingonul HP, Robertson RL, *et al*. Multi-component apparent diffusion coefficients in human brain: relationship to spin-lattice relaxation. *Magn Reson Med* 2000;**44** (2):292–300.

23. Meier C, Dreher W, Lebrfritz D. Diffusion in compartmental systems. I. A comparison of an analytical model with simulations. *Magn Reson Med* 2003;**50** (3):500–9.

24. Falangola MF, Jensen JH, Babb JS, *et al*. Age-related non-Gaussian diffusion patterns in the prefrontal brain. *J Magn Reson Imag* 2008;**28** (6):1345–50.

25. Lu HZ, Jensen JH, Ramani A, Helpern JA. Three-dimensional characterization of non-gaussian water diffusion in humans using diffusion kurtosis imaging. *NMR Biomed* 2006;**19** (2):236–47.

26. Bennett KM, Hyde JS, Schmainda KM. Water diffusion heterogeneity index in the human brain is insensitive to the orientation of applied magnetic field gradients. *Magn Reson Med* 2006;**56** (2):235–9.

27. Ozarslan E, Basser PJ, Shepherd TM, *et al*. Observation of anomalous diffusion in excised tissue by characterizing the diffusion-time dependence of the MR signal. *J Magn Reson* 2006;**183** (2):315–23.

28. Sukstanskii AL, Yablonskiy DA. Effects of restricted diffusion on MR signal formation. *J Magn Reson* 2002;**157** (1):92–105.

29. Sukstanskii AL, Ackerman JJH, Yablonskiy DA. Effects of barrier-induced nuclear spin magnetization inhomogeneities on diffusion-attenuated MR signal. *Magn Reson Med* 2003;**50** (4):735–42.

30. Stehling MK, Turner R, Mansfield P. Echo-planar imaging: magnetic-resonance imaging in a fraction of a second. *Science* 1991;**254** (5028):43–50.

31. Alsop DC. Phase insensitive preparation of single-shot RARE: application to diffusion imaging in humans. *Magn Reson Med* 1997;**38** (4):527–33.

32. Reese TG, Heid O, Weisskoff RM, Wedeen VJ. Reduction of eddy-current-induced distortion in diffusion MRI using a twice-refocused spin echo. *Magn Reson Med* 2003;**49** (1):177–82.

33. Haacke EM, Brown RW, Thompson MR, Venkatesan R. *Magnetic Resonance Imaging: Physical Principles and Sequence Design*. New York: Wiley-Liss; 1999.

34. Kilickesmez O, Yirik G, Bayramoglu S, Cimilli T, Aydin S. Non-breath-hold high *b*-value diffusion-weighted MRI with parallel imaging technique: apparent diffusion coefficient determination in normal abdominal organs. *Diagnost Intervent Radiol* 2008;**14** (2):83–7.

35. Zech CJ, Herrmann KA, Dietrich O, *et al*. Black-blood diffusion-weighted EPI acquisition of the liver with parallel imaging: comparison with a standard T2-weighted sequence for detection of focal liver lesions. *Investig Radiol* 2008;**43** (4):261–6.

36. Nasu K, Kuroki Y, Kuroki S, *et al*. Diffusion-weighted single shot echo planar imaging of colorectal cancer using a sensitivity-encoding technique. *Jap J Clin Oncol* 2004;**34** (10):620–6.

37. Weih KS, Driesel W, von Mengershausen M, Norris DG. Online motion correction for diffusion-weighted segmented-EPI and FLASH imaging. *Magn Reson Materials Phys Biol Med* 2004; **16** (6):277–83.

38. Atkinson D, Porter DA, Hill DLG, Calamante F, Connelly A. Sampling and reconstruction effects due to motion in diffusion-weighted interleaved echo planar imaging. *Magn Reson Med* 2000;**44** (1):101–9.

39. Butts K, deCrespigny A, Pauly JM, Moseley M. Diffusion-weighted interleaved echo-planar imaging with a pair of orthogonal navigator echoes. *Magn Reson Med* 1996;**35** (5):763–70.

40. Ordidge RJ, Helpern JA, Qing ZX, Knight RA, Nagesh V. Correction of motional artifacts in diffusion-weighted MR-images using navigator echoes. *Magn Reson Imag* 1994;**12** (3):455–60.

41. Spuentrup E, Buecker A, Koelker C, Guenther RW, Stuber M. Respiratory motion artifact suppression in diffusion-weighted MR imaging of the spine. *Eur Radiol* 2003;**13** (2):330–6.

42. Asbach P, Hein PA, Stemmer A, *et al.* Free-breathing echo-planar imaging based diffusion-weighted magnetic resonance imaging of the liver with prospective acquisition correction. *J Comput Assist Tomogr* 2008;**32** (3):372–8.

43. Murtz P, Flacke S, Traber F, *et al.* Abdomen: Diffusion-weighted MR imaging with pulse-triggered single-shot sequences. *Radiology* 2002;**224** (1):258–64.

44. Erturk SM, Alberich-Bayarri A, Herrmann KA, Marti-Bonmati L, Ros PR. Use of 3.0-T MR imaging for evaluation of the abdomen. *Radiographics* 2009;**29** (6):1547–64.

45. Ivancevic MK, Kwee TC, Takahara T, *et al.* Diffusion-weighted MR imaging of the liver at 3.0 tesla using Tracking Only Navigator Echo (TRON): a feasibility study. *J Magn Reson Imag* 2009;**30** (5):1027–33.

46. Manenti G, Di Roma M, Mancino S, *et al.* Malignant renal neoplasms: correlation between ADC values and cellularity in diffusion weighted magnetic resonance imaging at 3 T. *Radiologia Med* 2008;**113** (2):199–213.

47. Gibbs P, Pickles MD, Turnbull LW. Diffusion imaging of the prostate at 3.0 tesla. *Investig Radiol* 2006;**41** (2):185–8.

48. de Bazelaire CMJ, Duhamel GD, Rofsky NM, Alsop DC. MR imaging relaxation times of abdominal and pelvic tissues measured in vivo at 3.0 T: preliminary results. *Radiology* 2004;**230** (3):652–9.

49. Meiboom S, Gill D. Modified spin-echo method for measuring nuclear relaxation times. *Rev Sci Instrum* 1958;**29**:688–91.

50. Norris DG. Selective parity RARE imaging. *Magn Reson Med* 2007;**58** (4):643–9.

51. Williams CFM, Redpath TW, Norris DG. A novel fast split-echo multi-shot diffusion-weighted MRI method using navigator echoes. *Mag Reson Med* 1999;**41** (4):734–42.

52. Deng J, Omary RA, Larson AC. Multishot diffusion-weighted SPLICE PROPELLER MRI of the abdomen. *Magn Reson Med* 2008;**59** (5):947–53.

53. Le Roux P. Non-CPMG fast spin echo with full signal. *J Magn Reson* 2002;**155** (2):278–92.

54. Norris DG, Driesel W. Online motion correction for diffusion-weighted imaging using navigator echoes: application to RARE imaging without sensitivity loss. *Magn Reson Med* 2001;**45** (5):729–33.

55. Pipe JG, Farthing VG, Forbes KP. Multishot diffusion-weighted FSE using PROPELLER MRI. *Magn Reson Med* 2002;**47**:42–52.

56. Deng J, Miller FH, Salem R, Omary RA, Larson AC. Multishot diffusion-weighted PROPELLER magnetic resonance imaging of the abdomen. *Investig Radiol* 2006;**41** (10):769–75.

57. Gmitro AF, Kono M, Theilmann RJ, *et al.* Radial GRASE: implementation and applications. *Magn Reson Med* 2005;**53** (6):1363–71.

58. Lo GG, Ai V, Chan JKF, *et al.* Diffusion-weighted magnetic resonance imaging of breast lesions: first experiences at 3 T. *J Comput Assist Tomogr* 2009;**33** (1):63–9.

59. Nolte UG, Finsterbusch J, Frahm J. Rapid isotropic diffusion mapping without susceptibility artifacts: whole brain studies using diffusion-weighted single-shot STEAM MR imaging. *Magn Reson Med* 2000;**44** (5):731–6.

60. Cremillieux Y, WheelerKingshott CA, Briguet A, Doran SJ. STEAM-Burst: a single-shot, multi-slice imaging sequence without rapid gradient switching. *Magn Reson Med* 1997;**38** (4):645–52.

61. Steidle G, Schick F. Echoplanar diffusion tensor imaging of the lower leg musculature using eddy current nulled stimulated echo preparation. *Magn Reson Med* 2006;**55** (3):541–8.

62. Jeong EK, Kim SE, Kholmovski EG, Parker DL. High-resolution DTI of a localized volume using 3D single-shot Diffusion-Weighted STimulated Echo-Planar Imaging (3D ss-DWSTEPI). *Magn Reson Med* 2006;**56** (6):1173–81.

63. Buxton RB. The diffusion sensitivity of fast steady-state free precession imaging. *Magn Reson Med* 1993;**29** (2):235–43.

64. Carney CE, Wong STS, Patz S. Analytical solution and verification of diffusion effect in SSFP. *Magn Reson Med* 1991;**19** (2):240–6.

65. Zur Y, Bosak E, Kaplan N. A new diffusion SSFP imaging technique. *Magn Reson Med* 1997;**37** (5):716–22.

66. Bosak E, Harvey PR. Navigator motion correction of diffusion weighted 3D SSFP imaging. *Magn Reson Materials Phys Biol Med* 2001;**12** (2–3):167–76.

67. Miller KL, Pauly JM. Nonlinear phase correction for navigated diffusion imaging. *Magn Reson Med* 2003;**50** (2):343–53.

68. Miller KL, Hargreaves BA, Gold GE, Pauly JM. Steady-state diffusion-weighted imaging of in vivo knee cartilage. *Magn Reson Med* 2004;**51** (2):394–8.

69. Wu EX, Buxton RB. Effect of diffusion on the steady-state magnetization with pulsed field gradients. *J Magn Reson* 1990;**90** (2):243–53.

70. Jeong EK, Kim SE, Parker DL. High-resolution diffusion-weighted 3D MRI, using diffusion-weighted driven-equilibrium (DW-DE) and multishot segmented 3D-SSFP without navigator echoes. *Magn Reson Med* 2003;**50** (4):821–9.

71. Jiang HY, van Zijl PCM, Kim J, Pearlson GD, Mori S. DtiStudio: Resource program for diffusion tensor computation and fiber bundle tracking. *Comput Meth Programs Biomed* 2006;**81** (2):106–16.

72. Burdette JH, Elster AD, Ricci PE. Acute cerebral infarction: quantification of spin-density and T2 shine-through phenomena on diffusion-weighted MR images. *Radiology* 1999;**212** (2):333–9.

73. Song SK, Sun SW, Ramsbottom MJ, *et al.* Dysmyelination revealed through MRI as increased radial (but unchanged axial) diffusion of water. *Neuroimage* 2002;**17** (3):1429–36.

74. Pajevic S, Pierpaoli C. Color schemes to represent the orientation of anisotropic tissues from diffusion tensor data: application to white matter fiber tract mapping in the human brain. *Magn Reson Med* 1999;**42** (3):526–40.

75. Kan JH, Heemskerk AM, Ding ZH, *et al.* DTI-based muscle fiber tracking of the quadriceps mechanism in lateral patellar dislocation. *J Magn Reson Imag* 2009;**29** (3):663–70.

76. Notohamiprodjo M, Glaser C, Herrmann KA, *et al.* Diffusion tensor imaging of the kidney with parallel imaging: Initial clinical experience. *Investig Radiol* 2008;**43** (10):677–85.

77. Glass HI, De Garreta C. Quantitative limitations of exponential curve fitting. *Phys Med Biol* 1971; **16** (1):119–30.

78. Shrager RI, Weiss GH, Spencer RGS. Optimal time spacings for T-2 measurements: monoexponential and biexponential systems. *NMR Biomed* 1998; **11** (6):297–305.

79. Jones DK, Basser PJ. "Squashing peanuts and smashing pumpkins": how noise distorts diffusion-weighted MR data. *Magn Reson Med* 2004;**52** (5):979–93.

80. Dehmeshki J, Ruto AC, Arridge S, *et al.* Analysis of MTR histograms in multiple sclerosis using principal components and multiple discriminant analysis. *Magn Reson Med* 2001;**46** (3):600–9.

81. Lin FC, Yu CS, Jiang TZ, *et al.* Discriminative analysis of relapsing neuromyelitis optica and relapsing-remitting multiple sclerosis based on two-dimensional histogram from diffusion tensor imaging. *Neuroimage* 2006;**31** (2):543–9.

82. Kim S, Pickup S, Hsu H, Poptani H. Diffusion tensor MRI in rat models of invasive and well-demarcated brain tumors. *NMR Biomed* 2008;**21** (3):208–16.

83. Zhang JY, van Zijl PCM, Laterra J, *et al.* Unique patterns of diffusion directionality in rat brain tumors revealed by high-resolution diffusion tensor MRI. *Magn Reson Med* 2007;**58** (3):454–62.

84. Taouli B, Koh DM. Diffusion-weighted MR imaging of the liver. *Radiology* 2010;**254** (1):47–66.

85. Taouli B, Tolia AJ, Losada M, *et al.* Diffusion-weighted MRI for quantification of liver fibrosis: preliminary experience. *Am J Roentgenol* 2007;**189** (4):799–806.

86. Dale BM, Braithwaite AC, Boll DT, Merkle EM. Field strength and diffusion encoding technique affect the apparent diffusion coefficient measurements in diffusion-weighted imaging of the abdomen. *Investig Radiol* 2010;**45** (2):104–8.

87. Kreeftenberg HG Jr, Mooyaart EL, Huizenga JR, Sluiter WJ, Kreeftenberg HG. Quantification of liver iron concentration with magnetic resonance imaging by combining T1-, T2-weighted spin echo sequences and a gradient echo sequence. *Netherl J Med* 2000;**56** (4):133–7.

88. Gomori J, Horev G, Tamary H, *et al.* Hepatic iron overload: quantitative MR imaging. *Radiology* 1991;**179** (2):367–9.

89. Patel J, Sigmund EE, Rusinek H, *et al.* Diagnosis of cirrhosis with intravoxel incoherent motion diffusion MRI and dynamic contrast-enhanced MRI alone and in combination: preliminary experience. *J Magn Reson Imag* 2010;**31** (3):589–600.

90. Zhang J, Sigmund E, Rusinek H, *et al.*, eds. Quantification of renal diffusion-weighted images using a bi-exponential model. *Proc 17th Scientific Meeting International Society for Magnetic Resonance in Medicine*: Honolulu; 2009.

91. Zhang JL, Sigmund EE, Chandarana H, *et al.* Variability of renal apparent diffusion coefficients: limitations of the monoexponential model for diffusion quantification. *Radiology* 2010;**254** (3): 783–92.

92. Kim S, Jain M, Harris AB, *et al.* T1 hyperintense renal lesions: characterization with diffusion-weighted MR imaging versus contrast-enhanced MR imaging. *Radiology* 2009;**251** (3):796–807.

93. Taouli B, Thakur RK, Mannelli L, *et al.* Renal lesions: characterization with diffusion-weighted imaging versus contrast-enhanced MR imaging. *Radiology* 2009;**251** (2):398–407.

94. Thoeny HC, De Keyzer F, Oyen RH, Peeters RR. Diffusion-weighted MR imaging of kidneys in healthy volunteers and patients with parenchymal diseases: *initial experience. Radiology* 2005;**235** (3):911–17.

95. Thoeny HC, Zumstein D, Simon-Zoula S, *et al.* Functional evaluation of transplanted kidneys with diffusion-weighted and BOLD MR imaging: initial experience. *Radiology* 2006;**241** (3):812–21.

96. Chandarana H, Hecht E, Taouli B, Sigmund E, eds. Diffusion tensor imaging of in vivo human kidney at 3 T: robust anisotropy measurement in the medulla. *Proc 16th Scientific Meeting International Society for Magnetic Resonance in Medicine*: Toronto; 2008.

97. Kim S, Naik M, Sigmund EE, Taouli B. Diffusion-weighted MR imaging of the kidneys and the urinary tract. *Magn Reson Imag Clin N Am* 2008;**16** (4):585–96.

98. Ries M, Jones RA, Basseau F, Moonen CTW, Grenier N. Diffusion tensor MRI of the human kidney. *J Magn Reson Imag* 2001;**14** (1):42–9.

99. Chandarana H, Lee V, Barash I, Sigmund E, eds. Understanding renal DTI at 3T: FA and MD changes with water loading. *Proc 17th Scientific Meeting International Society for Magnetic Resonance in Medicine*: Honolulu; 2009 April;.

100. Chandarana H, Lee V, Stoffel D, *et al.*, eds. Evaluation of normal and dysfunctional renal transplants using DTI. *Proc 17th Scientific Meeting International Society for Magnetic Resonance in Medicine*: Honolulu; 2009.

101. Zelhof B, Pickles M, Liney G, *et al.* Correlation of diffusion-weighted magnetic resonance data with cellularity in prostate cancer. *BJU Int* 2009; **103** (7):883–8.

102. Hosseinzadeh K, Schwarz SD. Endorectal diffusion-weighted imaging in prostate cancer to differentiate malignant and benign peripheral zone tissue. *J Magn Reson Imag* 2004;**20** (4):654–61.

103. Kim CK, Park BK, Han JJ, Kang TW, Lee HM. Diffusion-weighted imaging of the prostate at 3 T for differentiation of malignant and benign tissue in transition and peripheral zones: preliminary results. *J Comput Assist Tomogr* 2007;**31** (3):449–54.

104. Morgan VA, Kyriazi S, Ashley SE, DeSouza NM. Evaluation of the potential of diffusion-weighted imaging in prostate cancer detection. *Acta Radiol* 2007;**48** (6):695–703.

105. Xu JQ, Humphrey PA, Kibel AS, *et al.* Magnetic resonance diffusion characteristics of histologically defined prostate cancer in humans. *Magn Reson Med* 2009;**61** (4):842–50.

106. Takayama Y, Kishimoto R, Hanaoka S, *et al.* ADC value and diffusion tensor imaging of prostate cancer: changes in carbon-ion radiotherapy. *J Magn Reson Imag* 2008;**27** (6):1331–5.

107. Manenti G, Carlani M, Mancino S, *et al.* Diffusion tensor magnetic resonance imaging of prostate cancer. *Investig Radiol* 2007;**42** (6):412–19.

108. Sinha S, Sinha U. In vivo diffusion tensor imaging of the human prostate. *Magn Reson Med* 2004;**52** (3):530–7.

109. Gurses B, Kabakci N, Kovanlikaya A, *et al.* Diffusion tensor imaging of the normal prostate at 3 Tesla. *Eur Radiol* 2008;**18** (4):716–21.

110. Mulkern RV, Barnes AS, Haker SJ, *et al.* Biexponential characterization of prostate tissue water diffusion decay curves over an extended *b*-factor range. *Magn Reson Imag* 2006;**24** (5):563–8.

111. Shinmoto H, Oshio K, Tanimoto A, *et al.* Biexponential apparent diffusion coefficients in prostate cancer. *Magn Reson Imag* 2009;**27** (3):355–9.

Chapter 2

Diffusion-weighted MRI of the liver

Bachir Taouli and Dow-Mu Koh

Introduction

With recent advances in technology, diffusion-weighted MRI (DWI) is reaching potential for clinical use in the abdomen, particularly for the assessment of focal and diffuse liver diseases. DWI is an attractive technique for multiple reasons:

- It can potentially add useful information to conventional imaging sequences.
- It is quick (it could be performed within a breath-hold) and can be easily incorporated to existing protocols.
- It does not require intravenous contrast administration, thus is easy to repeat, and useful in patients with severe renal dysfunction at risk of nephrogenic systemic fibrosis (NSF).

This chapter will discuss the applications of DWI applied for the diagnosis of diffuse and focal liver diseases.

Liver diffusion imaging acquisition and processing

DWI acquisition techniques

Single-shot echo-planar imaging (SS EPI) is the most frequently used sequence in combination with fat-suppression (e.g., spectral attenuated inversion recovery or chemical excitation with spectral suppression)[1–4]. Most diffusion studies have been conducted on 1.5-T MR systems, although there is a growing interest in performing such studies with 3-T systems due to increased availability and potential for improved image quality[5–6]. DWI of the liver is usually performed prior to contrast material administration, although performing DWI after the administration of gadolinium-DTPA did not appear to significantly affect apparent diffusion coefficient (ADC) calculations in a prior study[7].

Imaging may be performed in breath-hold which attempts to freeze motion or in free breathing with multiple signal averaging to reduce the effects of motion. Image acquisition in free breathing may also be combined with respiratory triggering[8–9]. Breath-hold SS EPI of the liver is quick to perform and the whole liver can be evaluated in generally two breath-holds of less than 25 s each. However, the disadvantages of breath-hold imaging include poorer signal-to-noise ratio (SNR), greater sensitivity to distortion and ghosting artifacts, lower spatial resolution (with wider section thickness, 8 to 10 mm), and a limitation on the number of b-values that can be used. By comparison, free-breathing multiple averaging SS EPI is a versatile technique that can be implemented reasonably well across different vendor MR platforms. The liver is typically evaluated in 3 to 6 min. The use of multiple signal averages results in images with improved SNR. Consequently, thinner image sections (≥ 5 mm) can be obtained, and more b-values can be accommodated within the longer measurement. High-quality diffusion images of the liver can be obtained by free-breathing technique because cyclical respiration is a coherent motion that does not result in additional signal attenuation from the liver[10]. The disadvantages include slight image blurring, and assessment of lesion heterogeneity may be suboptimal because of volume averaging. Free-breathing DWI may be combined with respiratory triggering, either by navigator or bellows control. When successfully implemented, such a technique results in high-quality images with good anatomical detail (Figure 2.1). It has been shown that respiratory-triggered DWI

Extra-Cranial Applications of Diffusion-Weighted MRI, ed. Bachir Taouli. Published by Cambridge University Press.
© Cambridge University Press 2011.

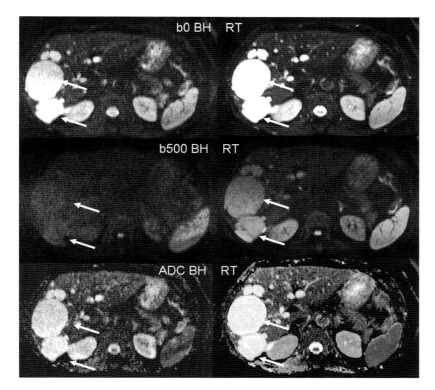

b0 BH RT

b500 BH RT

ADC BH RT

Figure 2.1 Breath-hold (BH) vs. respiratory-triggered (RT) SS EPI diffusion images in a 78-year-old female with liver cysts. RT acquisition (using navigator echo) (four averages) shows better image quality at $b = 0$ and $b = 500$ s/mm^2 (with better lesion delineation) and more homogeneous ADC maps compared to BH acquisition (two averages). There is strong signal drop of liver cysts (arrows) with corresponding high ADC values (3×10^{-3} mm^2/s). [Reproduced with permission from Taouli B, Koh DM. Diffusion-weighted MR imaging of the liver. *Radiology* 2010; **254**:47–66.]

improves liver detection compared to breath-hold DWI (sensitivity for lesion detection 93.7% vs. 84.3%)[11] and improves image quality, SNR, and ADC quantification[8]. However, the implementation of respiratory triggering increases the acquisition time (approximately 5 to 6 min), as the images are only acquired in part of the respiratory cycle. The longer acquisition time can increase the chance of patient movement in the scanner. Last but not least, there is a risk of pseudo-anisotropy artifact using respiratory triggering, which induces errors in the ADC calculation, especially in non-cirrhotic livers[12]. Interestingly, it has been found that there was no significant difference in the mean ADC values obtained using free-breathing or respiratory triggered acquisition schemes, although there was less scattering of ADC values associated with respiratory triggering schemes[13]. A recent study in volunteers has shown that the ADC values obtained using the free-breathing technique were more reproducible compared with breath-hold or navigator controlled image acquisitions[14]. Suggested image acquisition schemes using breath-hold and non-breath-hold techniques are summarized in Table 2.1.

Choice of b-values and sequence optimization

Because of the relatively short T2 relaxation time of the normal liver parenchyma (approximately 46 ms at 1.5 T and 24 ms at 3 T)[15], the b-values used for clinical imaging are typically no higher than 1000 s/mm^2. Applying a small diffusion weighting of $b < 100$–150 s/mm^2 nulls the intrahepatic vascular signal, creating black blood images, which improves the detection of focal liver lesions[6,11,16–17], while higher b-values ($\geq$500 s/mm^2) give diffusion information that helps focal liver lesion characterization[18–19] (Figure 2.2). Hence, when performing DWI in the liver, it is advantageous to perform imaging using both lower and higher b-values (e.g., using $b = 0$, $b \leq 100$, and $b \geq 500$ s/mm^2. Additional b-values can be considered in the context of research or clinical trials, or when the primary aim is to obtain an accurate ADC (e.g., for the assessment of liver fibrosis or cirrhosis). To ensure that the highest-quality images are consistently obtained, the imaging sequences should be optimized to maximize SNR and reduce artifacts which may arise from motion, eddy

Table 2.1 Suggested sequence parameters for performing diffusion-weighted MR imaging of the liver

	Breath-hold acquisition	Free-breathing or respiratory triggered acquisition
Field of view (RL × AP, mm)	350–400 × 262–300	350–400 × 262–300
Matrix size (Phase × Frequency encoding)	144 × 192	144 × 192
TR	≥1600–2000	2500–6000
TE[a]	Minimum (~71)	Minimum (~71–82)
EPI factor[b]	144	144
Phase encoding direction	AP	AP
Parallel imaging acceleration factor	2	2
Number of averages	2	≥ 5
Slice thickness (mm)	7–8	5–7
Number of slices	10	20
Direction of motion probing gradients[c]	Phase, frequency, and slice (Trace[d])	Phase, frequency, and slice (Trace)
Fat suppression	Yes	Yes
b-values (s/mm^2)	3 b-values: 0, 50–100, 500	4 b-values: 0, 50–100, 500, 700–1000
Acquisition time	23 s	2–3 min (free breathing), ≥3 min (respiratory triggering)

Notes: [a]Minimum TE depends on the system and the b values used, and should be kept fixed for all b values used in a study.
[b]EPI factor: number of k-space lines collected per excitation.
[c]Three directions are generally used for liver imaging, although more directions could be used (DTI)[51,61–67].
[d]Trace is the average image from three directions.
[Reproduced with permission from Taouli B, Koh DM. Diffusion-weighted MR imaging of the liver. *Radiology* 2010; **254**:47–66.]

currents, chemical shift, Nyquist ghosting, susceptibility effects[20], and the noise amplification from acceleration techniques[21].

Image display and processing

Trace diffusion images (average images between the images obtained with the three diffusion gradient directions) are displayed for each b-value acquired, together with an ADC map. High b-value images are assessed for areas of restricted diffusion, i.e., appearing in high signal intensity. Calculation of ADC values from the native b-value images is a semi-automated process on most commercial MR scanners or workstations. However, more sophisticated analyses may be possible off-line using developmental software to apply more complex algorithms to the data fitting (e.g., biexponential models based on IVIM)[22–27] (Figure 2.3).

Qualitative visual assessment

Visual assessment is helpful for disease detection and characterization by observing the differential signal attenuation between tissues on DWI. Cellular tissues, such as tumors or abscesses, will demonstrate restricted diffusion (high signal intensity) on the higher b-value (≥500 s/mm^2) images and lower ADC values. By contrast, cystic or necrotic tissues will show a greater degree of signal attenuation on the higher b-value diffusion images and return higher ADC values (Figures 2.1, 2.2, 2.4, 2.5, 2.6, and 2.7). However, the signal intensity observed on the diffusion image is dependent on both water proton diffusivity and tissue T2 relaxation time, which is a possible confounding factor. This means that a lesion may appear to show restricted diffusion on DWI, because of the long T2 relaxation time rather than the limited mobility of the water protons

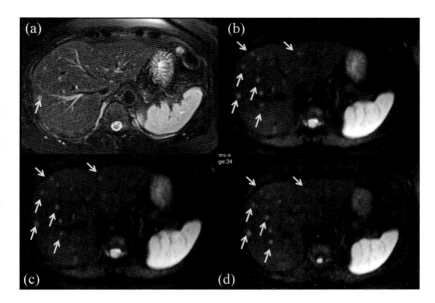

Figure 2.2 Liver metastases better detected with DWI compared to T2-WI. Axial fat suppressed fast spin-echo T2-weighted image (a) shows a small metastatic lesion (arrow). However, there are many more metastatic lesions (arrows) identified on axial fat suppressed SS EPI diffusion images ($b = 50$ [b], 500 [c], 1000 s/mm^2 [d]) in a 42-year-old female with breast cancer. The lesions are more easily detected on diffusion images, and remain bright on high b-value consistent with malignant lesions.

(T2 shine-through). This phenomenon can be observed in cysts and hemangiomas. The presence of T2 shine-through is recognized by correlating high b-value images with the ADC map. Areas demonstrating significant T2 shine-through rather than restricted diffusion will show high diffusivity on the ADC map and high ADC values (Figure 2.8). For this reason, diffusion images should be interpreted concurrently with the ADC map and all other available conventional imaging sequences.

Quantitative assessment

The ADC of the liver calculated from diffusion acquisition can be visually assessed from the ADC maps, or by drawing regions of interest (ROIs) on the ADC maps to record the mean or median ADC values in the tissue of interest. ADC is usually expressed in ($\times 10^{-3}$) mm^2/s and is being investigated by several research groups as a marker of tumor response to treatment. The ADC can also aid in the characterization of liver lesions, and for the diagnosis of liver fibrosis and cirrhosis. However, ADC quantification requires minimum acceptable SNR at higher b-values[28]. Using low SNR images for ADC quantification may artificially reduce the ADC.

Applications of liver DWI

These include liver lesion detection and characterization, assessment of tumor treatment response and diagnosis of liver fibrosis and cirrhosis.

Liver lesion detection and characterization

Several publications have reported the use of DWI for liver lesion detection[11,29–30]. Few of these studies have performed head-to-head direct comparison between DWI and T2-WI in terms of lesion detection. These studies have showed higher sensitivity in lesion detection with DWI[30–32] or showing comparable image quality with DWI using low b-values[17]. Black blood diffusion images (using low b-values) in which background signal of vessels in the liver parenchyma is suppressed allow for lesion detection, while images with higher b-values give diffusion information that enables lesion characterization. Zech et al.[32] compared DWI using $b = 50$ s/mm^2 with fat-suppressed T2WI, and observed better image quality, fewer artifacts, and better sensitivity for lesion detection with DWI sequence (83% vs. 61%). Bruegel et al.[31] compared respiratory-triggered DWI to five different T2-WI sequences (breath-hold fat-suppressed single-shot T2-WI FSE, breath-hold fat-suppressed FSE, respiratory-triggered fat-suppressed FSE, breath-hold short tau inversion recovery (STIR), and respiratory-triggered STIR) for the diagnosis of hepatic metastases at 1.5 T. DWI showed higher accuracy (0.91–0.92) compared to T2 TSE techniques (0.47–0.67). These differences were more significant for small metastatic lesions less than 1 cm in size. These studies have led to the claim that DWI is better and improved T2-WI sequence (Figures 2.2 and 2.4). In a recent study[33], the addition of DWI to Mangafodipir trisodium

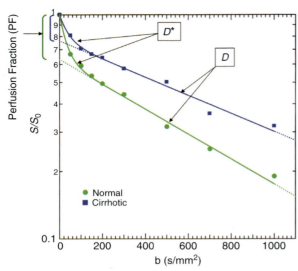

Figure 2.3 IVIM diffusion decay curves shown in a 70-year-old female patient with non-cirrhotic liver (green) and a 71-year-old female patient with cirrhosis related to chronic hepatitis C (blue). y-axis: ratio of signal intensity (SI) after application of diffusion gradient to baseline SI (in log scale) measured in liver parenchyma, x-axis: b-values (multiple b-values, 0–50–100–150–200–300–500–700–1000 s/mm^2 are used for sampling). The perfusion (or pseudo-diffusion) effect is seen as an early drop in SI observed with b-values lower than 200 s/mm^2. Perfusion fraction (PF) is measured as the difference between SI for b = 0 s/mm^2 and the intercept of the high b-value monoexponential fit. Pseudo-diffusion coefficient D* measures the curvature of the initial curve; true diffusion coefficient D is measured at b-values higher than 200 s/mm^2. ADC is measured using all b-values with a monoexponential fit. PF (%), D* ($\times 10^{-3}$ mm^2/s), D ($\times 10^{-3}$ mm^2/s), and ADC ($\times 10^{-3}$ mm^2/s) were all decreased in the cirrhotic patient (23.52, 24.02, 0.93, 1.22 in cirrhosis vs. 36.80, 29.78, 1.28, 2.05 in normal liver, respectively). [Reproduced with permission from Patel J, et al. Diagnosis of cirrhosis with intravoxel incoherent motion diffusion MRI and dynamic contrast-enhanced MRI alone and in combination: preliminary experience. J Magn Reson Imag 2010; 31:589–600.]

(MnDPDP)-enhanced MR significantly improved the diagnostic accuracy for detection of colorectal liver metastases compared with either technique alone. DWI was found to be of value in detecting small (<1 cm) metastases that mimicked intrahepatic vasculature and also in revealing lesions close to the edge of the liver. Hardie et al.[34] recently reported their experience for detection of liver metastases using DWI compared to gadolinium-enhanced T1-WI. Two observers retrospectively assessed 51 patients with extrahepatic malignancies. Ninety-three liver lesions (49 metastases, 44 benign lesions) were identified in 27 patients, 11 patients had no liver lesions, and 13 patients had innumerable metastatic and/or benign lesions. There was no difference in diagnostic performance between the two methods for either observer for the diagnosis of metastatic lesions per patient. For per-lesion analysis, sensitivity of DWI was equivalent to contrast-enhanced T1-WI for observer 1 (67.3% vs. 63.3%, $p = 0.67$), and lower for observer 2 (65.3% vs. 83.7%, $p = 0.007$). By pooling data from both observers, the sensitivity of DWI was 66.3% (65/98) and 73.5% (72/98) for CE T1-WI, not significantly different ($p = 0.171$). There were few cases in which DWI characterized metastases better than contrast-enhanced T1-WI (Figure 2.9). They concluded that DWI is a reasonable alternative to gadolinium-enhanced T1-WI for detection of liver metastases. However, they did not assess the additional value of DWI over contrast-enhanced T1-WI.

Although there is limited data on hepatocellular carcinoma (HCC) detection using DWI, studies have shown that addition of DWI to gadolinium-enhanced MRI or superparamagnetic iron oxide (SPIO)-enhanced MRI increases sensitivity for detection of HCCs. Thus combination of DWI with either gadolinium or SPIO-enhanced study outperforms single-contrast acquisition in detection of HCCs[35–36].

Visual assessment of diffusion images which include higher b-values (≥ 500 s/mm^2) can distinguish solid and cystic lesions. Quantitative ADC values can also be used to discriminate benign from malignant lesions as benign hepatic lesions have generally higher ADC values compared with malignant lesions, with variable degree of overlap[11,19,25,37–38]. Different ADC cut-offs (1.4–1.6×10^{-3} mm^2/s) have been described in the literature with reported sensitivity in the range of 74%–100% and specificity of 77%–100% (Table 2.2). The diagnostic performance of DWI reported in the study by Parikh et al.[11] (area under the curve, sensitivity, and specificity of 0.839, 74%, and 77%) likely reflects the realistic performance of ADC, since it assessed a large number of various benign and malignant lesions (including solid benign lesions and abscesses). However, there is considerable overlap between cellular benign hepatic lesions, such as focal nodular hypoplasia (FNH) and adenoma, and the malignant lesions like metastasis and HCC. Furthermore, mucinous or necrotic malignant tumors may have lower restriction to diffusion and hence high ADC and can be falsely diagnosed as benign lesions (Figure 2.10). These potential pitfalls of DWI must be kept in mind while using it for liver lesion characterization. The role of DWI in discriminating

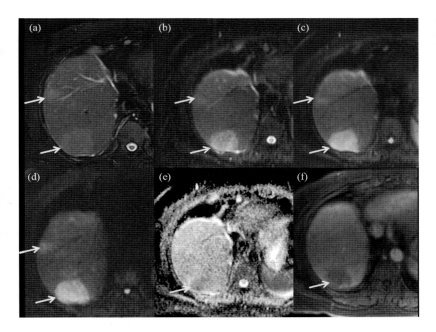

Figure 2.4 Detection and characterization of HCC with DWI. Axial fat suppressed fast spin-echo T2-weighted image (a) in a patient with hepatitis C related cirrhosis shows two liver lesions (arrows). The lesions are more conspicuous on axial fat-suppressed SS-EPI diffusion images ($b = 0$ [b], 50 [c], 500 s/mm² [d]). The ADC map shows decreased ADC in the largest posterior lesion, which is also hypovascular on the post-contrast T1-WI at the arterial phase.

	b0	High b	ADC
Benign lesion (e.g. cystic lesion)	○	●	○
Malignant lesion (e.g. Metastasis)	○	○	●
T2 shine-through (e.g. cyst-hemangioma)	○	○	○

Figure 2.5 Visual liver lesion characterization with DWI. This figure gives a simplified approach to lesion characterization using visual assessment of $b = 0$, higher b-value, and ADC maps. A benign fluid-containing lesion shows strong signal drop with high ADC, whereas a cellular malignant lesion shows no or minimal signal drop, with low ADC compared to surrounding liver parenchyma. A lesion with long T2 can sometimes show a T2 shine-through effect. [Reproduced with permission from Taouli B, Koh DM. Diffusion-weighted MR imaging of the liver. *Radiology* 2010;**254**:47–66.]

high-grade from low-grade HCC is also under investigation. In one recent study[39], moderately and poorly differentiated HCCs had significantly lower ADC compared to well differentiated HCCs and dysplastic nodules. Furthermore, in the same study authors demonstrated that all iso- to hypovascular lesions on gadolinium-enhanced examination which were also visible on DWI were poorly differentiated HCCs, whereas lesions not visible on DWI were low-grade HCCs or dysplastic nodules[39].

Diagnosis of liver fibrosis and cirrhosis with DWI

The diagnosis of early and moderate liver fibrosis is difficult with conventional MR imaging sequences and currently liver biopsy is considered the gold standard. Limitations of liver biopsy include not only morbidity but also sampling error due to heterogeneous spatial distribution of liver fibrosis. Several reports have suggested that ADC of the cirrhotic liver is lower than that of normal liver[18–19,40–41] Lewin *et al.*[42] compared DWI (using b-values of 400–800 s/mm²) to FibroScan© (sonographic elastography technique) and serum markers of fibrosis in 54 patients with chronic hepatitis C and 20 healthy volunteers. They observed an excellent performance of ADC for the prediction of moderate and severe fibrosis. Patients with moderate-to-severe fibrosis (F2–F4) had hepatic ADC values lower than those without or with mild fibrosis (F0–F1) and healthy volunteers (Figure 2.11): 1.10 ± 0.11 vs. 1.30 ± 0.12 vs. $1.44 \pm 0.02 \times 10^{-3}$ mm²/s, respectively. For the discrimination of patients with fibrosis stage F3–F4 from F0–F2, the areas under the curves (AUCs) were 0.92 for ADC, 0.92 for FibroScan©, 0.79–0.87 for blood tests. Sensitivity and specificity of ADC were 87% and 87%, respectively (using ADC cut-off of 1.21×10^{-3} mm²/s). In another study, although cirrhotic liver had much lower ADC compared to

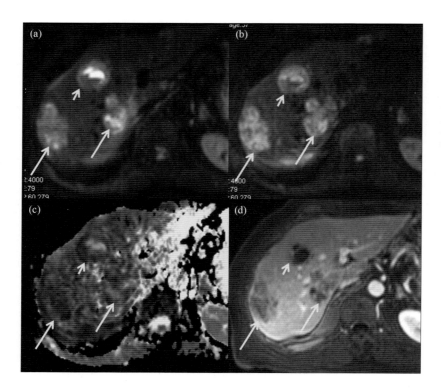

Figure 2.6 Neuroendocrine tumor metastases in a 70-year-old male. Axial SS EPI diffusion images ($b = 50$ [a] and $b = 500$ [b]), and ADC map (using 0–50–500 [c]) show multiple metastatic liver lesions with restricted diffusion (arrows), including a hemorrhagic necrotic lesion with internal fluid–fluid level (arrowhead). Axial fat-suppressed breath-hold post-contrast T1-WI (d) demonstrate mostly enhancing lesions except for the necrotic lesion.

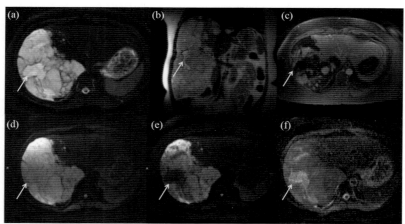

Figure 2.7 Giant hemangioma in a 42-year-old female. Breath-hold fat-suppressed axial T2-DWI (a), coronal single-shot T2 HASTE (b), and axial post-contrast fat suppressed T1-weighted images demonstrate a giant hemangioma replacing the entire right hepatic lobe with a small central cystic area (arrow). Axial SS EPI images ($b = 50$ [d]; $b = 500$ [e]) and ADC map (using 0–50–500 s/mm^2) demonstrate a bright lesion at $b = 50$, with some degree of signal loss, more pronounced in the central cystic area. The ADC map shows heterogeneous ADC distribution, with some areas with restricted diffusion.

normal non-cirrhotic liver, ADC was not able to reliably discriminate between low and high grade (F ≥ 2) fibrosis[43]. In this study approximately 35% of patients had undergone prior liver transplantation and it is unclear whether this may have been a confounding factor as effects of transplantation on liver ADC have not been well evaluated. Luciani *et al.*[26] acquired DW-MR with 10 *b*-values and performed biexponential fit as per intravoxel incoherent motion (IVIM) analysis. They demonstrated lower fast

diffusion component in cirrhotics compared to normal liver suggesting contribution of altered perfusion. In a recent study, Patel *et al.*[27] compared IVIM DWI with dynamic contrast-enhanced MRI (DCE-MRI) in 30 subjects (16 with non-cirrhotic liver, 14 with cirrhosis). They showed that PF (perfusion fraction), pseudo-diffusion coefficient (D^*), true diffusion coefficient (D), and ADC values were significantly lower in cirrhosis, whereas perfusion parameters assessed with DCE-MRI were also altered, without

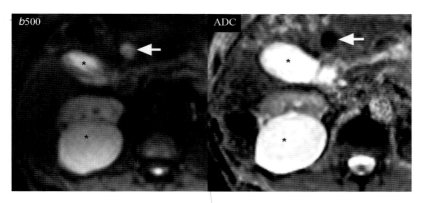

Figure 2.8 T2 shine-through effect with DWI. Axial fat-suppressed breath-hold SS EPI diffusion images in 60-year-old female with metastatic liver disease obtained for $b = 500s/mm^2$ and corresponding ADC map. The liver metastasis (arrow), the renal cyst, and the gallbladder (asterisks) show high signal intensity on the diffusion image. This is clarified on the ADC map, where the metastasis shows low diffusivity reflected by the low ADC, while the cyst and gallbladder show high ADC, not because of restricted water diffusion, but because of the long T2 relaxation time of the fluid (T2 shine-through). [Reproduced with permission from Taouli B, Koh DM. Diffusion-weighted MR imaging of the liver. *Radiology* 2010;**254**:47–66.]

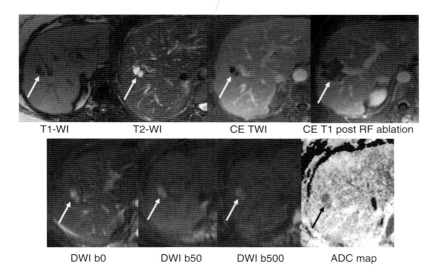

Figure 2.9 Mischaracterized metastatic lesion with contrast-enhanced imaging correctly characterized with DWI in a 63-year-old female patient with metastatic mucinous colon cancer. Axial out-of-phase T1-, fat-suppressed T2-, fat-suppressed T1-weighted contrast-enhanced (portal venous phase), T1-weighted contrast-enhanced (portal venous phase) post RF ablation (1 month later), and SS EPI diffusion-weighted images (for $b = 0$, 50, and 500 s/mm^2, and ADC map) show a bilobed right hepatic lobe lesion (arrow) interpreted incorrectly as benign using contrast-enhanced images, and correctly as metastasis using DWI. While the lesion has features suggestive of a benign bilobed cyst on T1-, T2-, and contrast-enhanced images, the lesion demonstrates restricted diffusion (persistent bright signal on the $b = 500$ image, and ADC visually lower than adjacent liver). The patient underwent subsequent RF ablation and right hepatectomy. [Reproduced with permission from Hardie AD, *et al*. Diagnosis of liver metastases: value of diffusion-weighted MRI compared with gadolinium-enhanced MRI. *Eur Radiol* 2010; **20**:1431–41.]

any correlation between IVIM and DCE-MRI parameters. The combination of ADC with DCE-MRI parameters provided 84.6% sensitivity and 100% specificity for diagnosis of cirrhosis. This should be confirmed in larger studies including intermediate stages of fibrosis (Figure 2.12), and should be compared with other methods such as MR elastography.

Assessment of tumor response to treatment

Studies in both animals and humans have shown that effective tumor treatment results generally in a rise in ADC, which can occur prior to measurable change in tumor size. A study by Koh *et al.*[44] in colorectal hepatic metastases demonstrated mean ADC increase

Table 2.2 Mean apparent diffusion coefficients (ADCs) of normal liver and focal liver lesions, ADC cut-offs, and sensitivity/specificity for diagnosing malignant lesions as reported in selected studies from the literature

	Namimoto[68]	Kim[18]a	Taouli[19]b	Bruegel[37]	Gourtsoyianni[38]	Parikh[11]
Number of patients/ lesions	51/59	126/79	66/52	102/204	38/37	53/211
b-values (s/mm^2)	30–1200	≤846	≤500	50–300–600	0–50–500–1000	0–50–500
ADC values						
Normal liver	0.69	1.02	1.83	1.24	1.25–1.31	
Metastases	1.15	1.06–1.11	0.94	1.22	0.99	1.50
HCCs	0.99	0.97–1.28	1.33	1.05	1.38	1.31
Hemangiomas	1.95	2.04–2.10	2.95	1.92	1.90	2.04
Cysts	3.05	2.91–3.03	3.63	3.02	2.55	2.54
Adenomas-FNHs			1.75	1.40		1.49
Benign lesions	1.95	2.49	2.45		2.55	2.19
Malignant lesions	1.04	1.01	1.08		1.04	1.39
ADC cut-off for diagnosis of malignant liver lesions^c		1.60	1.50	1.63	1.47	1.60
Sensitivity (%)		98	84	90	100	74
Specificity (%)		80	89	86	100	77

Notes: ^{a}ADCs for $b < 850$ s/mm^2 are given.
^{b}ADCs for $b = 0$–500 s/mm^2 are given.
^{c}Lesions with ADC below the proposed cut-off value are considered malignant while those with ADC above are considered benign.
[Reproduced with permission from Taouli B, Koh DM. Diffusion-weighted MR imaging of the liver. *Radiology* 2010; **254**:47–66.]

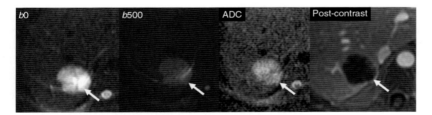

Figure 2.10 Pitfall of DWI: necrotic colon cancer metastasis post treatment. Transverse fat-suppressed breath-hold SS EPI diffusion images in a 62-year-old man with metastatic colon cancer treated with systemic chemotherapy, obtained using b-values of 0 and 500 s/mm^2 with corresponding ADC map and post-contrast image. The metastatic lesion is hyperintense at $b = 0$ s/mm^2, but shows no diffusion restriction with corresponding high ADC, in relation with its necrotic content, as shown on the post-contrast image. [Reproduced with permission from Taouli B, Koh DM. Diffusion-weighted MR imaging of the liver. *Radiology* 2010;**254**:47–66.]

in lesions that showed at least a partial response by the response criteria in solid tumors (RECIST) to chemotherapy. The rise in ADC was absent in lesions that showed either no change or disease progression by conventional RECIST criteria[44]. In another study[45], an early increase in ADC at 3–7 days after initiating chemotherapy was observed among responders but not in non-responders. Another interesting finding was that the colorectal metastases with a high pre-treatment ADC responded poorly to chemotherapy, suggesting that tumors that were more necrotic prior to treatment are more chemoresistant[44–45]. Clearly, these findings need to be validated in larger prospective studies, but nevertheless illustrate the potential

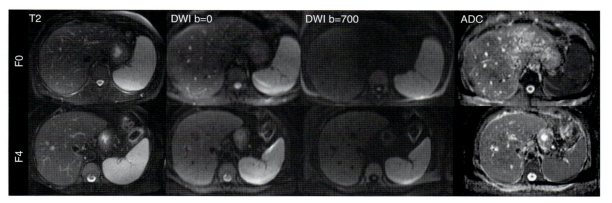

Figure 2.11 DWI for diagnosis of liver fibrosis. 52-year-old male with chronic hepatitis C without evidence of fibrosis at liver biopsy (F0 – top row) and 67-year-old female with cirrhosis secondary to chronic hepatitis C (F4 – bottom row). Breath-hold fat-suppressed TSE T2-weighted image and breath-hold fat-suppressed single-shot echoplanar diffusion-weighted images for $b = 0$ and $b = 700$ mm^2/s and ADC map (using $b = 0$ and $b = 700$ mm^2/s) are shown. In the patient without fibrosis, hepatic ADC was within normal range, measuring 1.6×10^{-3} s/mm^2, the liver appearing brighter than the spleen (which is known to have low ADC). In the cirrhotic patient, T2-weighted image shows minimal morphologic changes in relation with cirrhosis. However, hepatic ADC was decreased (reaching the spleen ADC), measuring 1.0×10^{-3} s/mm^2 (according to the ADC values described by Taouli et al. [41]). [Reproduced with permission from Taouli B, Ehman RL, Reeder SB. Advanced MRI methods for assessment of chronic liver disease. Am J Roentgenol 2009;**193**:14–27.]

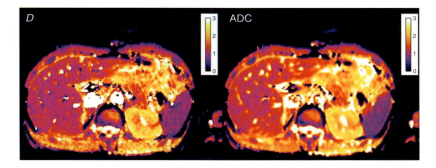

Figure 2.12 IVIM for diagnosis of liver fibrosis. 44-year-old female with chronic hepatitis C with stage 3 liver fibrosis at liver biopsy. D map (true diffusion coefficient obtained with biexponential fitting, left) and ADC map (right) obtained with seven b-values (0–1000 s/mm^2) show decreased D (1.03×10^{-3} mm^2/s) and ADC (1.12×10^{-3} mm^2/s). D is lower than ADC secondary to decreased perfusion contamination.

predictive value of the imaging quantitative ADC measurement. There are several reports on the use of DWI to evaluate HCC response to chemo- or radio-embolization[46–48]. These studies have demonstrated differences in ADC between viable and necrotic portions of HCCs post-treatment, and measurable differences before and after treatment. In our experience (28 HCCs in 21 patients)[49], ADC had a significant correlation with necrosis as assessed with histopathology ($r = 0.64$, $p < 0.001$) in patients who underwent treatment with transarterial chemoembolization prior to liver transplantation (Figure 2.13).

Limitations of DWI technique in the liver

Single-shot EPI DWI still suffers from limited image quality, including poor SNR, limited spatial resolution, and EPI-related artifacts (mainly distortion, ghosting, and blurring). Strategies to improve image quality are detailed in a recent review paper[50]. For example, parallel imaging should be used systematically to reduce susceptibility artifacts and decrease the echo time (TE), in order to improve SNR[51–53]. It is important to emphasize that DWI is an imaging technique that still often requires varying degrees of optimization to ensure consistent high-quality performance. To this end, we suggest that new clinical sites without experience with this technique should consider engaging the help of a clinical scientist, physicist, or vendor application specialist to assist in the optimization process.

Future directions

The value of DWI for tumor detection and tumor treatment response needs to be further assessed in

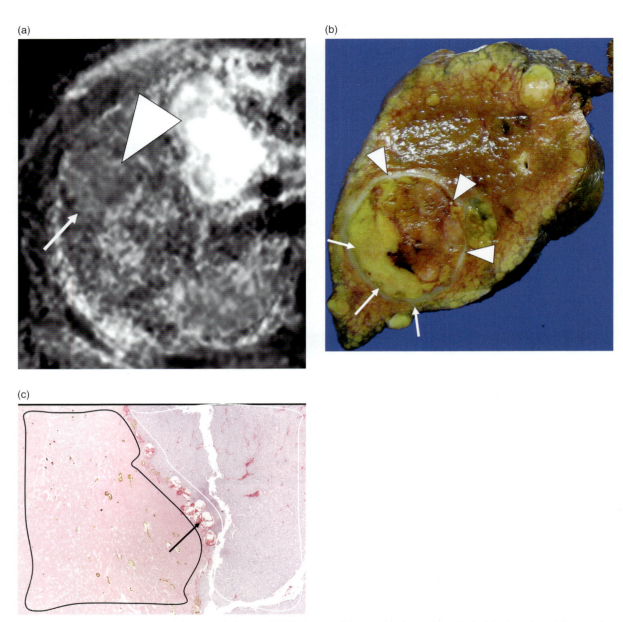

Figure 2.13 HCC post-transarterial chemoembolization (TACE). 51-year-old man with chronic hepatitis B cirrhosis and partially necrotic HCC post TACE. (a) Axial ADC map calculated from SS EPI diffusion images ($b = 0$–50–500 s/mm^2) shows posterior necrotic area (arrow) with higher ADC (2.21×10^{-3} mm^2/s) compared to anterior viable portion (arrowhead) (ADC 1.61×10^{-3} mm^2/s). (b) Gross coronal explant picture demonstrates 60% necrotic tumor (arrow), with viable (arrowhead) and necrotic portions (arrow) with similar spatial distribution as ADC map. (c) Microscopic picture (hematoxylin and eosin, $20 \times$ magnification) shows necrotic area (black line) and viable HCC (white line), as well as embolic material used for TACE (black arrow). [Reproduced with permission from Mannelli L, *et al*. Assessment of tumor necrosis of hepatocellular carcinoma after chemoembolization: diffusion-weighted and contrast-enhanced MRI with histopathologic correlation of the explanted liver. *Am J Roentgenol* 2009;**193**:1044–52.]

liver tumors treated locally or with systemic therapy, including newly developed antiangiogenic drugs. In addition, despite the increased availability of 3-T scanners, there is still limited data on the use of 3-T DWI of the liver[6,54]. High field imaging enables higher SNR[5–6,55–56]; however, EPI suffers from increased susceptibility artifacts at high field. A recent study has proposed DWI as a lower specific absorption rate (SAR) alternative to T2-WI at 3 T[6]. Non-EPI sequences may play a role at higher field; however, data on liver DWI are still sparse[57–58]. Finally, it might be interesting to assess the value of multiparametric imaging combining DWI with other functional MR imaging techniques such as dynamic contrast-enhanced MR imaging or MR elastography for assessment of diffuse liver disease and for tumor treatment response[59–60]. This should be ideally performed in a multicentric setting.

Conclusions

In the clinical setting, DWI can be used for liver lesion detection and lesion characterization, with better results compared to T2-WI and potential additional value to contrast-enhanced sequences. In the research setting, applications such as assessment of treatment response (especially in multicenter settings) and diagnosis of liver fibrosis and cirrhosis are promising; however, they require further confirmation. In addition to comparing DWI with conventional sequences, future studies should assess the value of combining DWI with conventional sequences. The radiologist has to be aware of potential pitfalls and limitations of the technique; and we suggest that diffusion images should be interpreted in conjunction with conventional sequences. In patients who cannot receive gadolinium contrast agents, DWI appears as a reasonable alternative technique to contrast-enhanced imaging.

References

1. Stehling MK, Turner R, Mansfield P. Echo-planar imaging – magnetic-resonance imaging in a fraction of a second. *Science* 1991;**254** (5028):43–50.

2. Butts K, Riederer SJ, Ehman RL, Felmlee JP, Grimm RC. Echo-planar imaging of the liver with a standard MR imaging system. *Radiology* 1993;**189** (1):259–64.

3. Turner R, Le Bihan D, Chesnick AS. Echo-planar imaging of diffusion and perfusion. *Magn Reson Med* 1991;**19** (2):247–53.

4. Turner R, Le Bihan D, Maier J, *et al.* Echo-planar imaging of intravoxel incoherent motion. *Radiology* 1990;**177** (2):407–14.

5. Braithwaite AC, Dale BM, Boll DT, Merkle EM. Short- and midterm reproducibility of apparent diffusion coefficient measurements at 3.0-T diffusion-weighted imaging of the abdomen. *Radiology* 2009; **250** (2):459–65.

6. van den Bos IC, Hussain SM, Krestin GP, Wielopolski PA. Liver imaging at 3.0 T: diffusion-induced black-blood echo-planar imaging with large anatomic volumetric coverage as an alternative for specific absorption rate-intensive echo-train spin-echo sequences: feasibility study. *Radiology* 2008;**248** (1):264–71.

7. Chiu FY, Jao JC, Chen CY, *et al.* Effect of intravenous gadolinium-DTPA on diffusion-weighted magnetic resonance images for evaluation of focal hepatic lesions. *J Comput Assist Tomogr* 2005;**29** (2):176–80.

8. Taouli B, Sandberg A, Stemmer A, *et al.* Diffusion-weighted imaging of the liver: comparison of navigator triggered and breathhold acquisitions. *J Magn Reson Imag* 2009;**30** (3):561–8.

9. Kandpal H, Sharma R, Madhusudhan KS, Kapoor KS. Respiratory-triggered versus breath-hold diffusion-weighted MRI of liver lesions: comparison of image quality and apparent diffusion coefficient values. *Am J Roentgenol* 2009;**192** (4):915–22.

10. Kwee TC, Takahara T, Ochiai R, Nievelstein RA, Luijten PR. Diffusion-weighted whole-body imaging with background body signal suppression (DWIBS): features and potential applications in oncology. *Eur Radiol* 2008;**18** (9):1937–52.

11. Parikh T, Drew SJ, Lee VS, *et al.* Focal liver lesion detection and characterization with diffusion-weighted MR imaging: comparison with standard breath-hold T2-weighted imaging. *Radiology* 2008;**246** (3):812–22.

12. Nasu K, Kuroki Y, Fujii H, Minami M. Hepatic pseudo-anisotropy: a specific artifact in hepatic diffusion-weighted images obtained with respiratory triggering. *Magma* 2007;**20** (4):205–11.

13. Nasu K, Kuroki Y, Sekiguchi R, Nawano S. The effect of simultaneous use of respiratory triggering in diffusion-weighted imaging of the liver. *Magn Reson Med Sci* 2006;**5** (3):129–36.

14. Kwee TC, Takahara T, Koh DM, Nievelstein RA, Luijten PR. Comparison and reproducibility of ADC measurements in breathhold, respiratory triggered, and free-breathing diffusion-weighted MR imaging of the liver. *J Magn Reson Imag* 2008;**28** (5):1141–8.

15. de Bazelaire CM, Duhamel GD, Rofsky NM, Alsop DC. MR imaging relaxation times of abdominal and pelvic tissues measured in vivo at 3.0 T: preliminary results. *Radiology* 2004;**230** (3):652–9.

16. Okada Y, Ohtomo K, Kiryu S, Sasaki Y. Breath-hold T2-weighted MRI of hepatic tumors: value of echo planar imaging with diffusion-sensitizing gradient. *J Comput Assist Tomogr* 1998;**22** (3):364–71.

17. Hussain SM, De Becker J, Hop WC, Dwarkasing S, Wielopolski PA. Can a single-shot black-blood T2-weighted spin-echo echo-planar imaging sequence with sensitivity encoding replace the respiratory-triggered turbo spin-echo sequence for the liver?

An optimization and feasibility study. *J Magn Reson Imag* 2005;**21** (3):219–29.

18. Kim T, Murakami T, Takahashi S, Hori M, Tsuda K, Nakamura H. Diffusion-weighted single-shot echoplanar MR imaging for liver disease. *Am J Roentgenol* 1999;**173** (2):393–8.

19. Taouli B, Vilgrain V, Dumont E, *et al.* Evaluation of liver diffusion isotropy and characterization of focal hepatic lesions with two single-shot echo-planar MR imaging sequences: prospective study in 66 patients. *Radiology* 2003;**226** (1):71–8.

20. Le Bihan D, Poupon C, Amadon A, Lethimonnier F. Artifacts and pitfalls in diffusion MRI. *J Magn Reson Imag* 2006;**24** (3):478–88.

21. Pruessmann KP, Weiger M, Scheidegger MB, Boesiger P. SENSE: sensitivity encoding for fast MRI. *Magn Reson Med* 1999;**42** (5):952–62.

22. Niendorf T, Dijkhuizen RM, Norris DG, van Lookeren Campagne M, Nicolay K. Biexponential diffusion attenuation in various states of brain tissue: implications for diffusion-weighted imaging. *Magn Reson Med* 1996;**36** (6):847–57.

23. Assaf Y, Cohen Y. Non-mono-exponential attenuation of water and *N*-acetyl aspartate signals due to diffusion in brain tissue. *J Magn Reson* 1998;**131** (1):69–85.

24. Le Bihan D, Breton E, Lallemand D, *et al.* Separation of diffusion and perfusion in intravoxel incoherent motion MR imaging. *Radiology* 1988;**168** (2):497–505.

25. Yamada I, Aung W, Himeno Y, Nakagawa T, Shibuya H. Diffusion coefficients in abdominal organs and hepatic lesions: evaluation with intravoxel incoherent motion echo-planar MR imaging. *Radiology* 1999;**210** (3):617–23.

26. Luciani A, Vignaud A, Cavet M, *et al.* Liver cirrhosis: intravoxel incoherent motion MR imaging – pilot study. *Radiology* 2008;**249** (3):891–9.

27. Patel J, Sigmund EE, Rusinek H, *et al.* Diagnosis of cirrhosis with intravoxel incoherent motion diffusion MRI and dynamic contrast-enhanced MRI alone and in combination: preliminary experience. *J Magn Reson Imag* 2010;**31** (3):589–600.

28. Gudbjartsson H, Patz S. The Rician distribution of noisy MRI data. *Magn Reson Med* 1995;**34** (6):910–14.

29. Nasu K, Kuroki Y, Nawano S, *et al.* Hepatic metastases: diffusion-weighted sensitivity-encoding versus SPIO-enhanced MR imaging. *Radiology* 2006;**239** (1):122–30.

30. Coenegrachts K, Delanote J, Ter Beek L, *et al.* Improved focal liver lesion detection: comparison of single-shot diffusion-weighted echoplanar and single-shot T2 weighted turbo spin echo techniques. *Br J Radiol* 2007;**80** (955):524–31.

31. Bruegel M, Gaa J, Waldt S, *et al.* Diagnosis of hepatic metastasis: comparison of respiration-triggered diffusion-weighted echo-planar MRI and five T2-weighted turbo spin-echo sequences. *Am J Roentgenol* 2008;**191** (5):1421–9.

32. Zech CJ, Herrmann KA, Dietrich O, *et al.* Black-blood diffusion-weighted EPI acquisition of the liver with parallel imaging: comparison with a standard T2-weighted sequence for detection of focal liver lesions. *Investig Radiol* 2008;**43** (4):261–6.

33. Koh DM, Brown G, Riddell AM, *et al.* Detection of colorectal hepatic metastases using MnDPDP MR imaging and diffusion-weighted imaging (DWI) alone and in combination. *Eur Radiol* 2008;**18** (5):903–10.

34. Hardie AD, Naik M, Hecht EM, *et al.* Diagnosis of liver metastases: value of diffusion-weighted MRI compared with gadolinium-enhanced MRI. *Eur Radiol* 2010;**20**:1431–41.

35. Nishie A, Tajima T, Ishigami K, *et al.* Detection of hepatocellular carcinoma (HCC) using super paramagnetic iron oxide (SPIO)-enhanced MRI: added value of diffusion-weighted imaging (DWI). *J Magn Reson Imag* 2010;**31** (2):373–82.

36. Xu PJ, Yan FH, Wang JH, Lin J, Ji Y. Added value of breathhold diffusion-weighted MRI in detection of small hepatocellular carcinoma lesions compared with dynamic contrast-enhanced MRI alone using receiver operating characteristic curve analysis. *J Magn Reson Imag* 2009;**29** (2):341–9.

37. Bruegel M, Holzapfel K, Gaa J, *et al.* Characterization of focal liver lesions by ADC measurements using a respiratory triggered diffusion-weighted single-shot echo-planar MR imaging technique. *Eur Radiol* 2008;**18** (3):477–85.

38. Gourtsoyianni S, Papanikolaou N, Yarmenitis S, *et al.* Respiratory gated diffusion-weighted imaging of the liver: value of apparent diffusion coefficient measurements in the differentiation between most commonly encountered benign and malignant focal liver lesions. *Eur Radiol* 2008;**18** (3):486–92.

39. Muhi A, Ichikawa T, Motosugi U, *et al.* High-b-value diffusion-weighted MR imaging of hepatocellular lesions: estimation of grade of malignancy of hepatocellular carcinoma. *J Magn Reson Imag* 2009; **30** (5):1005–11.

40. Aube C, Racineux PX, Lebigot J, *et al.* Diagnosis and quantification of hepatic fibrosis with diffusion weighted MR imaging: preliminary results. *J Radiol* 2004;**85** (3):301–6.

41. Taouli B, Tolia AJ, Losada M, *et al.* Diffusion-weighted MRI for quantification of liver fibrosis:

preliminary experience. *Am J Roentgenol* 2007;**189** (4):799–806.

42. Lewin M, Poujol-Robert A, Boelle PY, *et al.* Diffusion-weighted magnetic resonance imaging for the assessment of fibrosis in chronic hepatitis C. *Hepatology* 2007;**46** (3):658–65.

43. Sandrasegaran K, Akisik FM, Lin C, *et al.* Value of diffusion-weighted MRI for assessing liver fibrosis and cirrhosis. *Am J Roentgenol* 2009;**193** (6):1556–60.

44. Koh DM, Scurr E, Collins D, *et al.* Predicting response of colorectal hepatic metastasis: value of pretreatment apparent diffusion coefficients. *Am J Roentgenol* 2007;**188** (4):1001–8.

45. Cui Y, Zhang XP, Sun YS, Tang L, Shen L. Apparent diffusion coefficient: potential imaging biomarker for prediction and early detection of response to chemotherapy in hepatic metastases. *Radiology* 2008;**248** (3):894–900.

46. Kamel IR, Bluemke DA, Ramsey D, *et al.* Role of diffusion-weighted imaging in estimating tumor necrosis after chemoembolization of hepatocellular carcinoma. *Am J Roentgenol* 2003;**181** (3):708–10.

47. Deng J, Miller FH, Rhee TK, *et al.* Diffusion-weighted MR imaging for determination of hepatocellular carcinoma response to yttrium-90 radioembolization. *J Vasc Intervent Radiol* 2006;**17** (7):1195–200.

48. Kamel IR, Liapi E, Reyes DK, *et al.* Unresectable hepatocellular carcinoma: serial early vascular and cellular changes after transarterial chemoembolization as detected with MR imaging. *Radiology* 2009;**250** (2):466–73.

49. Mannelli L, Kim S, Hajdu CH, *et al.* Assessment of tumor necrosis of hepatocellular carcinoma after chemoembolization: diffusion-weighted and contrast-enhanced MRI with histopathologic correlation of the explanted liver. *Am J Roentgenol* 2009;**193** (4):1044–52.

50. Taouli B, Koh DM. Diffusion-weighted MR imaging of the liver. *Radiology* 2010;**254** (1):47–66.

51. Bammer R, Auer M, Keeling SL, *et al.* Diffusion tensor imaging using single-shot SENSE-EPI. *Magn Reson Med* 2002;**48** (1):128–36.

52. Bammer R, Keeling SL, Augustin M, *et al.* Improved diffusion-weighted single-shot echo-planar imaging (EPI) in stroke using sensitivity encoding (SENSE). *Magn Reson Med* 2001;**46** (3):548–54.

53. Taouli B, Martin AJ, Qayyum A, *et al.* Parallel imaging and diffusion tensor imaging for diffusion-weighted MRI of the liver: preliminary experience in healthy volunteers. *Am J Roentgenol* 2004;**183** (3):677–80.

54. Dale BM, Braithwaite AC, Boll DT, Merkle EM. Field strength and diffusion encoding technique affect the apparent diffusion coefficient measurements in diffusion-weighted imaging of the abdomen. *Investig Radiol* 2010;**45** (2):104–8.

55. Lee VS, Hecht EM, Taouli B, *et al.* Body and cardiovascular MR imaging at 3.0 T. *Radiology* 2007;**244** (3):692–705.

56. Barth MM, Smith MP, Pedrosa I, Lenkinski RE, Rofsky NM. Body MR imaging at 3.0 T: understanding the opportunities and challenges. *Radiographics* 2007;**27** (5):1445–62; discussion 62–4.

57. Deng J, Miller FH, Salem R, Omary RA, Larson AC. Multishot diffusion-weighted PROPELLER magnetic resonance imaging of the abdomen. *Investig Radiol* 2006;**41** (10):769–75.

58. Deng J, Omary RA, Larson AC. Multishot diffusion-weighted SPLICE PROPELLER MRI of the abdomen. *Magn Reson Med* 2008;**59** (5):947–53.

59. Hagiwara M, Rusinek H, Lee VS, *et al.* Advanced liver fibrosis: diagnosis with 3D whole-liver perfusion MR imaging: initial experience. *Radiology* 2008;**246** (3):926–34.

60. Talwalkar JA. Elastography for detecting hepatic fibrosis: options and considerations. *Gastroenterology* 2008;**135** (1):299–302.

61. Bammer R. Basic principles of diffusion-weighted imaging. *Eur J Radiol* 2003;**45** (3):169–84.

62. Bammer R, Augustin M, Strasser-Fuchs S, *et al.* Magnetic resonance diffusion tensor imaging for characterizing diffuse and focal white matter abnormalities in multiple sclerosis. *Magn Reson Med* 2000;**44** (4):583–91.

63. Chepuri NB, Yen YF, Burdette JH, *et al.* Diffusion anisotropy in the corpus callosum. *Am J Neuroradiol* 2002;**23** (5):803–8.

64. Dong Q, Welsh RC, Chenevert TL, *et al.* Clinical applications of diffusion tensor imaging. *J Magn Reson Imag* 2004;**19** (1):6–18.

65. Le Bihan D, Mangin JF, Poupon C, *et al.* Diffusion tensor imaging: concepts and applications. *J Magn Reson Imag* 2001;**13** (4):534–46.

66. Pierpaoli C, Jezzard P, Basser PJ, Barnett A, Di Chiro G. Diffusion tensor MR imaging of the human brain. *Radiology* 1996;**201** (3):637–48.

67. Taber KH, Pierpaoli C, Rose SE, *et al.* The future for diffusion tensor imaging in neuropsychiatry. *J Neuropsychiatry Clin Neurosci* 2002;**14** (1):1–5.

68. Namimoto T, Yamashita Y, Sumi S, Tang Y, Takahashi M. Focal liver masses: characterization with diffusion-weighted echo-planar MR imaging. *Radiology* 1997;**204** (3):739–44.

31

Chapter

3

Diffusion-weighted MRI of diffuse renal disease and kidney transplant

Frederik De Keyzer and Harriet C. Thoeny

Introduction

Since the early use of diffusion-weighted MRI (DWI) for detection of stroke in the brain, a whole evolution has taken place, resulting in the widespread use of this challenging technique outside the brain, particularly in oncology, where DWI has been shown to have potential for tumor detection, lesion characterization, and follow-up after treatment[1]. Another area where DWI has shown promising results is the kidney. This is not surprising, as the main renal functions are all related to movement of fluids, such as glomerular filtration, secretion, and both active and passive tubular reabsorption. Most pathologies occurring in the kidneys are in some way related to, or give rise to, changes in water mobility. As DWI provides contrast based on changes in water proton mobility, we expect that most renal pathologies can be detected and ultimately characterized using this innovative technique.

In this review, we will discuss the use of DWI for the detection and characterization of diffuse renal disease in native and transplanted kidneys. Renal masses will be discussed in a separate chapter.

DWI acquisition and processing applied to the kidneys

In theory, any MRI readout sequence can be adapted to provide diffusion-weighted images. All that needs to be done is to add two equally large, but opposite, magnetic field gradients between an initial 90° flip angle and the actual readout. Each application has different prerequisites and the DWI sequence needs to be optimally tailored for each of those. In this section, we will describe the prerequisites and some practical issues that need to be kept in mind when applying DWI to imaging of the kidneys.

Acquisition parameters

Due to the abundant presence of motion in the abdomen, ultrafast imaging sequences are generally preferred for renal imaging. Most anatomical MRI techniques in this organ are based on single-shot readout schemes, such as single-shot turbo spin echo, and single-shot gradient echo-planar imaging (EPI) sequences. DWI of the kidney has been almost exclusively performed using a spin-echo EPI technique (SE-EPI). Many groups have already used this sequence for the assessment of renal function. However, much variability in sequence parameters is observed in published studies on renal DWI, as summarized in Table 3.1.

The field of view (FOV) used during the scan depends on the orientation of the scan. For axial scans, the FOV is usually extended to include the entire abdomen, leading to a minimal dimension of 320 to 350 cm, depending on patient size. This has the benefits of inclusion of other structures in the abdomen and minimal anteroposterior artifacts due to respiration, and does not need additional saturation blocks, other than those to avoid inflow artifacts. However, for a good pixel resolution, a relatively large matrix, and subsequently a longer scan time, is needed. Coronal scans often need in-plane saturation blocks and can therefore be tailored closer to the kidney dimensions. At the same time, the coronal plane through the kidneys requires fewer slices to provide full kidney coverage, thereby strongly reducing scan time. The most important difference between the studies in the literature, and the reason why it is often so difficult to provide inter-study

Table 3.1 Reported b-values and breathing acquisition schemes for renal DWI reported in the literature

Study	b-values	Orientation	Acquisition scheme
Müller et al. (8)	2–395	Axial	Breath-hold + cardiac triggering
Müller et al. (17)	2–395	Axial	Breath-hold + cardiac triggering
Ichikawa et al. (21)	1.6–55	Axial	Breath-hold
Namimoto et al. (14)	30, 300	Axial	Breath-hold
Yamada et al. (22)	30–1100	Axial	Breath-hold
Fukuda et al. (19)	1.51–932	Axial	Breath-hold
Ries et al. (13)	0, 195, 390	Coronal	Breath-hold
Mürtz et al. (6)	50–1300	Axial	Breath-hold + pulse triggering
Chow et al. (23)	10, 300	Axial	Breath-hold
Jones et al. (16)	50–350	Coronal	Respiratory triggering
Cova et al. (24)	500	Axial	Breath-hold
Thoeny et al. (5)	0–1000	Axial	Free breathing
Thoeny et al. (20)	0–900	Coronal	Respiratory triggering
Xu et al. (18)	0, 500	Axial	Breath-hold
Yildirim et al. (15)	0–1000	Axial	Free breathing
Taouli et al. (26)	0, 400, 800	Axial	Breath-hold

comparisons, is the choice of b-values. These b-values indicate the amount of diffusion weighting present in the resulting images, and are a measure of the strength and/or timing of the two opposite gradients applied at the beginning of the sequence. From the literature, it is known that using high b-values provides information on the microscopic water motion in the extracellular extravascular space, which approximates the true diffusion of the tissue[2]. However, using lower b-values, an additional effect of vascular and tubular structures is seen, inducing stronger "guided" flow. This effect is usually called the perfusion contribution. Any combination of low and high b-values will therefore give mixed information, with a weighting towards the range where most b-values are used[3]. Therefore, we believe that reports in literature should make sure to clearly state the b-values used in order to correctly interpret the resulting apparent diffusion coefficient (ADC) values[2].

Respiration and pulsation effects

Imaging in a moving structure can generate partial volume effects, misregistration, and blurring. Vertical motion is significant in native kidneys, but mostly negligible in transplanted kidneys. The vertical motion between deep inspiration and deep expiration can amount to up to 39 mm for the upper pole and 43 mm for the lower pole of native kidneys, respectively[4]. This has important repercussions on coverage and interpretation of native kidney images. Fortunately, this movement is repetitive if the patient breathes normally, and can therefore be averaged out if scanned long enough. We have shown previously that ADC values of native kidneys were highly reproducible in volunteers who were scanned twice (with a 6-month interval) using a free-breathing approach, with a large number of b-values and averages in the axial imaging plane[5]. The in-plane blurring was also minimal, producing sharp kidney contours. On the other hand, blurring did occur at the lower and upper poles of the kidney due to the vertical motion of the kidney and the motion really becomes problematic if there are any lesions in the renal poles. Therefore, we suggest the use of respiratory triggered acquisition, even if imaging is performed in the axial plane.

When performing coronal diffusion acquisition, the in-plane motion would be significant, and could

Table 3.2 Comparison of free-breathing, respiratory triggered, and breath-hold image acquisition for renal diffusion imaging

	Breath-hold	Free breathing	Respiratory triggering
Scan duration	short	long	longest, depends on respiratory cycle
Kidney coverage	several acquisitions needed for full coverage	complete	complete
Suggested acquisition plane	coronal	axial/coronal	axial/coronal
Blurring	very low	moderate/high	low
Suppression of respiratory movement artifacts	high, depending on patient cooperation	moderate/high	high
Number of possible b-values	small	many	many
Spatial resolution	low	high	high
Possible in uncooperative patients	no	yes	yes, if breathing is regular

induce blurring at the renal edges. Therefore, coronal imaging of the kidneys should always be performed using respiratory triggered acquisition or in a breath-hold examination. A comparison of the three above-mentioned options based on personal experience is given in Table 3.2.

In axial acquisitions, pulsation artifacts can also become a problem if the artifact line crosses through the kidneys. This can usually be prevented by placing saturation blocks above and below the imaging slices, which saturate the incoming blood.

A study by Mürtz et al.[6] showed a significant influence of using pulse triggering on the resulting ADC values in the renal cortex. They compared ADC values calculated from three orthogonal directions with and without pulse triggering, and found in two of the three directions a significant difference in ADC values. This can be of importance when comparing examinations from different centers using pulse triggering versus non-pulse-triggered acquisitions.

Peristaltic bowel motion and air can also induce motion and susceptibility artifacts. In order to reduce bowel motion, administration of an antiperistaltic drug, e.g., 1 mg of glucagon intravenously could be used.

Several studies have focused on the reproducibility of ADC measurements in native kidneys[5,7–8], and have found low variability in repeated scans, indicating the robustness of the technique. Müller et al. did find that renal hydration state had a significant impact on the ADC measurement, with the higher hydration state having a higher renal ADC value[8]. A more recent study by Damasio et al., however, failed to confirm this finding[7]. The difference between these studies could be due to a different choice in b-values, as Müller et al. used b-values up to 400 s/mm^2, while Damasio et al. used b-values up to 800 s/mm^2.

Scanner and coil selection

DWI can be performed on any clinical 1.5-T or 3-T scanner. However, in order to acquire high-quality images with enough signal-to-noise ratio (SNR), state-of-the-art systems with high gradient capability are preferable. As standard diffusion images are acquired in single-shot (SS) and need a strong diffusion sensitization before the readout, the actual echo time (TE) is inherently quite high. This high TE leads to low signal in the resulting images, especially when the diffusion sensitization, indicated by the b-value, is set very high (for instance 1000 s/mm^2). High gradient strength allows diffusion sensitization in a much shorter time and at the same reduces the echo-spacing and the readout time. Both effects allow a decrease in TE, resulting in higher SNR.

However, even in state-of-the-art MR scanners, the SNR of SS EPI can be quite low, and this could be improved by the use of phased-array coils which enable the use of parallel imaging. The use of an anterior body coil combined with the built-in spine coil is in most cases sufficient. Provided that enough coil elements are available and that the coil element positions are spread out around the area of interest, parallel imaging can be very useful for renal DWI. This strongly reduces the time needed for the SS EPI readout, which benefits the imaging technique in two ways. First, movement artifacts are decreased because the total acquisition time per slice decreases. Second, the echo train length and TE are reduced, leading to higher SNR. The reduced echo train length also reduces the influence of susceptibility and leads to less distortion in the resulting image.

When going to higher field strengths, a dielectric cushion might be needed to minimize signal loss due to wavelength effects[9]. DWI of the kidney at 3 T is feasible, especially in transplanted kidneys. However, protocol optimization is necessary. A reduction in TE is required to minimize geometric distortion and retain adequate SNR. This reduction requires the use of parallel imaging techniques, and its resulting choice of receiver coils, as well as increasing the imaging bandwidth. A recent study on 3-T DWI of renal transplants indicated the feasibility of this technique and its sensitivity in respect of renal allograft rejection[10].

Adjustments for renal transplant imaging

As mentioned above, transplanted kidneys have much less movement than native kidneys, and as such their imaging can be performed with respiratory triggering or free-breathing. Coronal scans through the transplanted kidney seem to provide the best quality in a shorter time. Other parameters are similar to those for the imaging of native kidneys.

DWI quantification

Mono- vs. biexponential diffusion fitting

Diffusion is generally quantified by way of ADC calculation. This is based on fitting the signal intensities of images acquired with different diffusion sensitizing gradients (b-values) and a signal decay curve model. There are currently two main models used for diffusion quantification: monoexponential and biexponential models. The monoexponential model attempts to fit the measured data points with a formula of the form $S = S_0 \times e^{-b \times \mathrm{ADC}}$ and from this fit, the ADC value can then be calculated. It has been shown by Le Bihan *et al.* that this fit is sometimes quite poor, especially in the low b-value range, where it shows biexponential behavior[11]. For this reason,

the biexponential model with formula $S = S_0 \times [(1 - f) \times e^{-b \times D} + f \times e^{-b \times D^*}]$ was introduced. This model can then be used to calculate the true diffusion coefficient D, the pseudo-diffusion coefficient D^*, and the perfusion fraction f. The former model has been used by the majority of research groups[5,8,12–19]. A benefit of the monoexponential approach is that it is a very easy technique that can be implemented on most clinical scanners. It can be applied with as few as two b-values, and therefore does not require a long acquisition time. However, it has a number of drawbacks. It cannot differentiate between contributions of perfusion and diffusion in the free water pools, as it will make a combination of both contributions dependent on the choice of b values: for instance using only low b-values will result in a high ADC value, while using only high b-values will result in low ADC. This dependence makes it very difficult to compare between results of different studies, as differences in ADC values between the studies can be the result not only of different conditions, but also of different b-values used. The ADC values calculated using a biexponential diffusion fit are much less dependent on the choice of b-values, and a differentiation between perfusion influences and the true diffusion of the tissue becomes possible[2,20] provided that not only high but also several low b-values are applied. This provides extra information on the underlying microstructure of the tissue and might therefore help to differentiate renal pathologies. On the other hand, the biexponential model is more complex, with more variables that need to be estimated, which induces a much longer scan time and a larger mathematical variability. In kidney diffusion, the biexponential approach is becoming more and more important, due to the strong influence of perfusion and tubular flow on diffusion signal.

Standard diffusion vs. diffusion tensor imaging (DTI)

Diffusion-weighted acquisitions generally use a single diffusion sensitization direction[14] or a trace scan combining the three main directions[5,15,18]. However, this does not provide information on the directionality of the diffusion movement. In free water, movement of the water molecules is entirely random and movement in each direction is equally likely, so-called isotropy. However, cells, blood vessels and microstructures hamper free movement and introduce directionality of diffusion or anisotropy. It is common knowledge that the kidney is an anisotropic organ,

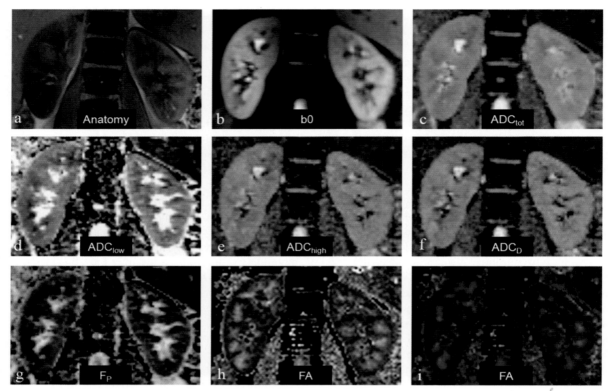

Figure 3.1 Example of diffusion images of native kidneys in a 22-year-old male volunteer. (a) Anatomical coronal T1-weighted image shows normal kidney size and differentiation. (b) Coronal respiratory triggered SS EPI diffusion image acquired using $b = 0$ s/mm². (c–e) ADC maps calculated using monoexponential fit including all b values ($b = 0$, 10, 20, 50, 100, 180, 300, 420, 550, 700 s/mm²) (c), only low b values ($b < 100$ s/mm²) (d), and only high b values ($b > 100$ s/mm²) (e). (f–g) Maps calculated using the biexponential fit: (f) ADC_D map (approximating true diffusion coefficient D), and (g) perfusion fraction (f_p) map. (h–i) (h: gray scale, i: color scale) of fractional anisotropy (FA) maps calculated from a diffusion tensor acquisition using respiratory triggering on the same volunteer, indicating directionality of the movement in the tissue in the medulla. The measured FA values were 0.45 in the medulla and 0.19 in the cortex.

especially in the medulla due to its radially oriented structures, and a standard diffusion-weighted acquisition will therefore not provide information regarding this anisotropy. Moreover, comparing studies that explore a different diffusion-weighted direction becomes nearly impossible with this approach. A few research groups have therefore attempted using diffusion tensor imaging (DTI) of the kidneys, with variable success[13]. DTI differs from standard diffusion-weighted imaging in the separate applications of diffusion-sensitizing gradients along different axes. The directionality of movement is examined by repeating a fast diffusion-weighted sequence along at least six different axes. This information is then used in the diffusion tensor, allowing visualization of the movement directions in three dimensions and calculation of the fractional anisotropy (FA) from

the eigenvalues of the diffusion tensor. This FA indicates the amount of anisotropy in the tissue, and ranges from 0 (equal diffusion in all directions) to 1 (completely unidirectional movement). The addition of directionality and anisotropy on DTI to the amount of diffusion on DWI might help in the characterization of tissue alterations and potentially the detection of renal malignancies. Of course, the fact that at least six separate diffusion-weighted images need to be acquired in DTI makes it inherently a lot longer to perform, and requires more advanced post-processing to obtain results. The clinical relevance and applicability of this technique is currently under investigation.

Example images of diffusion-weighted imaging and diffusion tensor imaging parameters are given in Figure 3.1.

Table 3.3 Reported ADC values of normal native kidneys in the literature. Higher ADC values are found when only low b values are used in the study and inversely low ADC values are found if higher b-values are used. Most studies show higher ADC in renal cortex compared to medulla

	b-values (s/mm^2)	ADC ($\times 10^{-3}$ mm^2/s)		
		Cortex	Medulla	Whole kidney
Müller et al. (8)	2, 8, 22, 32, 57, 89, 176, 395	3.5 ± 0.3^{a}	4.3 ± 0.5^{a}	—
Müller et al. (17)	2, 8, 22, 32, 57, 89, 176, 395	—	—	3.54 ± 0.47
Siegel et al. (12)	73, 370	2.39 ± 0.38	2.14 ± 0.38	—
Ichikawa et al. (21)	1.6, 16, 55	—	—	5.76 ± 1.36
Namimoto et al. (14)	30, 300	2.55 ± 0.62	2.84 ± 0.72	—
Yamada et al. (22)	30, 300, 900, 1100	—	—	1.55 ± 0.27
Fukuda et al. (19)	1.51, 55.3	—	—	4.31^{b}
	36.6, 317, 932	—	—	1.77^{b}
Ries et al. (13)	0, 195, 390	2.89 ± 0.28	2.18 ± 0.36	—
Mürtz et al. (6)	50, 300, 700, 1000, 1300	1.63 ± 0.14	—	—
Chow et al. (23)	10, 300	2.58 ± 0.05	2.09 ± 0.06	—
Cova et al. (24)	0, 500	—	—	1.72–2.65
Thoeny et al. (5)	0, 50, 100, 150, 200, 250, 300, 500, 750, 1000	2.03 ± 0.09	1.87 ± 0.08	—
Thoeny et al. (20)	0, 10, 20, 40, 60, 150, 300, 500, 700, 900	2.27 ± 0.12	2.17 ± 0.13	—
Xu et al. (18)	0, 500	—	—	2.87 ± 0.11
Yildirim et al. (15)	0, 111, 222, 333, 444, 556, 667, 778, 889, 1000	—	—	1.9 ± 0.1
Taouli et al. (26)	0, 400, 800	2.16 ± 0.37	1.90 ± 0.26	—

Notes: ^{a}ADC of dorsal cortex and medulla.
^{b}Central portion of the kidney.

DWI in diffuse diseases of native kidneys

Imaging-based diagnosis of diffuse renal pathology is often hampered by the lack of circumscribed lesions on conventional imaging, normal to only slightly enlarged or reduced kidneys, and the lack of normal kidney tissue for comparison. The latter is especially true when looking at a bilateral renal disease or at transplanted kidneys. Most non-invasive imaging modalities use kidney-size-based criteria and reduced or absent corticomedullary differentiation on T1-weighted imaging to detect diffuse renal pathology. DWI assessment, on the other hand, gives contrast based on underlying water mobility in renal tissue. This can be useful not only for detection and characterization of renal lesions, but also for diffuse renal diseases, provided they affect the mobility of the tissue water molecules. Here we will first discuss the normal ADC ranges in healthy kidneys, and compare these to the values observed in diffuse renal disease.

ADC values of healthy native kidneys

In order to use DWI for the assessment of renal pathologies, the range of normal ADC values needs to be established first. In the literature, a number of studies have reported ADC values for normal kidneys[5–6,8,12–15,17–24]. As seen in Table 3.3, there is much variability in ADC values between studies. Most of the discrepancies can be ascribed to the choice of different b-values. The use of low b-values generally increases the ADC value, while the use of high b-values generally results in lower ADC values. For instance, b-values ranging from 2 to 395 s/mm^2 resulted in mean renal ADC values of $3.5–4.3 \times 10^{-3}$ mm^2/s[8,17], while a range of 1.6–55 s/mm^2 yielded mean renal ADC values of 5.76×10^{-3} mm^2/s[21]; and finally a range of 50–1300 s/mm^2 resulted in mean values of 1.63×10^{-3} mm^2/s[6]. This variability detracts from the possibility of making inter-study comparisons. A pertinent choice of b-values before the start of the study is therefore imperative. Especially in multicenter studies or follow-up studies, a consensus on the choice of b-values and diffusion calculation needs to be reached and has to be respected in every comparable study. A first general consensus paper for oncologic applications with DWI has recently been published[25].

Prior studies have provided contradictory results regarding differences in ADC values between renal cortex and medulla. Several studies have found higher ADC values in the medulla than in the cortex[14,17]. However, recent studies including our own work found that medullary ADC values were actually lower than cortical values[5,12–13,20,23,26]. In more detail, ADC$_{avg}$ and ADC$_{high}$ values were significantly higher in the renal cortex than in the renal medulla; however, ADC$_{low}$ did not differ markedly between the two. While ADC$_{avg}$ is calculated using the entire range of b-values between 0 and 1000 s/mm^2 and is therefore influenced by both diffusion and perfusion effects, the ADC$_{low}$ calculated from only the low b-values ($b \leq 100$ s/mm^2) reflects mostly perfusion and the ADC$_{high}$ calculated from only high b-values (between 500 and 1000 s/mm^2) approximates pure diffusion. The difference in ADC$_{high}$ is thus probably due to the presence of more free diffusion-inhibiting structures in the medulla; this might be offset by a greater amount of perfusion or anisotropy in the medulla leading to a loss of the difference in ADC$_{low}$[5]. Unfortunately, not all researchers made separate assessments of cortical and medullary ADC values, most likely due to low spatial resolution of diffusion acquisitions. An example ADC map of healthy native kidneys is shown in Figure 3.1. Two studies from our group showed no differences between right and left kidney in healthy adults[5,20].

It is also possible to use DWI to evaluate fetal kidneys. Savelli et al.[27] showed a negative correlation between fetal renal ADC and gestational age. Between gestational ages of 17 and 36 weeks, fetal renal ADC decreased from 1.32 to 1.07×10^{-3} mm^2/s in normal fetal kidneys. A second group comprising pathologic kidneys in this study presented with very variable ADC values, although a trend could be seen that pathologic kidneys had lower ADC than normal ones

of comparable gestational age[27]. In children, a trend of increasing ADC could be seen with age[16]. As Jones et al. used a different b-value set as compared to Savelli et al. ($b = 50, 200, 350$ vs. $b = 0, 200, 700$ s/mm^2 respectively), a direct comparison of ADC values is difficult. However, a clear increase in ADC from 1.50 to 2.50×10^{-3} mm^2/s was reported between the ages of 0 and 18 years.

DWI findings in diffuse native renal diseases

Diffuse diseases of native kidneys can be subdivided into three groups: pre-renal disease, renal disease, and post-renal disease. Pre-renal disease is present when there is an impairment of the blood supply to the kidneys, such as in renal artery stenosis (RAS). On the other hand, post-renal disease is related to urinary tract obstruction, causing secondary damage to the kidney. Examples of post-renal disease are ureteral obstruction, with eventually consequent hydronephrosis and even pyonephrosis. Third, renal diseases are intrinsic to the kidney with no etiology related to either blood supply or urine outflow. In this category are classified acute and chronic renal failure and pyelonephritis. In the paragraphs below, we discuss how these separate pathologies can be assessed using DWI.

Renal artery stenosis (RAS)

Several studies have reported the use of DWI in RAS[14–15,18]. Namimoto et al. examined seven kidneys with RAS in six patients. They found a significant lower ADC value in the cortex of kidneys with RAS when compared to normal kidneys (1.55 ± 0.39 vs. $2.55 \pm 0.62 \times 10^{-3}$ mm^2/s, respectively). Also, ADC of the medulla of kidneys with RAS was lower than that of normal kidneys (2.24 ± 0.62 vs. $2.84 \pm 0.72 \times 10^{-3}$ mm^2/s), although this difference was not significant. They attributed the stronger effect to the higher blood perfusion in the cortex, which is impaired in RAS[14].

In 55 patients, Xu et al. also found a decreased ADC in impaired kidneys as compared to normal kidneys[18]. In their study, they did not do a straightforward comparison between ADC values of kidneys with RAS and normal kidneys, but rather correlated ADC values with split glomerular filtration rate (GFR) on scintigraphy. A subdivision according to the GFR into levels of renal impairment showed a

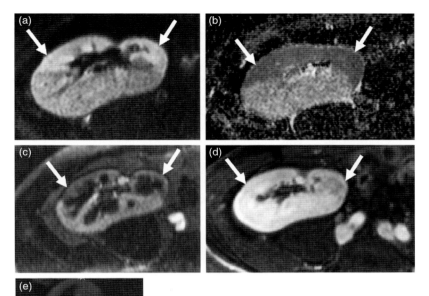

Figure 3.2 56-year-old woman with segmental ischemia of kidney transplant caused by high-grade renal artery stenosis. Axial SS EPI diffusion-weighted images demonstrate segmental restricted diffusion involving the anterior aspect of the transplanted kidney (arrows) on images at $b = 800$ s/mm^2 (a) and ADC map (b) compared with the remainder of the renal parenchyma. Axial contrast-enhanced fat-suppressed T1-weighted images obtained at the corticomedullary (c) and nephrographic (d) phases demonstrate decreased perfusion in the corresponding area consistent with ischemia. Coronal reconstruction of MR angiography (e) demonstrates severe stenosis of the anterior branch of the transplant renal artery (arrow). (With permission from Kim S *et al. Magn Reson Imag Clin N Am* 2008;**16**:585–96).

trend of decreasing ADC with increasing impairment. While normal kidneys had an ADC of $2.87 \pm 0.11 \times 10^{-3}$ mm^2/s, ADC of kidneys with RAS decreased to $2.55 \pm 0.17 \times 10^{-3}$ mm^2/s in mild impairment, to $2.29 \pm 0.10 \times 10^{-3}$ mm^2/s in moderate impairment, and down to $2.20 \pm 0.11 \times 10^{-3}$ mm^2/s in severely impaired kidneys[18]. These reported ADC values are higher than most other research groups; this is due to the use of a relatively small maximal b-value, as they used 0 and 500 s/mm^2 in this study. Individual comparison of ADC and GFR indicated a moderate positive correlation ($r < 0.709$). In a recent study by Yildirim *et al.*[15], similar results to those in the study by Xu *et al.* were observed with lower ADC values in kidneys with RAS compared to normal kidneys. Yildirim *et al.* found ADC values of $1.9 \pm 0.1 \times 10^{-3}$ mm^2/s and $1.7 \pm 0.2 \times 10^{-3}$ mm^2/s for normal and impaired kidneys, respectively. A nice illustration of RAS can be found in the review paper by Kim *et al.* (Figure 3.2)[28].

Acute and chronic renal failure

Recent studies[5,14] have assessed DWI of acute and chronic renal failure, and found significantly lower ADC values in kidneys with renal failure. In eight patients with chronic renal failure (CRF), Namimoto *et al.*[14] reported ADC values of $0.81 \pm 0.47 \times 10^{-3}$ mm^2/s and $1.59 \pm 0.79 \times 10^{-3}$ mm^2/s for cortex and medulla, respectively. This was lower than the values for acute renal failure (ARF) in four patients ($1.83 \pm 0.14 \times 10^{-3}$ mm^2/s and $1.76 \pm 0.50 \times 10^{-3}$ mm^2/s), which in turn was significantly lower than ADC of normal kidneys ($2.55 \pm 0.62 \times 10^{-3}$ mm^2/s and $2.84 \pm 0.72 \times 10^{-3}$ mm^2/s). The b-values used in that study were 30 and 300 s/mm^2. Namimoto *et al.* suggested that decreased ADC may be attributed to the presence of

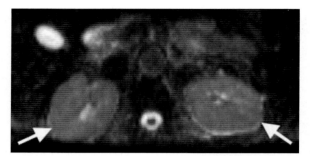

Figure 3.3 67-year-old man with acute renal failure due to interstitial nephritis. Axial renal ADC map calculated from SS EPI images using b values of 0, 50, 100, 150, 200, 250, 300, 500, 750, and 1000 s/mm^2. Both kidneys (arrows) are mildly enlarged, with low ADC ($\times 10^{-3}$ mm^2/s; right kidney: cortex 1.38, medulla 1.48; left kidney: cortex 1.51, medulla 1.52) (With permission from Thoeny HC *et al. Radiology* 2005;**235**:911–17).

fibrosis in CRF and to renal ischemia and subsequent cell swelling in ARF[14]. Similar findings were observed by our study[5], in which 11 patients were not subdivided into CRF and ARF groups, but rather according to their serum creatinine (sCr) levels into groups with sCr above or below 2.5 mg/dl (six patients below and five above this threshold). Using a large range of b-values (0, 50, 100, 150, 200, 250, 300, 500, 750, and 1000 s/mm^2), we found that healthy volunteers had the highest renal ADC values ($2.03 \pm 0.09 \times 10^{-3}$ mm^2/s and $1.87 \pm 0.08 \times 10^{-3}$ mm^2/s for cortex and medulla, respectively), followed by the patients with sCr below 2.5 mg/dl ($1.90 \pm 0.18 \times 10^{-3}$ mm^2/s and $1.79 \pm 0.14 \times 10^{-3}$ mm^2/s). The lowest ADC values were found in the patients with sCr above 2.5 mg/dl ($1.73 \pm 0.24 \times 10^{-3}$ mm^2/s and $1.61 \pm 0.26 \times 10^{-3}$ mm^2/s for cortex and medulla, respectively). Interestingly, the mean sCr values in the study of Namimoto *et al.* were 5.20 mg/dl for the CRF group and 3.65 mg/dl for the ARF group. Therefore, both studies indicate a lower ADC value for kidneys with the highest sCr values, an intermediate value for the kidneys with intermediate sCr values, and the highest ADC values in normal kidneys. An example ADC map of a patient with acute renal failure secondary to interstitial nephritis is given in Figure 3.3.

Pyelonephritis

Pyelonephritis is frequently observed in young female patients and children in native kidneys or in transplanted kidneys, and up till now requires contrast-enhanced computed tomography (CT) or MRI for confirmatory diagnosis. Large-scale studies have not been performed on the evaluation of pyelonephritis with DWI. We show a case of pyelonephritis (Figure 3.4), where the renal cortex showed a 44% lower ADC value in the pathologic kidney, and a 31.7% lower ADC value in the medulla compared to the contralateral normal kidney, probably due to zones of inflammation involving the medulla and cortex[5]. If this can be proven in a larger-scale study, this patient group would strongly benefit as no contrast agent or exposure to radiation is required.

Pyonephrosis–hydronephrosis

The differentiation of pyonephrosis and hydronephrosis has a high clinical impact because pyonephrosis needs immediate intervention due to the high risk of sepsis. In a small study including 12 patients with a dilated collecting system (four with pyonephrosis and eight with hydronephrosis) a significantly higher ADC was measured in the collecting system in patients with hydronephrosis ($2.98 \pm 0.65 \times 10^{-3}$ mm^2/s) compared to pyonephrosis ($0.64 \pm 0.35 \times 10^{-3}$ mm^2/s)[29]. Similar results were observed in another study confirming the potential of DWI in this particular clinical setting[24]. An illustration of a patient with both pyonephrosis and hydronephrosis is shown in Figure 3.5.

Ureteral obstruction

Ureteral obstruction can be secondary to a calculus or to intrinsic or extrinsic tumors. In case of a dilated collecting system, the diagnosis of ureteral obstruction is generally straightforward with any imaging technique. However, a non-dilated collecting system does not necessarily exclude obstruction (in acute cases), whereas a dilated collecting system (for instance in transplanted kidneys) does not necessarily correspond to obstruction. The diagnosis of acute obstruction is often difficult by imaging or clinical examination and current laboratory parameters. In a recent study by our group[30], 21 patients with acute ureteral obstruction due to ureteral stones were prospectively evaluated with DWI. No significant differences were observed between the ADC$_T$ (ADC total: ADC calculated from all 10 native diffusion-weighted images acquired using b-values between 0 and 900 s/mm^2) of either the medulla (2.20 ± 0.14 and $2.20 \pm 0.18 \times 10^{-3}$ mm^2/s, respectively) or the cortex (2.32 ± 0.13 and $2.35 \pm 0.13 \times 10^{-3}$ mm^2/s, respectively) of the obstructed and non-obstructed kidneys. Compared

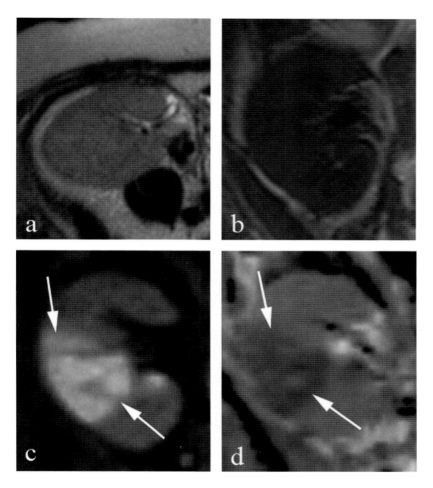

Figure 3.4 62-year-old woman with focal pyelonephritis of kidney transplant (patient presented with fever of unknown origin). Axial single-shot turbo spin echo and coronal T1-weighted spoiled gradient echo morphological images without contrast agent injection of the transplanted kidney (a–b) do not clearly show abnormal findings. However, on the diffusion image acquired using b value of 900 s/mm² (c), there is a large area of restricted diffusion appearing with decreased ADC on the ADC map (d) (arrow). This finding is highly suspicious for focal pyelonephritis, which was confirmed by urine analysis.

to control kidneys, only medullary ADC_T was slightly increased in the obstructed kidney ($p < 0.04$). However, ADC_D (approximating the true diffusion coefficient, D) in the medulla of both the obstructed and non-obstructed kidneys was significantly higher compared to controls (2.01 ± 0.16 and 1.99 ± 0.20 vs. $1.89 \pm 0.12 \times 10^{-3}$ mm²/sec, $p < 0.008$ and $p < 0.03$, respectively). The perfusion fraction (f_p) of the obstructed kidney was significantly lower in the cortex (20.2 ± 4.8 vs. $24.0 \pm 5.8\%$, respectively, $p < 0.002$) and slightly lower in the medulla (18.3 ± 5.9 vs. $20.7 \pm 6.4\%$, respectively, $p = 0.05$) compared to non-obstructed kidneys. These results suggest the potential of DWI to detect changes in perfusion and diffusion during acute obstruction as exemplified in patients with ureteral stones[30] (Figure 3.6). Table 3.4 summarizes the ADC changes observed in native kidneys as reported in the literature.

DWI in transplanted kidneys

In patients with end-stage renal disease, renal transplantation is the preferred treatment option due to the improved quality of life and better prognosis. Thanks to advances in surgical techniques and immunosuppressive therapy, long-term kidney graft survival has improved, reported to be about 90% during the first year after transplantation. However, early graft dysfunction is encountered in nearly 30% of renal allografts. Early and specific detection of medical problems in renal transplant recipients is of utmost importance to start accurate treatment or to change therapeutic strategies. Surgical complications, including lymphoceles, RAS, renal vein thrombosis, ureteral strictures, urinomas, and hematomas can relatively easily be evaluated by conventional MR sequences or even by ultrasound depending on the expertise of the

Table 3.4 Overview of ADC changes reported in the literature in diseased native kidneys

Pathology	ADC changes		Collecting system
	Cortex	Medulla	
Chronic renal failure	↓↓	↓↓	–
Acute renal failure	↓	↓	–
Renal artery stenosis	↓	no change	–
Chronic ureteric obstruction	↓	↓	–
Acute ureteric obstruction	↓	↓	~
Pyonephrosis	–	–	↓↓
Pyelonephritis	↓	↓	–

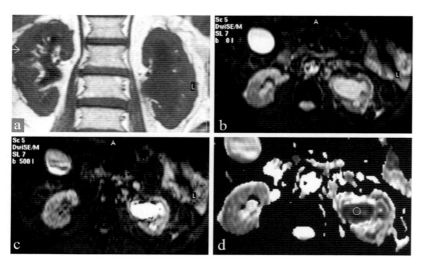

Figure 3.5 Hydronephrosis of the right kidney and pyonephrosis of the left kidney. Coronal fast SE T1-weighted (a) and axial SS EPI for $b = 0$ s/mm^2 (b) images show bilateral hydronephrosis, mild on the right and moderate on the left. (c) Axial SS EPI diffusion image for $b = 500$ s/mm^2 shows signal attenuation of right renal pelvis, and marked persistent hyperintensity of the left renal pelvis, indicative of restricted diffusion secondary to necrotic content and pus. (d) ADC map shows high ADC of the right pelvic content and low ADC of the left pelvic content (3.39 vs. 0.77×10^{-3} mm^2/s). (With permission from Cova M *et al. Br J Radiol* 2004;**77**:851–7).

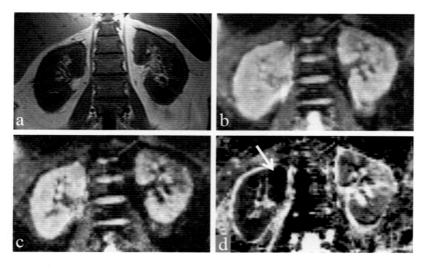

Figure 3.6 37-year-old man with acute flank pain due to right ureteral stone. Coronal (a) T1-weighted anatomical image, (b) ADC map calculated from a monoexponential fit of all b values (0, 10, 20, 40, 60, 150, 300, 500, 700, and 900 s/mm^2) and (c–d) ADC$_D$, approximating true diffusion of the tissue, and perfusion fraction maps of the kidneys, calculated from a biexponential fit on the same data. Note the normal collecting system on the T1-weighted images (a) on both sides. There is however a reduced perfusion fraction in the upper pole of the right kidney (arrow) secondary to acute obstruction, without significant ADC changes.

radiologist. Medical complications, including acute and chronic rejection, acute tubular necrosis (ATN), and delayed graft function, however, are difficult to diagnose and biopsy with histopathologic evaluation is still the only reliable technique to diagnose and differentiate these entities. In addition to being invasive and having the risk of complications such as bleeding, infection, fistulas, and rarely graft loss, sampling error is another important limitation of renal biopsy. Therefore, DWI might be a promising non-invasive technique to provide structural and functional information on diffusion and perfusion provided that these entities can be separated.

There are limited data on the use of DWI in kidney transplants. To date, one study has investigated the reproducibility of renal ADC of transplanted kidneys in rats by using spin-echo SS EPI at 7 T[31]. In this acute rejection model, ADC values in cortex and medulla decreased significantly (by more than 35%, $p < 0.01$) during angiotensin II-induced reduction in renal blood flow. This significant difference might be explained by the fact that relatively low b values (5, 20, 42, 72, 142, and 269 s/mm^2) with ADC consequently highly influenced by perfusion effects were applied in this study. When comparing renal allografts early after transplantation to native kidneys, allografts exhibited decreased ADC values and isografts demonstrated similar ADC values compared to native kidneys[31]. The authors of this study concluded that DWI has the potential to non-invasively monitor early graft rejection after kidney transplantation.

However, only one study analyzing the feasibility and reproducibility of DWI in transplanted kidneys in humans has been published[20]. In this study, 15 patients with renal allografts and stable kidney function and the same number of age- and sex-matched healthy volunteers underwent DWI of the kidneys at 1.5 T. DWI was performed in the coronal plane applying a multisection sequence with ten b-values (0, 10, 20, 40, 60, 150, 300, 500, 700, and 900 s/mm^2). The gradients were applied in three orthogonal directions and subsequently averaged to minimize the influence of anisotropy. Furthermore, parallel imaging (factor of 2) was used and respiratory triggering with TR of 3200 ms and TE of 71 ms was performed to reduce motion artifacts. The application of a large range of b-values allowed for biexponential fitting and yielded not only the ADC$_T$ calculated automatically out of all b-values, but also two additional parameters: f represents the perfusion fraction (i.e., the proportion of microcirculation of blood and movement in predefined structures, such as tubular flow) and ADC$_D$ (approximating the true diffusion coefficient, D) reflects predominately pure diffusion[20]. We observed that in transplanted kidneys, ADC$_T$, ADC$_D$, and perfusion fraction were almost identical in the medulla and the cortex. In contrast, all diffusion parameters in native kidneys were significantly higher in the cortex than in the medulla. The lack of corticomedullary difference in diffusion parameters of transplanted kidneys in contrast to native kidneys is probably due the fact that transplanted kidneys are denervated and may also be secondary to the effects of immunosuppressive drugs. Furthermore, medullary diffusion parameters were almost identical in transplanted and native kidneys, whereas cortical ADC$_T$ and ADC$_D$ values were substantially higher in native kidneys. In the same study, it was shown that these results of diffusion parameters

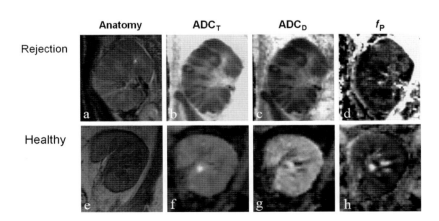

Figure 3.7 Representative images of transplanted kidneys in a 52-year-old male patient with biopsy-proven acute rejection (a–d) and of a 51-year-old male patient with a normally functioning kidney transplant (e–h). (a,e) Coronal T1-weighted anatomical images, and (b,f) coronal ADC maps calculated using a monoexponential fit on the diffusion-weighted images of all b values ($b = 0$, 10, 20, 40, 60, 150, 300, 500, 700, and 900 s/mm^2), (c,g) ADC$_D$ map approaching pure diffusion, and (d,h) perfusion fraction calculated using a biexponential fit of the diffusion-weighted images. All diffusion parameters are lower in acute rejection compared to normal kidney transplant.

in transplanted kidneys were highly reproducible[20] with coefficients of variation below 3.2% within subjects and below 4.8% between subjects for ADC_T and ADC_D. The perfusion fraction was less reproducible with within-subject coefficients of variation of 8.6% and 15.1% for cortex and medulla, respectively.

As has been demonstrated in this study of patients with renal allografts, DWI is promising for monitoring disease and eventually even for early detection of graft deterioration thanks to its highly reproducible parameters. Our early experience in a small number of patients with histologically proven acute rejection compared to a group of allograft recipients early after transplantation showed reduced microcirculation and/or tubular flow in renal allografts with acute rejection (Figure 3.7). One patient with acute tubular necrosis was included in the study, with lower values of ADC_T and in particular perfusion fraction compared to patients with stable renal function[10].

Therefore, one might conclude that DWI has the potential to obtain information on renal allograft function non-invasively. However, further data with histopathologic correlation are needed to confirm these findings.

Limitations and future directions

Renal DWI is an upcoming technique, but several pitfalls still hamper its widespread use for characterization of renal pathology. The large amount of movement in the kidney is a problem that can be addressed, although with upsides and downsides for each solution. Although DWI offers remarkable sensitivity to changes in diffusivity of the water protons, with renal pathology usually presenting with lower ADC, this method potentially lacks specificity for the characterization of renal pathology. The current move from predominantly monoexponential models to a biexponential model is a good first step and might be able to separate the diffusion changes from the perfusion changes in renal pathology. However, more sophisticated models or combination with other imaging techniques such as arterial spin labeling (ASL), blood oxygen level dependent (BOLD) MRI or DTI might help in a more comprehensive approach for various kidney diseases. Larger-scale studies with histopathologic correlation should be performed in order to establish DWI as a marker of renal function in clinical practice.

Conclusions

DWI is a method sensitive to early structural and functional changes in native and transplanted kidneys with different underlying pathologic conditions, with potential for single kidney function assessment. The standard monoexponential fitting of diffusion data has been able to detect many renal diseases in native kidneys. Unfortunately, to date, renal ADC changes are not very specific in terms of underlying pathology. Alternative models such as biexponential fitting can be used to obtain detailed information on both diffusion and perfusion changes separately and could result in better differentiation of the various diffuse renal pathologies in the future, although further studies are required. Combination of DWI with other imaging techniques such as BOLD, DTI, and ASL could also be beneficial for a more comprehensive characterization of renal pathology.

Acknowledgements

The authors would like to thank Tobias Binser for the interesting and motivating discussions during the preparation of this chapter.

Harriet Thoeny was supported by research grant #320000–113512 of the Swiss National Science Foundation for Research and by Carigest SA, Switzerland.

References

1. Thoeny HC, De Keyzer F. Extracranial applications of diffusion-weighted magnetic resonance imaging. *Eur Radiol* 2007;**17**:1385–93.

2. Le Bihan D. Intravoxel incoherent motion perfusion MR imaging: a wake-up call. *Radiology* 2008;**249**:748–52.

3. Thoeny HC, De Keyzer F, Boesch C, Hermans R. Diffusion-weighted imaging of the parotid gland: influence of the choice of *b*-values on the apparent diffusion coefficient value. *J Magn Reson Imag* 2004;**20**:786–90.

4. Schwartz LH, Richaud J, Buffat L, Touboul E, Schlienger M. Kidney mobility during respiration. *Radiother Oncol* 1994;**32**:84–6.

5. Thoeny HC, De Keyzer F, Oyen RH, Peeters RR. Diffusion-weighted MR imaging of kidneys in healthy volunteers and patients with parenchymal diseases: initial experience. *Radiology* 2005;**235**:911–17.

6. Mürtz P, Flacke S, Träber F, *et al.* Abdomen: diffusion-weighted MR imaging with pulse-triggered single-shot sequences. *Radiology* 2002;**224**:258–64.

7. Damasio MB, Tagliafico A, Capaccio E, *et al.* Diffusion-weighted MRI sequences (DW-MRI) of the

kidney: normal findings, influence of hydration state and repeatability of results. *Radiol Med* 2008;**113**:214–24.

8. Müller MF, Prasad PV, Bimmler D, Kaiser A, Edelman RR. Functional imaging of the kidney by means of measurement of the apparent diffusion coefficient. *Radiology* 1994;**193**:711–15.

9. Dietrich O, Reiser MF, Schoenberg SO. Artifacts in 3-T MRI: physical background and reduction strategies. *Eur J Radiol* 2008;**65**:29–35.

10. Eisenberger U, Thoeny HC, Binser T, *et al.* Evaluation of renal allograft function early after transplantation with diffusion-weighted MR imaging. *Eur Radiol* 2010; **20**:1374–83.

11. Le Bihan D, Breton E, Lallemand D, *et al.* Separation of diffusion and perfusion in intravoxel incoherent motion MR imaging. *Radiology* 1988;**168**:497–505.

12. Siegel CL, Aisen AM, Ellis JH, Londy F, Chenevert TL. Feasibility of MR diffusion studies in the kidney. *J Magn Reson Imag* 1995;**5**:617–20.

13. Ries M, Jones RA, Basseau F, Moonen CT, Grenier N. Diffusion tensor MRI of the human kidney. *J Magn Reson Imag* 2001;**14**:42–9.

14. Namimoto T, Yamashita Y, Mitsuzaki K, *et al.* Measurement of the apparent diffusion coefficient in diffuse renal disease by diffusion-weighted echo-planar MR imaging. *J Magn Reson Imag* 1999;**9**:832–7.

15. Yildirim E, Kirbas I, Teksam M, *et al.* Diffusion-weighted MR imaging of kidneys in renal artery stenosis. *Eur J Radiol* 2008;**65**:148–53.

16. Jones RA, Grattan-Smith JD. Age dependence of the renal apparent diffusion coefficient in children. *Pediatr Radiol* 2003;**33**:850–4.

17. Müller MF, Prasad P, Siewert B, *et al.* Abdominal diffusion mapping with use of a whole-body echo-planar system. *Radiology* 1994;**190**:475–8.

18. Xu Y, Wang X, Jiang X. Relationship between the renal apparent diffusion coefficient and glomerular filtration rate: preliminary experience. *J Magn Reson Imag* 2007;**26**:678–81.

19. Fukuda Y, Ohashi I, Hanafusa K, *et al.* Anisotropic diffusion in kidney: apparent diffusion coefficient measurements for clinical use. *J Magn Reson Imag* 2000;**11**:156–60.

20. Thoeny HC, Zumstein D, Simon-Zoula S, *et al.* Functional evaluation of transplanted kidneys with diffusion-weighted and BOLD MR imaging: initial experience. *Radiology* 2006;**241**:812–21.

21. Ichikawa T, Haradome H, Hachiya J, Nitatori T, Araki T. Diffusion-weighted MR imaging with single-shot echo-planar imaging in the upper abdomen: preliminary clinical experience in 61 patients. *Abdom Imag* 1999;**24**:456–61.

22. Yamada I, Aung W, Himeno Y, Nakagawa T, Shibuya H. Diffusion coefficients in abdominal organs and hepatic lesions: evaluation with intravoxel incoherent motion echo-planar MR imaging. *Radiology* 1999;**210**:617–23.

23. Chow LC, Bammer R, Moseley ME, Sommer FG. Single breath-hold diffusion-weighted imaging of the abdomen. *J Magn Reson Imag* 2003;**18**:377–82.

24. Cova M, Squillaci E, Stacul F, *et al.* Diffusion-weighted MRI in the evaluation of renal lesions: preliminary results. *Br J Radiol* 2004;**77**:851–7.

25. Padhani AR, Liu G, Loh DM, *et al.* Diffusion-weighted magnetic resonance imaging as a cancer biomarker: consensus and recommendations. *Neoplasia* 2009;**11**:102–25.

26. Taouli B, Thakur RK, Mannelli L, *et al.* Renal lesions: characterization with diffusion-weighted imaging versus contrast-enhanced MR imaging. *Radiology* 2009;**251**:398–407.

27. Savelli S, Di Maurizio M, Perrone A, *et al.* MRI with diffusion-weighted imaging (DWI) and apparent diffusion coefficient (ADC) assessment in the evaluation of normal and abnormal fetal kidneys: preliminary experience. *Prenat Diagnos* 2007;**27**:1104–11.

28. Kim S, Naik M, Sigmund E, Taouli B. Diffusion-weighted MR imaging of the kidneys and the urinary tract. *Magn Reson Imag Clin N Am* 2008;**16**:585–96.

29. Chan JH, Tsui EY, Luk SH, *et al.* MR diffusion-weighted imaging of kidney: differentiation between hydronephrosis and pyonephrosis. *Clin Imag* 2001;**25**:110–13.

30. Thoeny HC, Binser T, Roth B, Kessler TM, Vermathen P. Noninvasive assessment of acute ureteral obstruction using diffusion-weighted MRI: a prospective study. *Radiology* 2009;**252**:721–8.

31. Yang D, Ye Q, Williams DS, Hitchens TK, Ho C. Normal and transplanted rat kidneys: diffusion MR imaging at 7 T. *Radiology* 2004;**231**:702–9.

Chapter

4

Diffusion-weighted MRI of focal renal masses

Sooah Kim and Bachir Taouli

Introduction

Characterization of renal masses mainly relies on the presence or absence of enhancement on contrast-enhanced computed tomography (CT) or magnetic resonance (MR) imaging[1]. With MRI, enhancement can be assessed by measuring signal intensity changes[2] or visually without or with image subtraction[3]. There is a growing interest in the application of diffusion-weighted MRI (DWI) in body imaging for multiple reasons: DWI can provide structural and functional information without any intravenous (IV) contrast administration, thus it is easy to implement and repeat, and is very attractive in patients at risk for nephrogenic systemic fibrosis (NSF).

The signal and contrast in DWI are based on the thermally driven random motion of water and micro-capillary perfusion in tissues, and are usually quantified by calculating the apparent diffusion coefficient (ADC). The ADC is dependent on different factors such as molecular architecture, interactions, and temperature in free fluid. The protons' motion is hindered or restricted by different components such as cell membranes, cellular density, or macromolecules in tissues. This is manifested by an ADC that is reduced from the bulk value. In general, the clinical implications of ADC change depend upon the tissue under investigation; an anomalous rise in ADC can indicate increased edema, cystic changes, and necrosis; while an anomalous reduction in ADC might indicate ischemia, infection, or tumor. As such, diffusion measures should be taken in context with other imaging sequences to ensure an accurate diagnosis. The most commonly employed imaging method in clinical MRI scanners is single-shot echo-planar imaging (SS EPI) sequence with a bipolar gradient diffusion preparation.

Potentially DWI can provide additional information over conventional MR sequences, or it could be useful in combination with conventional MR sequences; and could potentially be used as an alternative to contrast-enhanced sequences in patients with chronic renal insufficiency, at risk of NSF.

In this chapter, we provide an overview on diffusion acquisition techniques, current available data, limitations, and future directions applied for the assessment of renal masses. Diffuse renal disease is discussed in a separate chapter.

Acquisition parameters for DWI of the kidneys

Breath-hold, free breathing, or respiratory-triggered (using a navigator echo) SS EPI diffusion-weighted sequences can be obtained before intravenous contrast injection using a 1.5-T or higher system, with the suggested following parameters: axial or coronal acquisition, fat suppression, tridirectional gradients using the following b-values: 0 (used as a reference image), 400/500 (intermediate), and 800/1000 (high) s/mm^2. The choice of b-values is somehow arbitrary and depends on the equipment used and the radiologist's experience. Lower b-values generate higher ADC values, owing to the contribution of intravoxel incoherent motion (IVIM) effects other than diffusion such as perfusion or flow phenomena, as opposed to higher b-values, which enable "pure" diffusion weighting, at the expense of lower residual signal. Maximum b-values ≥ 800 s/mm^2 are suggested to reduce the effects of IVIM, whenever possible. In addition, the use of at least three b-values provides a more precise ADC fit. Suggested acquisition parameters as used in our institution are summarized in Table 4.1.

Table 4.1 Suggested acquisition parameters of fat-suppressed SS EPI diffusion-weighted imaging sequence for assessment of renal masses

Acquisition parameter	Breath-hold acquisition	Free breathing or respiratory-triggered acquisition
TR (ms)	$\geq$1800	$\geq$2300 (free breathing) or 1 respiratory cycle (RT)
TE (ms)	Minimum	Minimum
Section thickness (mm)	7	5–6
Intersection gap (mm)	1.4	1.4
b values (s/mm^2)	0, 400, 800	At least 3 (0, 400, 800)
Matrix	128 × 128 (or 192)	144 × 192
Field of view (mm)	325–460	325–460
Number of averages	1–2	3–4
Parallel imaging acceleration factor	2	2
Acquisition plane	Axial or coronal	Axial or coronal
Acquisition time	<22 s	Minimum 120 s

Pixel-based ADC maps (integrating all b-values) can be generated using a commercial workstation. Values of ADC are calculated with a linear regression analysis of the function $S = S_0 \times \exp(-b \times \text{ADC})$, where S is the signal intensity (SI) after application of the diffusion gradient, and S_0 is the SI at $b = 0$ s/mm^2.

Applications of DWI for the characterization of focal renal masses

The diagnosis of renal neoplasm is usually based on the presence of enhancement on CT or MRI, and image subtraction has been shown to be superior to signal intensity measurement for the diagnosis of renal cell carcinoma (RCC)[3]. There is however a strong clinical need for alternatives to gadolinium-enhanced sequences for renal lesion characterization for the patients at risk for NSF[4–6]. There are a large number of studies describing renal DWI[7–18]; however, there are limited data on the use of DWI for renal lesion characterization[19–25]. These studies found that solid or malignant lesions generally have lower ADC with restricted diffusion compared to benign or cystic lesions, since the motion of water molecules is restricted in tissues with a high cellularity.

In the study by Cova et al.[19], 20 renal lesions were evaluated (13 simple cysts and 7 solid benign/malignant lesions) with DWI using b-values of 0–500 s/mm^2, with no cystic RCCs or complex cysts evaluated. Solid tumors showed mean ADC of $1.55 \pm 0.20 \times 10^{-3}$ mm^2/s. In another study which included solid and cystic RCCs, Squillaci et al.[20] also demonstrated lower ADC values in solid renal tumors ($n = 19$, including 12 RCCs) compared to simple cysts ($n = 20$): 1.7 ± 0.48 vs. $3.65 \pm 0.09 \times 10^{-3}$ mm^2/s, higher ADC in cystic RCCs compared to solid RCCs, and decreased ADC in angiomyolipomas (AMLs) ($1.46 \pm 0.09 \times 10^{-3}$ mm^2/s). Yoshikawa et al.[21] evaluated a total of 67 renal lesions (including 12 RCCs, ADC = 2.49 ± 0.72, AMLs [$n = 8$] 1.81 ± 0.41, cysts [$n = 42$] 3.82 ± 0.39, and complicated cysts [$n = 5$] 2.78 ± 0.71 using $b = 0$–600 s/mm^2), and found similar results as in the above-mentioned studies[19–20] (ADCs of renal cysts were significantly higher than those of RCCs). They found however no significant difference between ADCs of RCCs vs. complicated cysts and renal parenchyma. Zhang et al.[22] reported the use of DWI in solid and partially cystic renal masses ($n = 25$). Their ADC measurement method consisted of first taking large regions of interest (ROIs) fitting the whole lesion, and then segmenting lesions into necrotic/cystic and solid components based on contrast-enhanced imaging. Their findings extended those reported previously, with the addition of finding lower ADC values in cystic/necrotic portions of neoplasms compared to simple cysts.

47

Recently, Taouli et al.[23] reported the diagnostic performance of DWI compared to contrast-enhanced MRI in 109 renal masses (81 benign lesions and 28 RCCs) in 64 patients. The distribution of ADCs in benign and malignant renal lesions is shown in Figure 4.1. The distribution of ADC values (mean ± SD, × 10^{-3} mm²/s) at DWI performed with b values of 0, 400, and 800 s/mm² was as follows: simple cysts (category I from the Bosniak classification)[26] (highest ADC 2.78 ± 0.45, Figure 4.2), category II (2.47 ± 0.64), category IIF (1.85 ± 0.71), category III–IV (1.83 ± 0.85); as well as oncocytomas (1.91 ± 0.97), RCCs (including solid and cystic, 1.41 ± 0.61), and AMLs (0.74 ± 0.45). The ADCs of RCCs (1.41 × 10^{-3} mm²/s) were significantly lower than those of benign renal lesions (2.23 × 10^{-3} mm²/s, $p < 0.0001$).

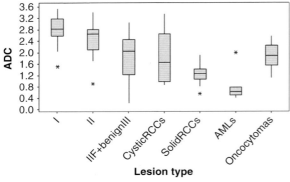

Figure 4.1 Box plot distribution of ADC values (using b values of 0, 400, and 800 s/mm²) in 109 renal lesions (in 64 patients): cystic lesions categorized by using Bosniak classification (categories I, II, IIF, and benign III lesions; malignant category III and IV lesions [cystic RCCs]), solid benign lesions (AMLs and oncocytomas), and solid RCCs. * Outliers. Top and bottom of each box represent 25% and 75% percentile of ADC values, respectively. Horizontal line inside each box represents median ADC value. [Reproduced with permission from Taouli B, et al. Renal lesions: characterization with diffusion-weighted imaging versus contrast-enhanced MR imaging. Radiology 2009;251:398–407.]

Using a cut-off ADC ≤ 1.92 × 10^{-3} mm²/s, the area under the ROC curve (AUC), sensitivity, and specificity of DWI for the diagnosis of RCCs were 0.856, 86%, and 80%, respectively (when excluding AMLs). The corresponding AUC, sensitivity, and specificity of contrast-enhanced T1-weighted imaging were 0.944, 100%, and 89%, respectively (Figure 4.3). AMLs were found to have the lowest ADCs (Figure 4.4); the decreased ADC could be explained by the muscular and fat components. Cystic RCCs (Figure 4.5) demonstrate higher ADC values compared to solid tumors due to their cystic components. In addition, Taouli et al.[23] found lower ADC in papillary RCCs (Figure 4.6) compared to non-papillary RCCs (mostly clear cell carcinomas): 1.12 ± 0.18 vs. 1.62 ± 0.73 ($p = 0.048$), and a significant difference in ADC between the cystic and the solid components of cystic RCCs ($p = 0.001$). They found that the ADCs (×10^{-3} mm²/s) of oncocytomas (Figure 4.7) were higher than those of solid RCCs (1.91 ± 0.97 vs. 1.54 ± 0.69, $p = 0.0097$).

Kim et al.[24] compared the diagnostic performance of contrast-enhanced T1-weighted imaging (using image subtraction and enhancement ratio) compared to DWI for the characterization of non-fat-containing T1 hyperintense renal lesions (64 lesions, including 38 benign T1 hyperintense cysts and 26 RCCs in 41 patients). The calculated AUC was 0.846 for ADC, 0.882 for enhancement ratio at the nephrographic phase, 0.865 for enhancement ratio at the excretory phase, and 0.861 for image subtraction. An enhancement ratio threshold of 15% for the diagnosis of RCC at the excretory phase, as described previously[27], demonstrated sensitivity of 65% and specificity of 93%. There was no significant difference between the three methods for the diagnosis of RCC (Figure 4.8). The combination of DWI and subtraction resulted in an AUC, sensitivity, and specificity of

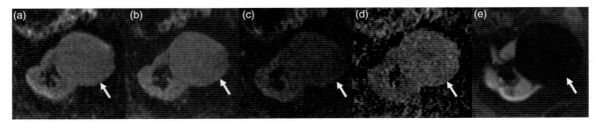

Figure 4.2 73-year-old man with simple left renal cyst. Axial SS EPI diffusion-weighted images demonstrate a 7-cm left renal lesion with free diffusion: it is hyperintense on b = 0 (a), with strong signal drop at b = 400 (b), and b = 800 (c), with high ADC (d) of 3.1 × 10^{-3} mm²/s, compatible with a benign cyst. Axial post-contrast T1-weighted image (e) confirms lack of lesion enhancement.

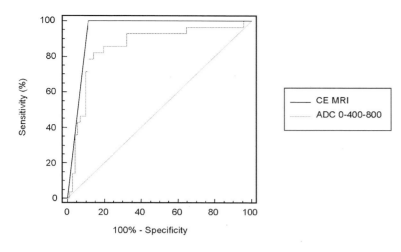

Figure 4.3 Receiver operating characteristic curves for ADC (at b-values of 0, 400, and 800 s/mm^2) and contrast-enhanced MRI used as predictors of malignancy in 99 non-fat-containing renal lesions in 62 patients. [Reproduced with permission from Taouli B, *et al.* Renal lesions: characterization with diffusion-weighted imaging versus contrast-enhanced MR imaging. *Radiology* 2009;**251**:398–407.]

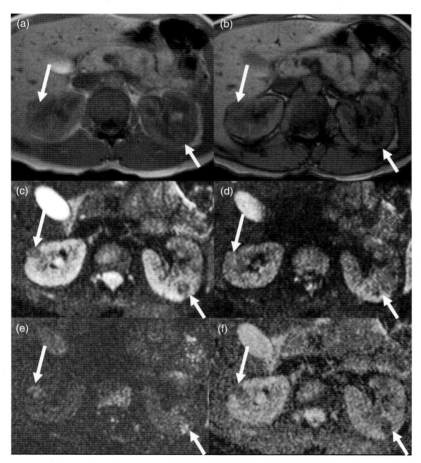

Figure 4.4 39-year-old woman with tuberous sclerosis and multiple bilateral renal angiomyolipomas (AMLs). Axial breath-hold in-phase (a) and opposed-phase (b) T1-weighted images show multiple fat-containing AMLs in both kidneys. Axial SS EPI diffusion-weighted images show that the largest AMLs (arrows) are hypointense compared to kidney parenchyma on $b = 0$ (c), isointense on $b = 400$ (d), and hyperintense on $b = 800$ (e) images. The ADC map (f) shows low ADC in both dominant AMLs (ADC of AML in right kidney was 1.18×10^{-3} mm^2/s, and that of left kidney was 1.27×10^{-3} mm^2/s). These lesions would have been diagnosed as malignant with DWI only.

0.893, 87%, and 92%, respectively, with significantly improved reader confidence compared with subtraction alone ($p = 0.041$) and slightly but not significantly ($p = 0.4254$) improved accuracy compared with image subtraction alone (accuracy, 89.8% vs. 86.7%). The same study showed that T1 hyperintense cysts (which

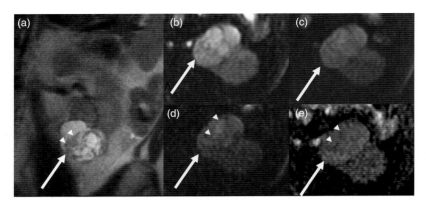

Figure 4.5 62-year-old man with cystic renal cell carcinoma of the left kidney. Coronal breath-hold half-Fourier acquisition single-shot turbo spin-echo (HASTE) T2-weighted image demonstrates a predominantly cystic multiseptated left renal mass (arrow) with solid components (arrowheads) (a). Axial SS EPI diffusion-weighted images at $b = 0$ (b), $b = 400$ (c), and $b = 800$ (d) show strong signal attenuation of the lesion, except for the small solid portions. Mean ADC (e) of the whole lesion was 2.78×10^{-3} mm²/s, while the ADC was lower in the solid portions (1.75×10^{-3} mm²/s) compared to the cystic portion.

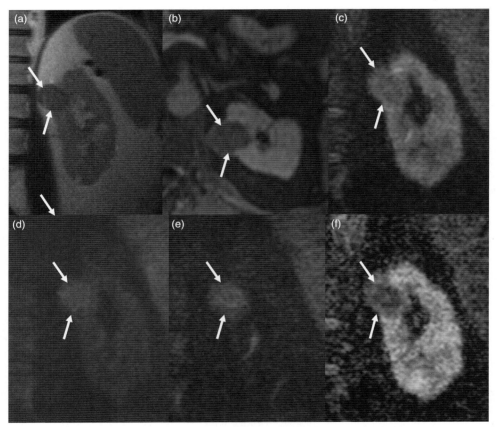

Figure 4.6 77-year-old man with papillary renal cell carcinoma of the left kidney. Coronal breath-hold half-Fourier acquisition single-shot turbo spin-echo (HASTE) T2-weighted image (a) shows a hypointense left renal mass (arrows). The mass shows mild enhancement on axial breath-hold contrast-enhanced fat-suppressed T1-weighted image (b). Coronal SS EPI diffusion-weighted images demonstrate that the lesion has restricted diffusion: it is hypointense on $b = 0$ (c), and becomes progressively hyperintense on $b = 400$ (d) and $b = 800$ (e) images compared to renal parenchyma. ADC map (f) shows low ADC (0.76×10^{-3} mm²/s) consistent with a malignant lesion.

include proteinaceous and hemorrhagic cysts) have slightly lower ADCs compared to simple cysts, probably related to a T2 effect, and to restricted diffusion in hemorrhage or high protein component as described in brain hematomas[28]. However, the ADCs of T1 hyperintense benign cysts were still higher than those of T1 hyperintense RCCs: 2.50 ± 0.53 vs. 1.75 ± 0.57, $p < 0.0001$.

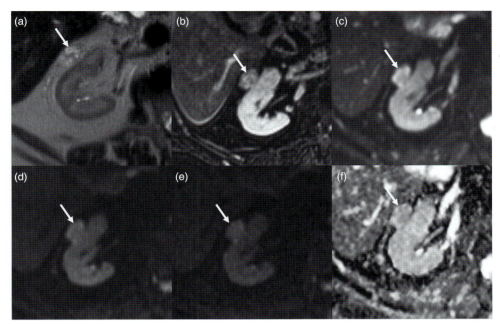

Figure 4.7 76-year-old woman with right renal oncocytoma. Axial breath-hold half-Fourier acquisition single-shot turbo spin-echo sequence (HASTE) T2- (a) and contrast-enhanced subtracted fat-suppressed T1-weighted images (b) show an exophytic T2 hyperintense right renal mass (arrow) with evidence of enhancement on subtraction consistent with a neoplasm, which was subsequently diagnosed as an oncocytoma by partial nephrectomy. Axial SS EPI diffusion-weighted images demonstrate that the lesion is hyperintense at $b = 0$ (c), $b = 400$ (d), and $b = 800$ (e). The ADC map (f) shows intermediate ADC (1.80×10^{-3} mm²/s).

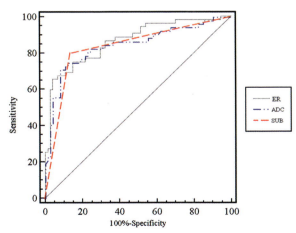

Figure 4.8 Receiver operating characteristic curves show the diagnostic utility of ADC compared with that of subtraction (SUB) and enhancement ratio (ER) in the excretory phase for the diagnosis of renal cell carcinoma in T1 hyperintense lesions. There were no significant differences between the values obtained with the three measurement techniques ($p > 0.3$). [Reproduced with permission from Kim S, et al. T1 hyperintense renal lesions: characterization with diffusion-weighted MR imaging versus contrast-enhanced MR imaging. *Radiology* 2009;**251**:796–807.]

In a recently published study, Sandrasegaran et al.[25] also found that the ADC values of the benign lesions were significantly higher than those of malignant lesions, with higher ADC in benign cysts compared to cystic RCCs. However, as opposed to the study by Taouli et al.[23], they found no significant difference between ADCs of clear-cell cancers and non-clear-cell cancers. They also observed lower ADC in high-grade clear-cell RCCs compared to low-grade clear-cell RCCs (1.77 vs. 1.95×10^{-3} mm²/s, without reaching significance).

Limitations of DWI

There are several limitations to the technique that may impact its widespread use: the ADC values are highly dependent on the parameters and the scanner used, thus there is a need for standardization of acquisition parameters and post-processing methods between centers. More histopathologic correlation data are needed for better use of DWI in renal masses. Another limitation is the limited sensitivity and specificity of ADC measurement for the diagnosis of renal neoplasm, as ADC can be decreased in renal abscesses (Figure 4.9) and pyelonephritis (Figure 4.10), and elevated in cystic RCCs. And last but not least, there is a need for improving image

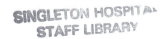

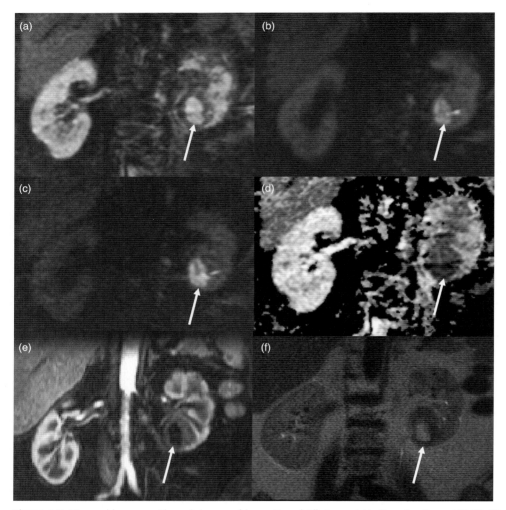

Figure 4.9 60-year-old woman with renal abscess, a false positive of diffusion-weighted imaging. Coronal SS EPI diffusion-weighted images demonstrate a hyperintense lesion with a peripheral hypointense rim (arrow) at $b = 0$ in the lower pole of the left kidney (a). The lesion demonstrates restricted diffusion: it is hyperintense at $b = 400$ (b) and strongly hyperintense at $b = 800$ (c). The ADC map (d) shows low ADC (1.01×10^{-3} mm^2/s) compared to the remainder of the renal parenchyma. Coronal contrast-enhanced fat-suppressed T1- (e) and coronal half-Fourier acquisition single-shot turbo spin-echo (HASTE) T2-weighted images (f) demonstrate a centrally necrotic lesion with peripheral T2 hypointense enhancing rim consistent with renal abscess, subsequently confirmed by percutaneous aspiration. Restricted diffusion is related to pus formation.

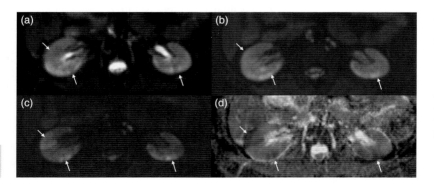

Figure 4.10 64-year-old woman with bilateral pyelonephritis. Axial SS EPI diffusion-weighted images demonstrate multifocal bilateral patchy renal lesions hypointense at $b = 0$ (a), iso- to slightly hyperintense at $b = 400$ (b), and hyperintense at $b = 800$ (c) compared to renal parenchyma (arrows). ADC map (d) shows decreased ADC compared to the remainder of normal renal parenchyma.

quality, for example using a combination of 3T, parallel imaging, and navigator echo acquisition.

Future directions

Studies assessing the ADC changes with response to treatment, for example post local ablation of RCC, are needed. Evaluation of ADC using selected ROIs within lesions is prone to sampling bias. Therefore, histogram analysis of ADC values is also worth investigating in heterogeneous cystic renal lesions. Another interesting application is the use of IVIM DWI[29] which could separate the effects of diffusion and perfusion by using a wide range of *b*-values. Finally, the role of DWI in the prediction of histologic subtypes of RCC and for the determination of tumor grade remains to be confirmed in larger studies.

Conclusion

DWI is a promising technique for the assessment of focal renal disease with multiple potential applications. The ability to perform DWI without intravenous gadolinium contrast agents is also a major advantage of DWI. However, more supporting data comparing DWI to contrast-enhanced imaging and pathology are needed.

References

1. Israel GM, Bosniak MA. Renal imaging for diagnosis and staging of renal cell carcinoma. *Urol Clin N Am* 2003;**30** (3):499–514.

2. Ho VB, Allen SF, Hood MN, Choyke PL. Renal masses: quantitative assessment of enhancement with dynamic MR imaging. *Radiology* 2002;**224** (3):695–700.

3. Hecht EM, Israel GM, Krinsky GA, *et al.* Renal masses: quantitative analysis of enhancement with signal intensity measurements versus qualitative analysis of enhancement with image subtraction for diagnosing malignancy at MR imaging. *Radiology* 2004;**232** (2):373–8.

4. Grobner T. Gadolinium: a specific trigger for the development of nephrogenic fibrosing dermopathy and nephrogenic systemic fibrosis? *Nephrol Dial Transplant* 2006;**21** (4):1104–8.

5. Sadowski EA, Bennett LK, Chan MR, *et al.* Nephrogenic systemic fibrosis: risk factors and incidence estimation. *Radiology* 2007;**243** (1): 148–57.

6. Boyd AS, Zic JA, Abraham JL. Gadolinium deposition in nephrogenic fibrosing dermopathy. *J Am Acad Dermatol* 2007;**56** (1):27–30.

7. Muller MF, Prasad PV, Bimmler D, Kaiser A, Edelman RR. Functional imaging of the kidney by means of measurement of the apparent diffusion coefficient. *Radiology* 1994;**193** (3):711–15.

8. Siegel CL, Aisen AM, Ellis JH, Londy F, Chenevert TL. Feasibility of MR diffusion studies in the kidney. *J Magn Reson Imag* 1995;**5** (5):617–20.

9. Namimoto T, Yamashita Y, Mitsuzaki K, *et al.* Measurement of the apparent diffusion coefficient in diffuse renal disease by diffusion-weighted echo-planar MR imaging. *J Magn Reson Imag* 1999; **9** (6):832–7.

10. Ichikawa T, Haradome H, Hachiya J, Nitatori T, Araki T. Diffusion-weighted MR imaging with single-shot echo-planar imaging in the upper abdomen: preliminary clinical experience in 61 patients. *Abdom Imag* 1999;**24** (5):456–61.

11. Fukuda Y, Ohashi I, Hanafusa K, *et al.* Anisotropic diffusion in kidney: apparent diffusion coefficient measurements for clinical use. *J Magn Reson Imag* 2000;**11** (2):156–60.

12. Ries M, Jones RA, Basseau F, Moonen CT, Grenier N. Diffusion tensor MRI of the human kidney. *J Magn Reson Imag* 2001;**14** (1):42–9.

13. Chan JH, Tsui EY, Luk SH, *et al.* MR diffusion-weighted imaging of kidney: differentiation between hydronephrosis and pyonephrosis. *Clin Imag* 2001; **25** (2):110–13.

14. Murtz P, Flacke S, Traber F, *et al.* Abdomen: diffusion-weighted MR imaging with pulse-triggered single-shot sequences. *Radiology* 2002;**224** (1):258–64.

15. Chow LC, Bammer R, Moseley ME, Sommer FG. Single breath-hold diffusion-weighted imaging of the abdomen. *J Magn Reson Imag* 2003;**18** (3):377–82.

16. Thoeny HC, De Keyzer F, Oyen RH, Peeters RR. Diffusion-weighted MR imaging of kidneys in healthy volunteers and patients with parenchymal diseases: initial experience. *Radiology* 2005;**235** (3):911–17.

17. Xu Y, Wang X, Jiang X. Relationship between the renal apparent diffusion coefficient and glomerular filtration rate: preliminary experience. *J Magn Reson Imag* 2007;**26** (3):678–81.

18. Notohamiprodjo M, Glaser C, Herrmann KA, *et al.* Diffusion tensor imaging of the kidney with parallel imaging: initial clinical experience. *Investig Radiol* 2008;**43** (10):677–85.

19. Cova M, Squillaci E, Stacul F, *et al.* Diffusion-weighted MRI in the evaluation of renal lesions: preliminary results. *Br J Radiol* 2004;**77** (922):851–7.

20. Squillaci E, Manenti G, Di Stefano F, *et al.* Diffusion-weighted MR imaging in the evaluation of renal tumours. *J Exp Clin Cancer Res* 2004;**23** (1):39–45.

21. Yoshikawa T, Kawamitsu H, Mitchell DG, et al. ADC measurement of abdominal organs and lesions using parallel imaging technique. *Am J Roentgenol* 2006;**187** (6):1521–30.

22. Zhang J, Tehrani YM, Wang L, *et al.* Renal masses: characterization with diffusion-weighted MR imaging: a preliminary experience. *Radiology* 2008;**247** (2): 458–64.

23. Taouli B, Thakur RK, Mannelli L, *et al.* Renal lesions: characterization with diffusion-weighted imaging versus contrast-enhanced MR imaging. *Radiology* 2009;**251**:398–407.

24. Kim S, Jain M, Harris AB, *et al.* T1 hyperintense renal lesions: characterization with diffusion-weighted MR imaging versus contrast-enhanced MR imaging. *Radiology* 2009;**251** (3):796–807.

25. Sandrasegaran K, Sundaram CP, Ramaswamy R, *et al.* Usefulness of diffusion-weighted imaging in the evaluation of renal masses. *Am J Roentgenol* 2010; **194** (2):438–45.

26. Israel GM, Bosniak MA. MR imaging of cystic renal masses. *Magn Reson Imag Clin N Am* 2004; **12** (3):403–12.

27. Ho VB AS, Hood MN, Choyke PL. Renal masses: quantitative assessment of enhancement with dynamic MR imaging. *Radiology* 2002;**224** (3): 695–700.

28. Silvera S, Oppenheim C, Touze E, *et al.* Spontaneous intracerebral hematoma on diffusion-weighted images: influence of T2-shine-through and T2-blackout effects. *Am J Neuroradiol* 2005;**26** (2):236–41.

29. Le Bihan D, Breton E, Lallemand D, *et al.* Separation of diffusion and perfusion in intravoxel incoherent motion MR imaging. *Radiology* 1988;**168** (2): 497–505.

Chapter 5

Diffusion-weighted MRI of the pancreas

Tomoaki Ichikawa, Ali Muhi, Utaroh Motosugi, and Katsuhiro Sano

Introduction

Pancreatic cancer is one of the leading causes of cancer-related death in the world with a poor 5-year survival rate. Despite recent advances in cross-sectional imaging, such as multidetector-row computed tomography (MDCT) or magnetic resonance (MR) imaging techniques, advanced disease at time of initial presentation results in a low rate of surgical interventions (10–20%) which is the cause of high mortality[1]. CA19–9 is a sensitive tumor marker for diagnosis of pancreatic carcinoma but lacks specificity. Endoscopic ultrasound (EUS) is regarded as the modality of choice in patients with a high index of clinical suspicion and negative MDCT, but is invasive and operator dependent. Currently, contrast-enhanced MDCT is the primary imaging modality for the detection and staging of pancreatic adenocarcinoma. A meta-analysis of 86 studies revealed sensitivity and specificity of 84% and 82% for MRI versus 91% and 85% for helical CT for detection of pancreatic adenocarcinoma[2]. MRI and fluoro-D-glucose positron emission tomography (FDG-PET) are complementary modalities to CT. Although contrast-enhanced CT achieves generally high sensitivity and specificity for the detection of pancreatic carcinoma, for staging and determination of resectability of the tumor, it is less specific in differentiating benign and malignant lesions[3–4]. The differentiation of pancreatic adenocarcinoma from mass-forming pancreatitis is difficult because both share morphological characteristics at imaging[5]. In the light of the limitations in diagnostic performance of the current imaging techniques, there is a compelling need for establishing an imaging technique as a cancer-screening method to provide high sensitivity for the detection and characterization of pancreatic tumors, and for the differentiation of tumors from benign inflammatory processes.

Diffusion-weighted MRI (DWI) is a recently developed imaging technique that has shown preliminary but promising results for detecting most types of malignancies outside the brain. Diffusion is a term used to describe random translational molecular motion, and is arbitrary and irregular. Diffusion is thermodynamic in origin and is usually quantified by the apparent diffusion coefficient (ADC), which describes the amount of water diffusion in the intracellular, extracellular, intravascular, and transmembranous compartments, as well as microcapillary perfusion. The increased cell density in tumors results in decrease of extracellular space, and a subsequent decrease in proton mobility leading to the restricted diffusion[6]. DWI is quite different from conventional imaging techniques, in that it can detect and quantify water motion in tissues that reflect tissue cellularity and cell membrane integrity. Recent technical developments in MRI, including the use of parallel imaging techniques, have improved the image diffusion quality and allowed the use of higher b-values in the abdomen[7].

Preliminary but promising results show that high b-value DWI showing high sensitivity for the detection of certain types of abdominal malignancies, such as colorectal cancers, pancreatic cancers, or hepatic metastases, have been already obtained[8–14]. Since most malignant lesions had restricted diffusion, i.e., high signal intensity on DWI and low ADC value, calculating the ADC value can be used to distinguish benign from malignant lesions.

DWI acquisition and processing applied to the pancreas

The magnetic field inhomogeneity and the motion arising from different organs (lungs, diaphragm, heart, and bowel) could degrade abdominal diffusion

Extra-Cranial Applications of Diffusion-Weighted MRI, ed. Bachir Taouli. Published by Cambridge University Press.
© Cambridge University Press 2011.

Table 5.1 DWI sequence parameters proposed for the evaluation pancreatic lesions[14,20,22–26,30–31,36,38–39]

Technique	Breath-hold	Free-breathing	Respiratory trigger
TR (ms)	2500	2000–10 000	1 respiratory cycle
TE (ms)	123	61.6–85	72
Field of view (mm)	300–380	400–480	300–455
Matrix size	188 × 150	128 × 256	128 × 256
Fat suppression	CHESS/STIR/water excitation		
Parallel imaging factor	2		
Number of averages	1	38	6
Section thickness/gap (mm)	6–8/0–1	4–6/0–1	4–6/0–1
Direction of motion-probing gradients	Phase, frequency, slice		
b-values (s/mm^2)	30, 300, 900	0, 50, 400, 500, 600, 1000	0, 500, 1000

images. Recent technological developments in MRI, including echo-planar imaging (EPI), parallel imaging techniques, and the use of respiratory triggering and cardiac gating, have helped overcome some of these problems. Parallel imaging enables shorter echo time and reduced echo-train length which shorten the acquisition time and improve signal-to-noise ratio (SNR). DWI is commonly performed using single-shot (SS) spin-echo EPI with parallel imaging acquisition (e.g., SENSE, GRAPPA) to minimize acquisition time, with preserved SNR and reduced motion-related artifacts, without affecting ADC calculation[15–17].

Currently, three imaging protocols can be used for SS EPI DWI of the pancreas: (1) breath-hold DWI, (2) free-breathing DWI, and (3) respiratory-triggered DWI. The selection of the protocol is dependent on available magnet time and the goal of imaging (i.e., whether quantitative or qualitative data are expected). Suggested parameters are summarized in Table 5.1.

Breath-hold single-shot DWI This acquisition has the advantage of being quick, with less blurriness compared to free-breathing acquisition. Disadvantages include lower SNR and limited spatial resolution, and limited number of b-values used for sampling. In addition, cardiac pulsation can cause artifacts in breath-hold technique, which can be minimized by the use of cardiac pulse triggering, which in turn increases acquisition time, and is therefore not often used clinically.

Free-breathing and respiratory-triggered DWI Increased signal averaging enables the acquisition of thinner slices and the use of multiple b-values, and produces better image quality, with improved SNR and ADC quantification (through the use of multiple b-values). However, the ADC of small lesions may be inaccurate due to image blurring. The advantage of free-breathing acquisition compared to respiratory-triggered technique is the possibility of using it in uncooperative patients.

Respiratory-triggered DWI shares all the advantages of free-breathing DWI, with the additional following advantages: minimized motion artifacts resulting in improved detection rate of small lesions, and decreased slice misalignment for creating maximum intensity projection (MIP) images and/or fusion images.

At our institution, we prefer the use of respiratory-triggered over breath-hold DWI, because the former provides better image quality and SNR without compromise in the calculated ADC values[18].

Fat suppression The use of fat suppression with SS EPI is essential to reduce chemical shift-induced ghosting. Takahara et al.[7] suggested the use of short tau inversion recovery (STIR), which enables more robust fat suppression. Chemical fat selective saturation (e.g., spectral selected attenuation with inversion recovery [SPAIR] or chemical shift selective [CHESS]) may be more useful because these methods produce better SNR, due to longer repetition time (TR), compared to STIR technique. Even if CHESS or SPAIR techniques are selected, an inversion recovery pulse may be employed to suppress undesirable background signal.

T2 shine-through effect T2 shine-through effect occurs as a result of high signal intensity returned from tissues with long intrinsic T2 relaxation times. Visual assessment alone may falsely ascribe the high signal intensity observed on DWI to restriction of water diffusion. Application of high b-values (e.g., 1000 s/mm^2) helps minimize T2 shine-though. On low and medium b-values (e.g., 100, 500 s/mm^2), T2 shine-through is difficult to avoid but may be overcome by assessing and calculating the ADC.

Choice of b-values A number of factors influence the selection of the b-values including the DWI technique used, expected SNR, and whether DWI is used for qualitative or quantitative analysis. Using higher (>800 s/mm^2) vs. intermediate b-values (e.g., 400–600 s/mm^2) is associated with lower SNR, but with reduction of T2 shine-through and perfusion effect. An ADC calculated using only low b-values (<100 s/mm^2) is sensitive to intravoxel capillary perfusion, while ADC calculations using higher b-values (e.g., 500 to 1000 s/mm^2) are relatively perfusion insensitive and reflect tissue cellularity and integrity of cellular membranes.

Image processing Diffusion images can be qualitatively assessed using multiplanar reconstruction (MPR) or (MIP). Takahara et al.[7] has reported an effective display with the use of MIP images with black-and-white inversion of contrast. Black-and-white inverse display of DWI can produce significant visual effects (similar to PET images) for lesion detection. Conventional display is more useful for lesion characterization or comparison with T2-weighted images. Thus, display methods should be used properly according to the purpose of the examinations. Although diffusion images are ideal for lesion detection, soft-tissue anatomy is often not well visualized, due to low SNR and limited spatial resolution. Fusion of diffusion images with conventional images obtained in the same MR session could help localize diffusion findings, and can improve the diagnostic value compared with each imaging technique alone.

ADC quantification ADC values are obtained most of the time by placing regions of interest (ROIs) over the lesion or pancreatic parenchyma on ADC maps obtained automatically with commercial workstations provided by major vendors. ADC is calculated using a monoexponential fit: $ADC = \ln[SI_1/SI_2] / [b_2 - b_1]$, where ln is the natural logarithm, and SI_1 and SI_2 are the signal intensity measurements obtained for low b-value and high b-value diffusion images, respectively.

ROIs should be placed within the confines of the lesion or pancreatic parenchyma. For heterogeneous lesions, the ROIs should include the entire lesion and should not exclude various components with different attenuation. Care should be taken to avoid artifacts within the regions of interest.

DWI results in acute and chronic pancreatitis

The diagnosis and assessment of severity of acute pancreatitis are usually made with contrast-enhanced CT, and MRI is rarely used in these patients at the acute phase. There is very limited data on the use of DWI in acute pancreatitis. A case report has described the appearance of acute pancreatitis on DWI as diffuse bright signal of the pancreas and reduction in the ADC[19]. Our experience (based on six cases) is similar (Fig. 5.1). The high signal on DWI usually returns to normal after the resolution of inflammation.

The diagnosis of chronic pancreatitis is usually based on contrast-enhanced CT, endoscopic retrograde cholangiopancreatography (ERCP), MR cholangiopancreatography (MRCP), or EUS. Findings on conventional diagnostic imaging may be normal in mild cases of chronic pancreatitis. ERCP has been considered to be the best available test for making the diagnosis of chronic pancreatitis. However, ERCP is relatively invasive, requires patient sedation, and may cause acute pancreatitis by itself. High b-value DWI has evolved as an additional imaging modality, which measures changes in the tissue water diffusion. Recent reports have described lower ADC in chronic pancreatitis compared to normal pancreas, which may be explained by fibrosis, chronic inflammation and reduction of pancreatic exocrine tissue[20–22]. In addition, Balci et al.[22] found a strong correlation between ADC and pancreatic exocrine function as well as with Cambridge score in chronic pancreatitis. They described a mean ADC value of $1.52 \pm 0.13 \times 10^{-3}$ mm^2/s in patients with endoscopically abnormal pancreatic exocrine function and a mean ADC of $1.78 \pm 0.07 \times 10^{-3}$ mm^2/s in normal patients. Akisik et al.[20–21] measured pancreatic ADC before and after secretin injection, and found that mean pre-secretin and maximum post-secretin ADCs were lower in patients with mild or severe chronic pancreatitis compared to healthy individuals, but did not vary between mild and severe chronic pancreatitis. They found no correlation between the percentage of increase in ADC

(a)

(b)

(c)

(d)

(e)

(f)

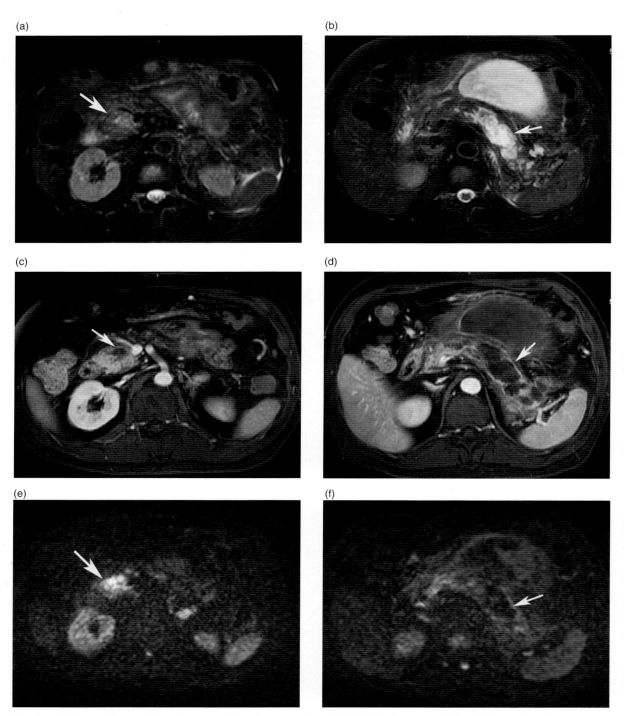

Figure 5.1 46-year-old man with acute pancreatitis and large pseudocyst. (a, b) Axial fat-suppressed T2-weighted imaging shows massive necrosis (white arrow) of the pancreatic head and body and large pseudocyst anterior to the pancreas (black arrow). (b, c) There is no enhancement of the pancreatic necrosis or pseudocyst on the pancreatic phase of contrast-enhanced MRI. (c, d) Axial DWI at $b = 1000$ s/mm^2, the pancreatic necrosis returns low signal intensity except for the pancreatic head, while the pseudocyst returns low–slight signal intensity.

after secretin administration (range from 22% for controls to 25% for patients with mild pancreatitis) and peak time with the severity of inflammation (range from 4.3 min for patients with severe pancreatitis to 5 min for patients with mild pancreatitis) and they concluded that ADC response to secretin administration is less useful[20]. This is in contradiction to the previous report by Erturk et al. who found no difference in the mean ADC value before secretin administration, and suggested that a peak time of ADC 4 min after administration of secretin as a cut-off value, with a sensitivity of 100% and specificity of 94.7%, differentiates between healthy individuals (peak before 4 min) and patients with or at risk of chronic pancreatitis (no peak or peak after 4 min, respectively)[23]. This should be further clarified by additional studies.

Pancreatic ductal adenocarcinoma

Pancreatic ductal adenocarcinoma is the most common pancreatic malignant tumor, forming about 80% of total pancreatic tumors. The tumor occurs most commonly in the head (60–62%), while 26% occurs at the pancreatic body, and 12% involves the pancreatic tail. Clinical symptoms such as abdominal pain, jaundice, and weight loss develop late in the disease and depend on the site of the tumor. Tumors in the body and tail produce late symptoms.

The treatment and outcome have not significantly changed in the recent years possibly due to late presentation at the time of diagnosis. Early diagnosis and accurate staging of pancreatic cancer is crucial in determining the treatment of choice. Differentiation from pancreatitis and benign tumors is particularly important because the prognosis of pancreatic adenocarcinoma is very poor, and it is curable only by surgical resection. Recent advances in imaging techniques have contributed to the accurate diagnosis of pancreatic cancer, but still the diagnosis is usually late. Contrast-enhanced CT, ERCP, MRI, and EUS are commonly used modalities in the detection of pancreatic adenocarcinoma.

DWI has emerged as an additional modality, which is sensitive to changes in water diffusion in pancreatic tissue. Our group has reported sensitivity of 92% and specificity of 96% for the detection of pancreatic ductal adenocarcinoma using DWI (Fig. 5.2)[14]. Recently, Kartalis et al.[24] found that DWI has a similar accuracy to conventional MRI for the diagnosis of pancreatic cancer. They reported

similar sensitivity and specificity (92% and 97%) to our study for the diagnosis of malignant pancreatic lesions. Takeuchi et al.[25] and Matsuki et al.[26] reported that all pancreatic cancers displayed high signal on DWI.

DWI can be performed as an adjunct to conventional MRI study. Furthermore, diffusion images can be fused with conventional images to achieve better anatomic resolution. DWI has the potential to become the imaging method of choice for screening patients with symptoms suggestive of pancreatic adenocarcinoma. Moreover, this technique can also be used for screening of patients who have hereditary predisposition for pancreatic cancer such as patients with hereditary pancreatitis, multiple endocrine neoplasia type 1, and Gardner syndrome.

Although CT and MRI are advantageous in providing precise anatomical delineation of pancreatic tumors, they are less specific in differentiating malignant and benign lesions[3–4,27]. Kim et al.[5] reported that the intrapancreatic fibrotic changes (such as in chronic pancreatitis), are visualized on CT and MRI, but cannot be distinguished from pancreatic adenocarcinoma. The most definite factor to differentiate between the two entities is the presence of spread, whether extensive local spread or distant metastasis.

Despite the few reports describing the usefulness of DWI with its high sensitivity and specificity in detecting pancreatic carcinoma[14,24–26,28], differentiation from inflammatory lesions is still challenging. Most of previous reports demonstrate that pancreatic cancers have lower ADC values than the normal pancreas[24–26,28–32].

In our experience, ADC value of pancreatic adenocarcinomas was significantly higher than that of acute mass-forming pancreatitis (1.02 ± 0.17 vs. $0.81 \pm 0.19 \times 10^{-3}$ mm^2/s) (Fig. 5.3). A cut-off ADC value $\geq 0.9 \times 10^{-3}$ mm^2/s was used to differentiate pancreatic carcinoma from mass-forming pancreatitis (acute and chronic) with 87% sensitivity and 75% specificity. Pancreatic adenocarcinomas and mass-forming pancreatitis during acute phase could be distinguished from the mass-forming pancreatitis during the chronic phase ($1.37 \pm 0.17 \times 10^{-3}$ mm^2/s) by visual assessment on high b-value DWI; the former show high signal intensity on high b-value DWI, whereas the latter displays slight iso-hyperintensity relative to the pancreatic parenchyma. Using cut-off ADC values $\geq 1.33 \times 10^{-3}$ mm^2/s ($b = 0$–500) and $\geq 1.19 \times 10^{-3}$ mm^2/s ($b = 0$–1000), Lee et al.[30]

(a)

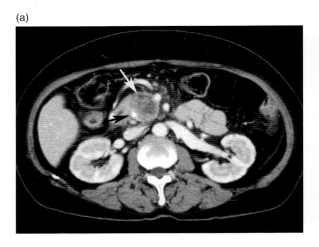

(b)

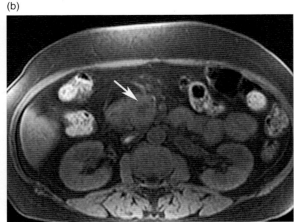

(c)

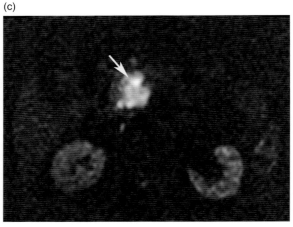

Figure 5.2 66-year-old woman with pancreatic adenocarcinoma. (a) Axial contrast-enhanced CT at the pancreatic parenchymal phase shows a hypovascular mass in the pancreatic head (white arrow). The tumor abuts the superior mesenteric vein. A stent is seen in the common bile duct (black arrow). (b) Axial pre-contrast fat-suppressed T1-weighted image shows that the tumor is partially hypointense relative to pancreatic parenchyma. (c) Axial fat-suppressed SS EPI DWI at $b = 1000$ s/mm^2 shows corresponding hyperintensity relative to the pancreatic parenchyma (arrow). Tumor ADC was 1.1×10^{-3} mm^2/s while ADC of pancreatic parenchyma was 1.5×10^{-3} mm^2/s.

reported sensitivities ranging from 72.3% to 87% and specificities ranging from 69.2% to 76.9% for differentiating pancreatic carcinoma and mass-forming pancreatitis. Fattahi *et al.* found that the mean ADC value of pancreatic carcinoma (1.46 ± 0.18 mm^2/s) was significantly lower than the remaining pancreas ($2.11 \pm 0.32 \times 10^{-3}$ mm^2/s), mass-forming focal pancreatitis ($2.09 \pm 0.18 \times 10^{-3}$ mm^2/s), and pancreatic gland in the control group ($1.78 \pm 0.07 \times 10^{-3}$ mm^2/s)[31]. They also described that mass-forming focal pancreatitis was visually indistinguishable from the remaining pancreas whereas pancreatic carcinoma was hyperintense relative to the remaining pancreas but they did not describe whether the ADC values were measured during acute or chronic phases of the inflammation. Thus, DWI could be of value in differentiating adenocarcinoma from benign mass-forming pancreatitis. The ADC

values of various pancreatic solid lesions are summarized in Table 5.2.

Previous reports indicate that DWI shows high sensitivity and specificity for the detection of liver metastases[33–35]. In our experience, lymph node metastases show high signal intensity on DWI and return low ADC (range from 0.52 to 2.4×10^{-3} mm^2/s). However, the value of ADC in differentiating benign and malignant nodes is limited because both reactive and malignant lymph nodes show high signal intensity on DWI.

Because only few pancreatic cancers are resectable, accurate pre-operative evaluation of resectability is essential. Factors that preclude a curative resection include invasion of major vessels, involvement of the perivascular neural plexus, invasion of adjacent organs, and distant metastases. The use of thin slice

(a)

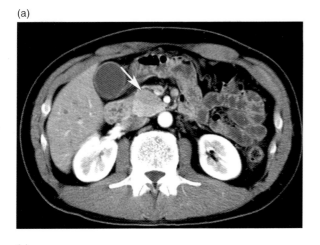

(b)

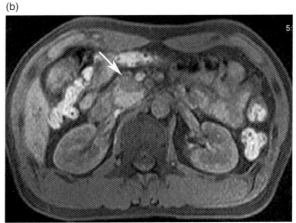

(c)

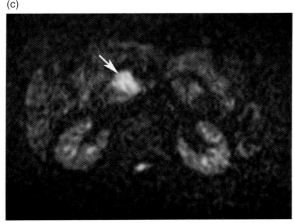

Figure 5.3 47-year-old woman with mass-forming autoimmune pancreatitis. (a) Axial contrast-enhanced CT during at the pancreatic parenchymal phase shows a poorly defined hypovascular mass in the pancreatic head (arrow). (b) Axial fat-suppressed T1-weighted image shows a hypointense tumor. (c) Axial fat-suppressed SS EPI DWI at $b = 1000$ s/mm^2 shows that the tumor is hyperintense (arrow), and therefore cannot be differentiated from adenocarcinoma. However, the ADC was 0.7×10^{-3} mm^2/s, lower than the adenocarcinoma showed in Fig. 5.2. Despite the lower ADC, the tumor is still surgical, and the patient underwent a Whipple procedure which showed mass-forming pancreatitis.

contrast-enhanced CT and reformatted images is superior to DWI for prediction of resectability. DWI, at best, is a complementary technique in this regard.

In summary, DWI can be useful for visual detection of pancreatic cancer and ADC measurements may help as a supplement to other imaging modality to differentiate between pancreatic carcinoma and benign mass-forming pancreatitis.

Other solid pancreatic neoplasms
Neuroendocrine tumors

Neuroendocrine tumors of the pancreas (formerly called islet cell tumors) arise from the islets of Langerhans. Neuroendocrine tumors can be functioning or non-functioning, benign or malignant. The most common types are insulinoma, gastrinoma, and non-functioning tumors. The clinical symptoms are either related to hormone secretion or related to invasion of adjacent structures and distant metastases by malignant tumors. They can be isolated or associated with multiple endocrine neoplasia syndrome type 1, and they could be single or multiple. The diagnosis of functioning neuroendocrine tumors is usually made clinically.

The role of imaging is to determine the location, size, and number of tumors. In our experience, all neuroendocrine tumors that were evaluated with high b-value DWI show high signal intensity probably related to their cellularity and have an ADC value lower than that of pancreatic ductal adenocarcinoma (0.56 ± 0.29 vs. $1.02 \pm 0.17 \times 10^{-3}$ mm^2/s) (Fig. 5.4). Bakir et al.[36] reported that all neuroendocrine tumors demonstrated high signal intensity relative to

61

Table 5.2 Reported ADC values of solid pancreatic lesions

	Ichikawa et al. (unpubl data)	Bakir et al.[36]	Kartalis et al.[24]	Niwa et al.[40]	Fattahi et al.[31]	Matsuki et al.[26]	Muraoka et al.[28]	Takeuchi et al.[25]	Lee et al.[30]
b-values (s/mm²)	500, 1000	50, 400, 800	0, 500	0, 1000	0, 600	0, 800	0, 500	0, 800	0, 1000
Pancreatic adenocarcinoma	1.02 ± 0.17		1.40 ± 0.30	0.72 to 1.88	1.46 ± 0.18	1.44 ± 0.20	1.27 ± 0.52	1.38 ± 0.32	1.23 ± 0.18
Acute mass-forming pancreatitis	0.81 ± 0.19								
Chronic mass-forming pancreatitis	1.37 ± 0.17					2.31 ± 0.18		1.00 ± 0.18	
Mass-forming pancreatitis (unspecified)					2.09 ± 0.18				1.04 ± 0.18
Neuroendocrine tumor	0.56 ± 0.29	1.51 ± 0.35							1.30 ± 0.41
Solid pseudopapillary tumor (solid component)	1.3 ± 0.47							1.16 ± 0.36	1.16 ± 0.36

(a)

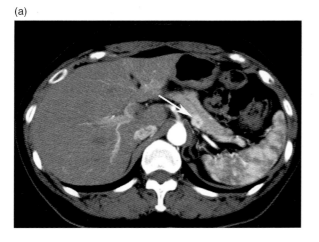

(b)

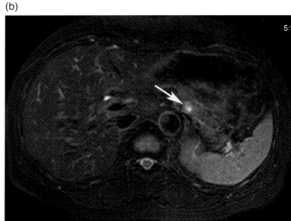

(c)

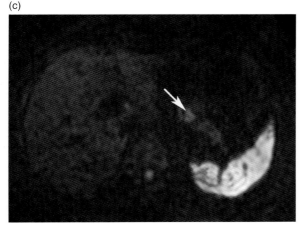

Figure 5.4 63-year-old woman with small neuroendocrine tumor of the pancreas (glucagonoma). (a) Axial contrast-enhanced CT at the pancreatic parenchymal phase shows a small hypervascular tumor in the pancreatic body with tiny central area of decreased enhancement. (b) Axial fat-suppressed T2-weighted image shows heterogeneous intermediate signal intensity lesion at the pancreatic body with central higher signal. (c) The tumor is hyperintense on axial fat-suppressed SS EPI DWI at $b = 1000$ s/mm^2.

the surrounding pancreatic parenchyma on diffusion images. They reported a mean ADC value of ($1.51 \pm 0.35 \times 10^{-3}$ mm^2/s) which was significantly higher than surrounding parenchyma ($0.76 \pm 0.15 \times 10^{-3}$ mm^2/s) and normal pancreas in normal volunteers ($0.80 \pm 0.06 \times 10^{-3}$ mm^2/s). Lee et al. reported ADC values of $1.62 \pm 0.60 \times 10^{-3}$ mm^2/s (ADC$_{500}$) and $1.30 \pm 0.41 \times 10^{-3}$ mm^2/s (ADC$_{1000}$) for neuroendocrine tumors which were lower than normal pancreas ($2.06 \pm 0.42 \times 10^{-3}$ mm^2/s [ADC$_{500}$] and $1.62 \pm 0.34 \times 10^{-3}$ mm^2/s [ADC$_{1000}$])[30]. The described variations in the ADC values may be related to the differences in the used b-value, tissue characteristics, or necrosis. High b-value DWI in conjunction with conventional MRI may be the modality of choice in the future for preoperative localization of functioning neuroendocrine tumors and may be a useful adjunct in the diagnosis of non-functioning neuroendocrine tumors.

Solid and papillary epithelial neoplasm

Solid and papillary epithelial neoplasm of the pancreas is a rare, non-functioning low-grade malignant tumor affecting mainly young women. It is usually large, well encapsulated, and undergoing hemorrhagic necrosis. Solid and papillary epithelial neoplasms typically arise from the tail of the pancreas but can arise from any portion of the pancreas. These tumors are usually large at diagnosis, with a mean diameter of 10 cm. The gross appearance is variable with tumors being solid, cystic, or mixed cystic and solid. Solid and papillary epithelial neoplasm is a low-grade malignancy that is curable with surgical excision. The solid component of solid and papillary neoplasm has high signal intensity on high b-value DWI probably reflecting the high cellularity of the solid component (Fig. 5.5). The cystic component shows iso- or hypointensity reflecting the increase in free water permitting free diffusion. In our experience, based on two cases, the ADC of the solid component is $1.3 \pm 0.47 \times 10^{-3}$ mm^2/s, while the mean ADC of the cystic component is $2.6 \pm 0.24 \times 10^{-3}$ mm^2/s. Based on six cases, Lee *et al.* reported an ADC of 1.43 ± 0.29 ($b = 0$–500) and $1.16 \pm 0.36 \times 10^{-3}$ mm^2/s ($b = 0$–1000) for solid and papillary epithelial neoplasms[30].

Cystic pancreatic lesions

Cystic pancreatic lesions include pseudocysts, serous cystic tumors, mucinous cystic tumors, intraductal papillary mucinous neoplasms (IPMNs), solid and papillary epithelial neoplasms, and cystic islet cell tumors. The mucinous cystic tumors are premalignant while the serous cystic tumor and pseudocysts are benign conditions. In our experience, molecular diffusion is strongly correlated with the viscosity of the fluid. Because diffusion is closely related to viscosity of the fluid, the characterization of cystic fluid may be possible with DWI. The ADC values of various pancreatic cystic lesions are summarized in Table 5.3.

Pseudocysts

A pseudocyst is a fluid collection consisting of necrotic material, proteinaceous debris, and enzymatic material that is confined by a fibrous capsule. Most cystic masses of the pancreas encountered in clinical practice are post-inflammatory pseudocysts. They develop most often as a complication of acute or chronic pancreatitis. In patients with no clear history of acute or chronic pancreatitis, differentiation of pseudocyst from cystic pancreatic tumor can be difficult.

In our experience, based on six cases, pseudocysts display iso- to intermediate signal intensity on high b-value DWI and return an ADC of $3.08 \pm 0.35 \times 10^{-3}$ mm^2/s (Fig. 5.1). Yamashita *et al.* reported an ADC of $3.2 \pm 1.3 \times 10^{-3}$ mm^2/s in 10 pseudocysts, which was significantly lower than those of serous cystadenomas or cerebrospinal fluid ($5.8 \pm 2.0 \times 10^{-3}$ mm^2/s)[37]. The high ADC reported by Yamashita *et al.* may be attributed to the low b-value used ($b = 300$ s/mm^2). Using

$b = 0$, 600 s/mm^2, Yoshikawa *et al.* found that pseudocysts have lower ADC ($3.60 \pm 0.69 \times 10^{-3}$ mm^2/s) than simple cysts ($3.96 \pm 0.14 \times 10^{-3}$ mm^2/s)[15]. Inan *et al.* found that six out of seven pseudocysts were isointense on DWI ($b = 0$–1000 s/mm^2), with an ADC value of $2.8 \pm 0.7 \times 10^{-3}$ mm^2/s which was lower than that of simple cysts ($3.3 \pm 0.7 \times 10^{-3}$ mm^2/s)[38]. This is to be expected, because of the high viscosity of the necrotic content of pseudocyst. Inan *et al.* found that pseudocysts and simple cysts have a significantly higher ADC than abscesses, hydatid cysts, and neoplastic cysts. Theoretically, the ADC value of pseudocysts is lower than that of serous cystadenomas, but this is not usually seen in clinical practice.

Intraductal papillary mucinous neoplasm

Intraductal papillary mucinous neoplasm (IPMN) has a primarily intraductal, papillomatous growth pattern, which is associated with excessive mucin secretion and results in progressive ductal dilatation or cyst formation. The tumor occurs in three forms: segmental or diffuse involvement of the main pancreatic duct and/or cystic involvement of branch ducts. IPMN is a premalignant condition which tends to affect elderly people. Accurate pre-operative diagnosis is important because the disease has excellent prognosis after surgical treatment. Yamashita *et al.* has reported that IPMN shows high signal intensity on DWI ($b = 300$ s/mm^2), and an ADC ($2.7 \pm 0.9 \times 10^{-3}$ mm^2/s) lower than that of serous cystadenomas ($5.8 \pm 2.0 \times 10^{-3}$ mm^2/s)[37]. The high signal intensity reported by Yamashita *et al.* is probably related to the use of low b-value. In our experience, based on 76 cases, all tumors display iso- or hypointensity relative to the pancreatic parenchyma with a mean ADC of $2.8 \pm 0.36 \times 10^{-3}$ mm^2/s (Fig. 5.6). Furthermore, high b-value DWI was useful to detect the solid component in two tumors, which shows high signal intensity on DWI and low ADC ($0.7 \pm 0.17 \times 10^{-3}$ mm^2/s) (Fig. 5.7). We also found that the ADC of IPMN was significantly higher than that of mucinous cystic neoplasm ($2.0 \pm 0.3 \times 10^{-3}$ mm^2/s). Thus, high b value DWI can occasionally help differentiate benign from malignant IPMN. The differentiation of IPMN from other cystic neoplasm on the basis of diffusion signal intensity and ADC measurement is however difficult if not impossible, and conventional imaging findings including MRCP remain essential for diagnosis.

(a)

(b)

(c)

(d)

(e)

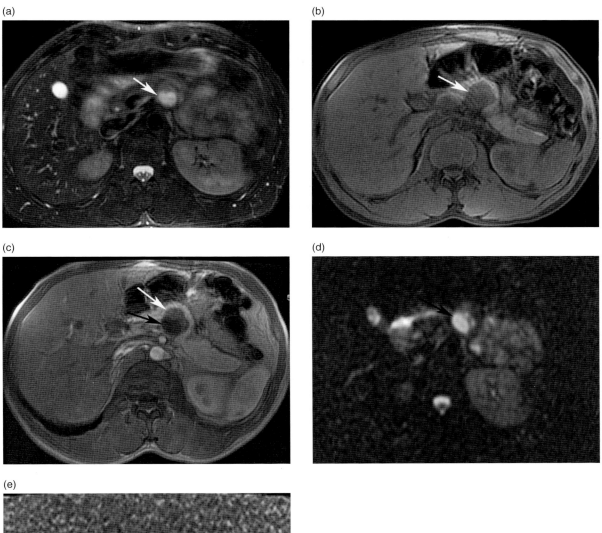

Figure 5.5 35-year-old-man with solid pseudopapillary tumor of the pancreas. (a) Axial fat-suppressed T2-weighted image shows heterogeneous lesion (arrow) of the pancreatic body with a hyperintense portion (cystic/necrotic component) and a solid portion in intermediate signal. (b) The tumor displays intermediate T1 signal on axial fat-suppressed pre-contrast T1-weighted image. (c) Axial fat-suppressed contrast-enhanced T1-weighted image shows mild enhancement of the solid portion (white arrow) and a posterior cystic portion (black arrow). (d) Axial SS EPI diffusion image at $b = 0$ s/mm^2 shows that cystic portion of tumor is hyperintense relative to adjacent pancreatic parenchyma (black arrow). (e) Axial SS EPI diffusion image at $b = 1000$ s/mm^2 shows that solid portion is hyperintense (white arrow) but the posterior cystic/necrotic portion now shows signal loss (black arrow).

Table 5.3 Reported ADC values of cystic pancreatic lesions

	Ichikawa *et al.* (unpubl data)	Irie *et al.*[39]	Inan *et al.*[38]	Yamashita *et al.*[37]
b-values (s/mm^2)	500, 1000	30, 300, 900	0, 500, 1000	30, 300
Intraductal papillary mucinous neoplasm	2.9 ± 0.36	2.8 ± 1.0		2.7 ± 0.9
Mucinous cystadenoma	2.0 ± 0.3		2.6 ± 1.1	
Mucinous cystadenocarcinoma			2.7 ± 0.7	
Serous cystadenoma	2.6 ± 0.28	2.9 ± 2.6	2.7 ± 0.2	5.8 ± 2.0
Pseudocyst	3.08 ± 0.35	2.9 ± 1.2	2.8 ± 0.7	3.2 ± 1.0
Simple cyst			3.3 ± 0.5	
Abscess			2.5 ± 0.2	
Hydatid cyst			2.6 ± 0.2	
Solid pseudopapillary tumor (cystic component)	2.6 ± 0.24			

(a)

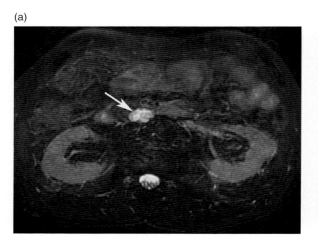

(b)

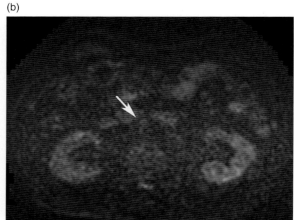

(c)

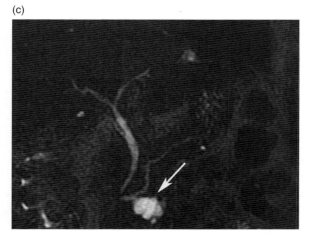

Figure 5.6 61-year-old man with branch duct intraductal papillary mucinous neoplasm (IPMN). (a) Axial fat-suppressed T2-weighted image demonstrates a lobulated cystic mass of the uncinate process of the pancreas. (b) Axial fat-suppressed SS EPI DWI at *b* = 1000 s/mm^2 shows that the tumor is hypointense compared to the surrounding pancreas. ADC value was 3.2 × 10^{-3} mm^2/s. (c) Coronal thick slice MRCP shows communication with the main pancreatic duct, diagnostic of branch duct IPMN.

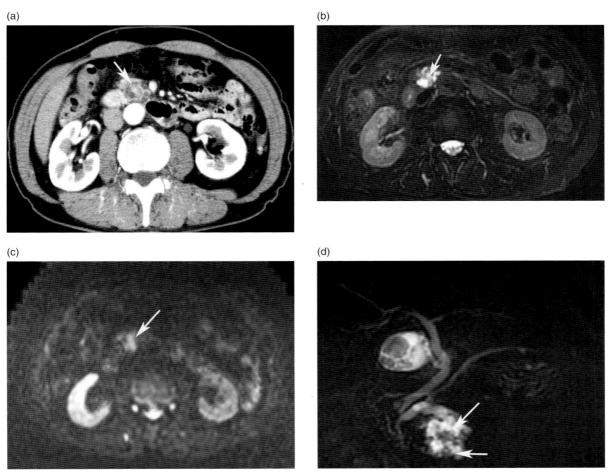

Figure 5.7 72-year-old man with malignant IPMN. (a) Axial contrast-enhanced CT at the pancreatic parenchymal phase shows a complex cystic mass of the pancreatic uncinate process with enhancing mural nodule (arrow). (b) Axial T2-weighted image shows lobulated cystic and solid mass with intermediate signal intensity mural nodule (arrow). (c) Axial fat-suppressed SS EPI DWI at $b = 1000$ s/mm^2 shows mural nodule in high signal intensity, suspicious for malignancy. (d) Coronal thick slice MR cholangiopancreatography demonstrates communication of the mass with the dilated main pancreatic duct. Solid nodules demonstrate low signal intensity (arrows).

Mucinous cystic neoplasms

Mucinous cystic neoplasms are rare cystic tumors of the pancreas. The large cystic spaces are lined by columnar, mucin-producing epithelium. Mucinous cystic neoplasms may be uni- or mutilocular. Secondary cysts along the internal wall are common. Solid papillary excrescences sometimes protrude from the wall into the interior of these tumors. The mucinous cystic neoplasms are premalignant or malignant tumors. The tumor occurs in middle-aged patients (median age 49 years), most commonly females. The clinical symptoms include epigastric pain or discomfort, which may radiate to the back, anorexia, weakness, and weight loss.

On high b-value DWI, the mucinous cystic tumors display iso- to intermediate signal intensity probably due to the high viscosity of the mucin content (Fig. 5.8). In our small experience (based on eight cases), mucinous cystic tumors showed mean ADC of $2.0 \pm 0.3 \times 10^{-3}$ mm^2/s, lower than that of serous cystadenomas. Inan *et al.* reported an ADC value of $2.6 \pm 1.1 \times 10^{-3}$ mm^2/s in mucinous cystic neoplasms, significantly lower than that of simple cysts and pseudocysts, but not different from serous cystadenomas[38]. DWI can also show the solid components as high signal intensity foci within the tumor with lower ADC value. Mucinous cystic tumors should always be resected because they are all

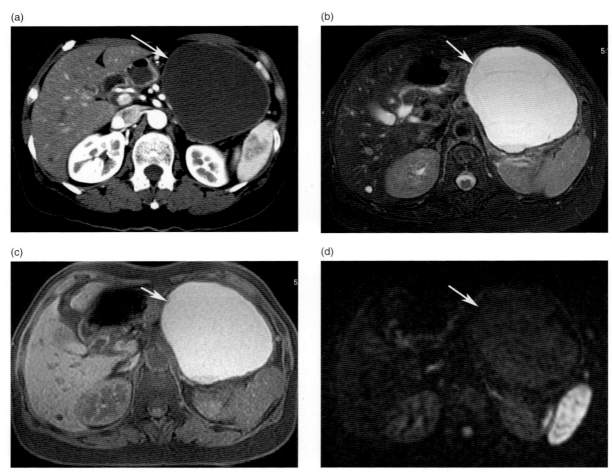

Figure 5.8 22-year-old woman with large mucinous cystadenoma. (a) Axial contrast-enhanced CT at the pancreatic parenchymal phase shows a large cystic tumor of the pancreatic body with no appreciable enhancement or solid component. (b) Axial fat-suppressed T2-weighted image shows high signal intensity cystic tumor in the pancreatic body with dependent fluid level. (c) Axial fat-suppressed T1-weighted image demonstrates high signal intensity of the tumor with fluid–fluid level in the dependent portion of the tumor, compatible with hemorrhage. (d) Axial fat-suppressed SS EPI DWI at $b = 1000$ s/mm^2 shows tumor to be hypointense, compatible with cystic lesion.

potentially malignant. More data are necessary to determine the role of ADC for diagnosing mucinous cystic neoplasms.

Serous cystadenomas

Serous cystadenomas (also called microcystic cystadenomas) are more commonly found in patients over 60 years and equally in men and women. Some patients present with non-specific complaint of abdominal pain or weight loss or more commonly lesions are diagnosed incidentally. Typical serous cystadenomas are composed of multiple small cysts containing glycogen with no mucin. The cysts vary in size from 0.2 to 2.0 cm, and the size of the tumors

ranges from 1.4 to 27 cm with a mean diameter of 10.8 cm. They most commonly occur in the pancreatic head. On high b-value DWI, serous cystadenomas display isointensity relative to the pancreatic parenchyma due to the free diffusion of molecules in the serous fluid (Fig. 5.9). Yamashita et al. reported an ADC value of $5.8 \pm 2.0 \times 10^{-3}$ mm[37], but in our experience serous cystadenomas tend to have a lower ADC than previously described (2.6×10^{-3} mm^2/s) (based on two cases). This discrepancy is probably due to the use of low b-value by Yamashita et al. ($b = 0$–300 s/mm^2). Inan et al. reported an ADC of $2.7 \pm 0.2 \times 10^{-3}$ mm^2/s ($n = 2$)[38]. Asymptomatic serous cystadenomas do

(a)

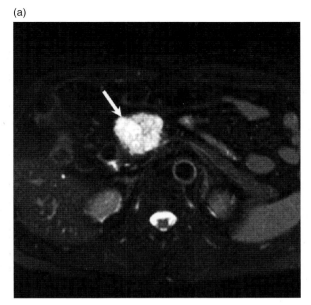

(b)

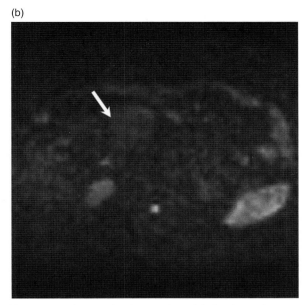

Figure 5.9 51-year-old male patient with serous cystadenoma. (a) Axial fat-suppressed T2-weighted image shows lobulated cystic lesion of the pancreatic head. (b) Axial fat-suppressed SS EPI DWI at $b = 1000$ s/mm^2 shows the tumor to be hypointense, without any hyperintense component. ADC measured 2.6×10^{-3} mm^2/s.

not require surgical excision because they are never malignant.

Limitations of DWI of the pancreas

The principal limitation of DWI is its low SNR, particularly on high b-values, and limited spatial resolution. Fusion or correlation of diffusion images with conventional MR images helps localize the findings more precisely. Combining morphological information from conventional MRI and functional information from DWI has the potential to improve the diagnostic value compared with each imaging alone, although data are lacking. DWI is also susceptible to a number of artifacts related to motion, and EPI-related artifacts. The respiratory-motion-related artifact can cause errors in ADC calculation of small lesions. To minimize respiratory-motion artifact, breath-hold or respiratory trigger technique can be employed. EPI is associated with ghosting artifacts, which are worst in the phase encoding direction, due to magnetization phase shifts. This can be managed by adjusting the receiver's bandwidth. DWI is also sensitive to susceptibility artifacts. Air in the gastrointestinal tract can cause susceptibility artifacts that obscure visualization of adjacent structures.

Conclusion

For solid pancreatic tumors, DWI can be useful for visual detection of pancreatic cancer and ADC measurements may help as a supplement to other imaging modalities to differentiate between pancreatic carcinoma and benign mass-forming pancreatitis. For cystic lesions of the pancreas, DWI may be useful to detect solid components within the cystic lesions. Differentiation between the different cystic lesions using DWI signal or ADC calculation alone is difficult if not impossible and correlation with other imaging modalities is mandatory.

References

1. Poston GJ, Williamson RC. Causes, diagnosis, and management of exocrine pancreatic cancer. *Compr Ther* 1990;**16** (1):36–42.

2. Bipat S, Phoa SS, van Delden OM, *et al.* Ultrasonography, computed tomography and magnetic resonance imaging for diagnosis and determining resectability of pancreatic adenocarcinoma: a meta-analysis. *J Comput Assist Tomogr* 2005; **29** (4):438–45.

3. Ho CL, Dehdashti F, Griffeth LK, *et al.* FDG-PET evaluation of indeterminate pancreatic masses. *J Comput Assist Tomogr* 1996;**20** (3):363–9.

4. Neff CC, Simeone JF, Wittenberg J, Mueller PR, Ferrucci JT Jr. Inflammatory pancreatic masses: problems in differentiating focal pancreatitis from carcinoma. *Radiology* 1984;**150** (1):35–8.

5. Kim T, Murakami T, Takamura M, *et al.* Pancreatic mass due to chronic pancreatitis: correlation of CT and MR imaging features with pathologic findings. *Am J Roentgenol* 2001;**177** (2):367–71.

6. Lyng H, Haraldseth O, Rofstad EK. Measurement of cell density and necrotic fraction in human melanoma xenografts by diffusion weighted magnetic resonance imaging. *Magn Reson Med* 2000;**43** (6):828–36.

7. Takahara T, Imai Y, Yamashita T, *et al.* Diffusion weighted whole body imaging with background body signal suppression (DWIBS): technical improvement using free breathing, STIR and high resolution 3D display. *Radiat Med* 2004;**22** (4):275–82.

8. Muller MF, Prasad P, Siewert B, *et al.* Abdominal diffusion mapping with use of a whole-body echo-planar system. *Radiology* 1994;**190** (2):475–8.

9. Taouli B, Vilgrain V, Dumont E, *et al.* Evaluation of liver diffusion isotropy and characterization of focal hepatic lesions with two single-shot echo-planar MR imaging sequences: prospective study in 66 patients. *Radiology* 2003;**226** (1):71–8.

10. Moteki T, Horikoshi H, Oya N, Aoki J, Endo K. Evaluation of hepatic lesions and hepatic parenchyma using diffusion-weighted reordered turboFLASH magnetic resonance images. *J Magn Reson Imag* 2002;**15** (5):564–72.

11. Moteki T, Horikoshi H. Evaluation of hepatic lesions and hepatic parenchyma using diffusion-weighted echo-planar MR with three values of gradient b-factor. *J Magn Reson Imag* 2006;**24** (3):637–45.

12. Sun XJ, Quan XY, Huang FH, Xu YK. Quantitative evaluation of diffusion-weighted magnetic resonance imaging of focal hepatic lesions. *World J Gastroenterol* 2005;**11** (41):6535–7.

13. Ichikawa T, Erturk SM, Motosugi U, *et al.* High *b*-value diffusion-weighted MRI in colorectal cancer. *Am J Roentgenol* 2006;**187** (1):181–4.

14. Ichikawa T, Erturk SM, Motosugi U, *et al.* High *b* value diffusion-weighted MRI for detecting pancreatic adenocarcinoma: preliminary results. *Am J Roentgenol* 2007;**188** (2):409–14.

15. Yoshikawa T, Kawamitsu H, Mitchell DG, *et al.* ADC measurement of abdominal organs and lesions using parallel imaging technique. *Am J Roentgenol* 2006; **187** (6):1521–30.

16. Taouli B, Martin AJ, Qayyum A, *et al.* Parallel imaging and diffusion tensor imaging for diffusion-weighted MRI of the liver: preliminary experience in healthy volunteers. *Am J Roentgenol* 2004;**183** (3):677–80.

17. Oner AY, Celik H, Oktar SO, Tali T. Single breath-hold diffusion-weighted MRI of the liver with parallel imaging: initial experience. *Clin Radiol* 2006;**61** (11):959–65.

18. Kandpal H, Sharma R, Madhusudhan KS, Kapoor KS. Respiratory-triggered versus breath-hold diffusion-weighted MRI of liver lesions: comparison of image quality and apparent diffusion coefficient values. *Am J Roentgenol* 2009;**192** (4):915–22.

19. Shinya S, Sasaki T, Nakagawa Y, *et al.* Acute pancreatitis successfully diagnosed by diffusion-weighted imaging: a case report. *World J Gastroenterol* 2008;**14** (35):5478–80.

20. Akisik MF, Aisen AM, Sandrasegaran K, *et al.* Assessment of chronic pancreatitis: utility of diffusion-weighted MR imaging with secretin enhancement. *Radiology* 2009;**250** (1):103–9.

21. Akisik MF, Sandrasegaran K, Jennings SG, *et al.* Diagnosis of chronic pancreatitis by using apparent diffusion coefficient measurements at 3.0-T MR following secretin stimulation. *Radiology* 2009; **252** (2):418–25.

22. Balci NC, Momtahen AJ, Akduman EI, *et al.* Diffusion-weighted MRI of the pancreas: correlation with secretin endoscopic pancreatic function test (ePFT). *Acad Radiol* 2008;**15** (10):1264–8.

23. Erturk SM, Ichikawa T, Motosugi U, Sou H, Araki T. Diffusion-weighted MR imaging in the evaluation of pancreatic exocrine function before and after secretin stimulation. *Am J Gastroenterol* 2006; **101** (1):133–6.

24. Kartalis N, Lindholm TL, Aspelin P, Permert J, Albiin N. Diffusion-weighted magnetic resonance imaging of pancreas tumours. *Eur Radiol* 2009;**19** (8): 1981–90.

25. Takeuchi M, Matsuzaki K, Kubo H, Nishitani H. High-*b*-value diffusion-weighted magnetic resonance imaging of pancreatic cancer and mass-forming chronic pancreatitis: preliminary results. *Acta Radiol* 2008;**49** (4):383–6.

26. Matsuki M, Inada Y, Nakai G, *et al.* Diffusion-weighed MR imaging of pancreatic carcinoma. *Abdom Imag* 2007;**32** (4):481–3.

27. Lammer J, Herlinger H, Zalaudek G, Hofler H. Pseudotumorous pancreatitis. *Gastrointest Radiol* 1985;**10** (1):59–67.

28. Muraoka N, Uematsu H, Kimura H, *et al.* Apparent diffusion coefficient in pancreatic cancer: characterization and histopathological correlations. *J Magn Reson Imag* 2008;**27** (6):1302–8.

29. Ichikawa T, Haradome H, Hachiya J, Nitatori T, Araki T. Diffusion-weighted MR imaging with single-shot echo-planar imaging in the upper abdomen:

preliminary clinical experience in 61 patients. *Abdom Imag* 1999;**24** (5):456–61.

30. Lee SS, Byun JH, Park BJ, *et al.* Quantitative analysis of diffusion-weighted magnetic resonance imaging of the pancreas: usefulness in characterizing solid pancreatic masses. *J Magn Reson Imag* 2008; **28** (4):928–36.

31. Fattahi R, Balci NC, Perman WH, *et al.* Pancreatic diffusion-weighted imaging (DWI): comparison between mass-forming focal pancreatitis (FP), pancreatic cancer (PC), and normal pancreas. *J Magn Reson Imag* 2009;**29** (2):350–6.

32. Moteki T, Sekine T. Echo planar MR imaging of the liver: comparison of images with and without motion probing gradients. *J Magn Reson Imag* 2004;**19** (1):82–90.

33. Parikh T, Drew SJ, Lee VS, *et al.* Focal liver lesion detection and characterization with diffusion-weighted MR imaging: comparison with standard breath-hold T2-weighted imaging. *Radiology* 2008;**246** (3):812–22.

34. Koh DM, Brown G, Riddell AM, *et al.* Detection of colorectal hepatic metastases using MnDPDP MR imaging and diffusion-weighted imaging (DWI) alone and in combination. *Eur Radiol* 2008; **18** (5):903–10.

35. Nasu K, Kuroki Y, Nawano S, *et al.* Hepatic metastases: diffusion-weighted sensitivity-encoding versus SPIO-enhanced MR imaging. *Radiology* 2006;**239** (1):122–30.

36. Bakir B, Salmaslioglu A, Poyanli A, Rozanes I, Acunas B. Diffusion weighted MR imaging of pancreatic islet cell tumors. *Eur J Radiol* 2009.

37. Yamashita Y, Namimoto T, Mitsuzaki K, *et al.* Mucin-producing tumor of the pancreas: diagnostic value of diffusion-weighted echo-planar MR imaging. *Radiology* 1998;**208** (3):605–9.

38. Inan N, Arslan A, Akansel G, Anik Y, Demirci A. Diffusion-weighted imaging in the differential diagnosis of cystic lesions of the pancreas. *Am J Roentgenol* 2008;**191** (4):1115–21.

39. Irie H, Honda H, Kuroiwa T, *et al.* Measurement of the apparent diffusion coefficient in intraductal mucin-producing tumor of the pancreas by diffusion-weighted echo-planar MR imaging. *Abdom Imag* 2002;**27** (1):82–7.

40. Niwa T, Ueno M, Ohkawa S, *et al.* Advanced pancreatic cancer: the use of the apparent diffusion coefficient to predict response to chemotherapy. *Br J Radiol* 2009;**82** (973):28–34.

Chapter 6

Diffusion-weighted MRI of the prostate

Sophie F. Riches and Nandita M. deSouza

Background

Epidemiology

Prostate cancer is the most frequently diagnosed carcinoma in men in the UK[1]. It occurs at an increasing rate with advancing age with most patients being over the age of 60 years at the time of diagnosis. The incidence of detected carcinoma of the prostate has increased dramatically due to new screening and biopsy techniques and varies dramatically with screening levels. In Western Europe, the age-standardized incidence rate is 61.6 per 100 000 compared with 119.9 in North America where screening is widespread; however, there is little variation in the mortality rates of 17.5 per 100 000 in Western Europe and 15.8 per 100 000 in North America[1]. There are also remarkable racial differences in incidence: in the USA the incidence rate is 40% lower in Asians and 50% higher in African Americans than in Whites, and the African American population also have the highest death rates from prostate cancer[1]. About 10% of cases are familial, with a significantly increased risk in men whose first-degree relatives have had the disease. Patients with a *BRACA2* mutation have a higher incidence of prostate cancer[1]. However, the vast majority of cases are sporadic.

The cause of prostatic carcinoma is unknown. Because of the distribution in incidence worldwide there is some suggestion but no proof yet that dietary fat may increase the risk of developing prostate adenocarcinoma by influencing levels of testosterone, which in turn affects the growth of the prostate. There is no evidence of a relationship between benign prostatic hyperplasia (BPH) and carcinoma.

Normal anatomy of the prostate

The adult prostate gland is a composite organ made up of several glandular and non-glandular components tightly fused within a common capsule. The prostate gland has four distinct glandular regions, two of which arise from different segments of the prostatic urethra: the peripheral, central, transitional, and anterior fibromuscular zones.

The peripheral zone comprises up to 70% of the normal prostate gland in young men. It forms the subcapsular portion of the posterior aspect of the prostate gland which surrounds the distal urethra. It is from this portion of the gland that more than 70% of prostatic cancers originate[2]. The central zone constitutes approximately 25% of the normal prostate gland and surrounds the ejaculatory ducts. Central zone tumors account for 25% of all prostate cancers. The transition zone is responsible for 5% of the prostate volume and is very rarely associated with carcinoma. It surrounds the proximal urethra and is the region of the prostate gland which grows throughout life leading to BPH. The anterior fibromuscular zone (or stroma) accounts for approximately 5% of the prostatic weight and is devoid of glandular components, and composed of muscle and fibrous tissue. This zonal anatomy is used to guide the classification of the zones visualized on T2-weighted imaging (T2-WI) MRI. On T2-WI a glandular peripheral zone is seen posteriorly and a heterogeneous signal intensity central gland is seen anteriorly which includes central and transitional zones (Fig. 6.1). The anterior fibromuscular zone is seen as a dense condensation of low T2 signal behind the high signal intensity retropubic fat pad.

Extra-Cranial Applications of Diffusion-Weighted MRI, ed. Bachir Taouli. Published by Cambridge University Press.
© Cambridge University Press 2011.

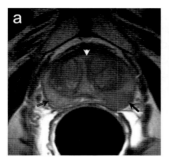
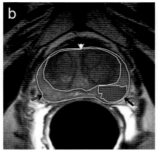
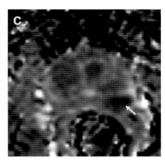

Figure 6.1 Patient with prostate cancer. Axial T2-weighted image (a) using an endorectal coil shows left-sided peripheral zone tumor (black arrow) in low signal intensity compared to the normal peripheral zone. The central gland (CG, arrowhead) is in mixed signal intensity. Regions of interest outlining the tumor, CG and non-malignant peripheral zone are shown on the same T2-weighted image (b). The tumor demonstrates restricted diffusion (black arrow) on the apparent diffusion coefficient (ADC) map (c) obtained with SS EPI sequence. [Reproduced with permission from deSouza et al. 2007[25].]

Histology of the prostate

The glandular architecture of the normal prostate consists of small, round acini amid loosely woven, randomly orientated stroma. The epithelium is arranged in glands around a central lumen with intervening stroma made up of smooth muscle and fibrous tissue. Microscopically, BPH can involve both glands and stroma, although the former is usually more prominent. The glands are well differentiated and still have some intervening stroma. In neoplasia, the glands of prostatic adenocarcinoma may still be recognizable as glands, but there is often little intervening stroma and the nuclei are hyperchromatic.

Histologically normal and tumor-containing tissues exhibit differences in microvascular and cellular content that result in differences in water movement within these tissues. Diffusion-weighted MRI (DW-MRI) exploits these differences to differentiate normal and cancer-containing tissues.

The need for imaging in prostate cancer

As with all cancers, once disease is suspected, it is essential to stage it prior to management decisions. At presentation, prostate cancer is broadly classified as localized, locally advanced, or metastatic. Locally advanced and metastatic disease are usually imaged with a combination of computerized tomography (CT) or conventional MRI of the pelvis and a bone scan. In these cases, disease within the prostate is delineated sufficiently well using standard T2-WI MRI sequences. It is in localized disease where there is an increasing range of management options and in treatment response assessment that information from new imaging techniques is being explored.

Treatment options for localized prostate cancer are many and varied, ranging from immediate radical surgery through to observation alone. On the one hand, radical prostatectomy has been shown in a good-quality randomized controlled trial to have an overall survival advantage compared with watchful waiting[3]. On the other hand, prostate cancer can often behave in an indolent fashion even without treatment, with no effect on either health or longevity. In such cases, radical treatment, with its risks of incontinence and impotence, could be worse than the "disease." So, the challenge of managing localized prostate cancer is to distinguish patients with clinically relevant cancers, who may benefit from radical treatment, from the remainder who do not need any intervention. There is a major unmet need for markers of prostate cancer behavior that could be used to inform the decision whether or not to undertake radical treatment.

The best current method of imaging prostate cancer is with endorectal T2-WI. Unfortunately the sensitivity of T2-WI alone varies from 60% to 82%, for disease detection within the gland with a specificity of around 55–70%[4,5]. Awareness of clinical data significantly improves reader detection of prostate cancer nodules with endorectal MRI, but there is no overall change in reader accuracy, because of an associated increase in false-positive findings[6]. MR spectroscopy (MRS) has also been used as an adjunct to imaging and improves accuracy of prostate cancer detection[7,8], but is time-consuming both for image acquisition and subsequent data processing and is not easy to implement in many centers. Although MRI is useful in disease staging[9], these functional MR indices to date have not been used for predicting disease outcome in prostate cancer.

An alternative to conventional T2-WI is to develop image contrast through "apparent diffusivity" (tissue water incoherent displacement over distances of 1–20 μm). DW-MRI has been used in both clinical and research settings for detecting cerebral as well as cancer-related pathologies. In the first instance, in order to understand the basis of diffusion-weighted contrast within the prostate, a clear knowledge of the macroscopic and microscopic anatomy of the prostate is essential. Images acquired with multiple b-values (a parameter combining gradient strength and duration) allow derivation of apparent diffusion coefficient (ADC) maps quantifying the degree of restriction of water diffusion. Figure 6.1 shows a conventional T2-weighted image of the prostate and the corresponding ADC map showing the malignant nodule as a low signal region of restricted diffusion.

Diffusion-weighted contrast methodology

Optimizing the signal-to-noise ratio

Endorectal vs. non-endorectal techniques

In MR examinations of the prostate, it is essential to maximize the signal-to-noise ratio (SNR) of diffusion-weighted data. One option is to use rigid or balloon coils placed endorectally in close proximity to the prostate which offer improved SNR over external coils[10], and will allow more accurate ADC calculations from fast echo-planar imaging (EPI) sequences. For T2-WI, early reports of artifacts and inferior visualization of the anterior portion of the prostate[11] have been overcome and detection is further improved with integrated endorectal and phased-array pelvic imaging (sensitivity: 78–79%, specificity: 56–58%, accuracy: 96%)[12]. However, compared with rigid coils[10], balloon coils filled with air tend to increase the distortion seen with EPI-based diffusion sequences due to the air/tissue boundary close to the prostate. Filling the balloon coil with substances of similar susceptibility to tissue can reduce these effects[13,14]; perfluorocarbon is more successful for diffusion imaging than barium as the bulk motion of the liquid within the coil is not visible due to the absence of hydrogen atoms. Endorectal coils may compress the posterior of the prostate gland, although different coil designs offer differing amounts of compression. Successful registration of endorectal diffusion images to histological whole-mount slides shows

regions of restricted diffusion can still be seen in areas of histologically confirmed tumor that are compressed by the coil[15]. Rigid coils compress the gland less and may be preferable if perfusion data are also being acquired. Local experience has found it to be advantageous to place a sandbag on the handle of the endorectal coil to weight it and reduce motion vibrations during the EPI sequence.

Alternatively, it is possible to acquire good-quality data using only phased-array coils by acquiring a greater number of signal averages or by using higher field strength (see next section). This offers the advantage of less patient preparation time and greater patient comfort, and allows images to be acquired that do not compress the prostate at all.

With either choice of coil set-up, superior images free from motion blurring require an injection of glucagon to freeze bowel motion. At our institution we routinely administer 20 mg of hyoscine-N-butylbromide (Boehringer Ingelheim Ltd, Bracknell, UK) intramuscularly to all patients immediately prior to scanning, which allows acquisition of motion-free images for around 30 min. Some centers also administer enemas to clear the bowel and rectum, although we have never found this advantageous.

Choice of field strength

As at 1.5 T, imaging the prostate at 3 T can be done using a pelvic array or an endorectal technique. At 3 T, pelvic array anatomic imaging offers similar image quality and diagnostic accuracy to endorectal imaging at 1.5 T[16,17]. Heijmink et al.[18] compared endorectal and pelvic array T2-WI at 3 T and found that although endorectal coil imaging gave more artifacts than pelvic array imaging, it improved image quality and increased detection sensitivity while maintaining specificity. As diffusion imaging is an inherently low SNR technique, the increased signal using an endorectal coil at 3 T allows an increase in spatial resolution or a decrease in scan time. On the other hand, in pelvic array DW-MRI at 3 T, parallel imaging techniques can be used to reduce the scan time whilst maintaining the SNR level obtainable at 1.5 T thus reducing the artifacts associated with motion. Figure 6.2 shows a T2-weighted image and an ADC map acquired at 3 T showing high levels of structure in the ADC map due to the increased SNR.

Severe magnetic susceptibility artifacts and distortion are also reported in the diffusion images from patients with dilated rectums when using pelvic array

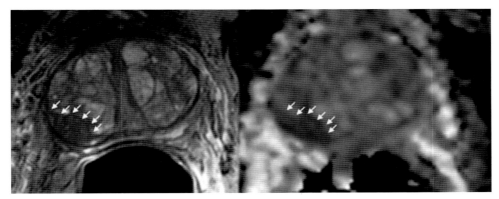

Figure 6.2 65-year-old man with prostate cancer (PSA 19.8 ng/ml, Gleason score 3 + 3). Axial T2-weighted image (left) and ADC map (right) obtained with a 3-T system and endorectal coil show tumor in the peripheral zone of right midgland (arrows). The increased SNR at 3 T should allow better tumor delineation and possibly better detection compared to 1.5 T.

coils alone at 3 T[19]. This effect is compounded by air-filled coils. For endorectal imaging, the increased chemical shift and susceptibility artifacts at higher field strengths therefore increase the necessity to use filled or rigid coils for DW-MRI; the latter offers the opportunity to further exploit endorectal array designs and parallel imaging techniques. An additional refocusing pulse has also been successfully used to reduce the increased distortion artifacts[20] from the use of an EPI sequence at 3 T.

Despite the superior morphologic visualization of the prostate in ADC maps reported at 3 T[19], ADC values obtained at 3 T for normal peripheral zone and malignant tissue[20] are similar to those acquired at 1.5 T. However, they have been shown to be repeatable only to within 15% in the central gland and 32% in the peripheral zone for both inter- and intra-session studies[21]. Regardless of this increased inter-subject variation in the data composed with 1.5 T, diagnostic accuracies are around 0.85 (sensitivity 82%, specificity 78%) using a cut-off ADC of 1.5×10^{-3} mm^2/s at 3 T[22] for tumor.

Technical considerations in DW-MRI of the prostate

Choice of sequence

As diffusion imaging is inherently sensitive to motion, large-scale bulk motion must be minimized to avoid masking the small-scale movement of water associated with diffusion gradients. Within the pelvis, the prostate exhibits slow movement due to bladder and rectal filling as well as faster periodic motion associated with peristalsis and respiration. Single-shot

EPI, which allows a whole slice to be imaged in a time-frame of minimal respiratory motion, has therefore been the most commonly used sequence in prostate diffusion imaging. However, distortion due to local field inhomogeneities, local fat causing chemical shift artifacts, and susceptibility artifacts from both the bone/tissue interfaces and air in balloon endorectal coils can lead to significant artifacts. This has prompted exploration of mean single-shot fast spin echo (FSE) sequences. However, FSE sequences result in reduced SNR due to sensitivity of the sequence to the phase incoherence caused by bulk motion during the preparation phase of the sequence[23]. Also, in comparison to EPI-based ADC maps which show the internal structure of the prostate clearly in a heavily distorted image, the FSE-based ADC maps show a marked reduction in geometrical distortions but exhibit general blurring and result in higher uncertainty in numerical ADC values. Figure 6.3 compares ADC maps reconstructed from DW-MRI data acquired with a single-shot FSE sequence and a single-shot EPI sequence. Whilst both sequences showed statistical differences between normal peripheral zone and central gland and prostate cancer, the EPI sequence gave higher ADC values than the FSE sequence (2.0 ± 0.2 vs. $1.6 \pm 0.3 \times 10^{-3}$ mm^2/s ($p < 0.001$) in peripheral zone, 1.5 ± 0.1 vs. $1.4 \pm 0.2 \times 10^{-3}$ mm^2/s in central gland, and 1.2 ± 0.3 vs. $1.0 \pm 0.2 \times 10^{-3}$ mm^2/s in cancer ($p < 0.01$)[23].

With the effectively infinite repetition time (TR) of an EPI sequence, the diffusion signal attenuation is compounded by T2 relaxation of the tissue, and with normal prostate tissue T2 values of ~100 ms, T2 "shine-through" is evident on diffusion weighted

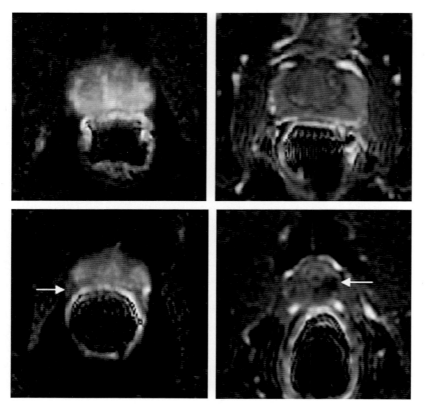

Figure 6.3 Axial ADC maps reconstructed from the DW-MRI data acquired from four different subjects using endorectal coil. Left column shows ADC maps reconstructed from the data acquired with the single-shot DW-FSE sequence and the right column from the data acquired with the single-shot DW-EPI sequence. Top row shows data acquired from subjects with negative biopsy results, whereas the bottom row shows data acquired from the subjects with biopsy-proven cancer. The hypointense areas on the ADC maps (arrows) correspond to the location of the tumors confirmed by the biopsy and/or prostatectomy results. [Reproduced with permission from Kozlowski et al. 2008[23].]

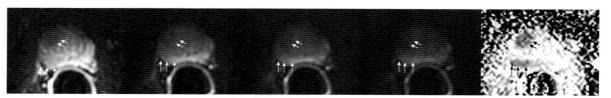

Figure 6.4 64-year-old man with prostate cancer: Single-shot EPI axial diffusion-weighted images of the prostate using b-values of 0, 300, 500, and 800 s/mm² (from left to right), with corresponding ADC map on the far right. Two tumors (anterior in central gland and right posterior peripheral zone, arrows) show restricted diffusion on the ADC map, and are more easily detected than on the native diffusion images.

images (acquired with the shortest possible echo time [TE], usually 60–100 ms). This can reduce the contrast between normal and malignant prostate tissue, making maps of the ADC more useful than DW-MRI images in identifying areas of restricted diffusion. Figure 6.4 shows regions of restricted diffusion on an ADC map clearer than correspondingly persistently bright areas on the DW-MRI images.

A third sequence which has been successfully used in the prostate is line-scan diffusion imaging (LSDI)[24], which uses serial snapshot acquisitions of tissue columns with little distortion or motion artifacts. However the line-scan technique has low SNR due to the reduction in tissue volume contributing to the signal. It also takes longer to acquire than EPI and FSE sequences.

Selection of b-values

Apparent diffusion coefficients (ADCs) are derived from the slope of signal intensity vs. b-value and provide quantitative information on the degree of restriction of water diffusion within tissues.

ADC values of malignant prostate have been shown to be significantly lower than in non-malignant peripheral zone[25–30]. Depending on the *b*-values used, the ADC can either represent a fast diffusion component including contribution from microcapillary perfusion or a slow component over a shorter diffusion path length corresponding to Brownian diffusion within the extracellular space. ADCs therefore are directly associated with coherent microvessel density and cellularity[31].

Although accurate derivation of the ADC is best performed by curve-fitting of the signal decay with multiple *b*-value samples, the need to reduce the time cost of diffusion imaging means that often only two *b*-values are employed to estimate the ADC, i.e., acquiring data with no diffusion gradient and at a single *b*-value. In order to minimize the error associated with this two-point estimation of the exponential signal loss, the *b*-value of the diffusion-weighted image must be optimized to account for the range of expected diffusion coefficients, the SNR of the images, and the T2 values of the tissues[32]. Applying *b*-value optimization schemes previously employed in the brain suggests an optimal difference in *b*-values of around $1.28/ADC$[32], with the ratio of the number of measurements using these two values of 1 : 3. Using reported ADC values in the prostate indicates that the second *b*-value should be between ~550 and 1000 s/mm^2. If optimal *b*-values are used, it has been shown that minimum variance in ADC estimates from multiple *b*-values can occur when using just two *b*-values in the calculation[33].

Studies comparing two-point estimation of prostate tissue ADC with $b = 0$, 1000 s/mm^2 and $b = 0$, 2000 s/mm^2 showed that ADC values decrease by >20% for normal tissue and >40% for malignant tissues when higher *b*-values are used, increasing the overlap in the ADC values of normal and malignant tissues[34]. However, for a constant number of signal averages, the ~20% reduction of SNR in prostate tissues at the higher *b*-values[34] exposes the ADC to errors due to insufficient SNR for accurate data fitting, and can lead to underestimation of the ADC[35].

If multiple *b*-value images are acquired with a single receive coil, it has been shown that a SNR greater than 7 (corrected for magnitude data) allows the variance of ADCs derived using the least-squares curve-fitting algorithm to be comparable to the more robust maximum likelihood derived values[36]. Transferring this value to routinely acquired clinical data is non-trivial, however, as the exact determination of comparable SNR is notoriously difficult with the

Table 6.1 Suggested acquisition parameters for 1.5-T endorectal DWI of the prostate as used in our institution

Sequence	Single-shot EPI
Acquisition plane	Axial
Phase encoding direction	Left–right
TR	4500
TE	Shortest (~66 ms)
Slice thickness	3 mm
b-values	0, 100, 300, 500, 800
Field of view	192 × 192
Matrix size	128 × 128 (reconstructed to 256 × 256)
Number of averages	5 at all *b* values
Acquisition time	~4 min 36 s

distribution of noise in phased-array images. All *b*-value images and signal decay curves should be reviewed carefully to assess the SNR in the high *b*-value images, especially in anterior regions of the prostate furthest from the endorectal coil when this coil is used alone. In order to overcome the decreased SNR at increased *b*-values, some clinical scanners allow increased signal averages at higher *b*-value images, although the variable SNR associated with different *b*-values in the resulting signal decay curve must still be accounted for by weighting the values in any curve-fitting algorithm.

Table 6.1 gives example parameters in use at our institution which give high SNR images at all *b*-values.

Deriving ADC maps
Monoexponential and biexponential fitting of data

The accuracy of two-point sampling schemes depends on the assumption that the signal decays monoexponentially with increasing *b*-values. However, it is proposed that at very low *b*-values the motion detected is dominated by the fast bulk motion associated with perfusion in the tissues. In order to remove the effect of the perfusion from the diffusion measurements, often three or more *b*-values are employed and the signal from the $b = 0$ s/mm^2 image is not used in the two-point calculation of the monoexponential ADC[37]. Data acquired with 11 *b*-values ranging from 0 to 800 s/mm^2 showed that removal of *b*-values less than 100 s/mm^2 from the monoexponential calculation resulted in an ADC equal to that predicted by a biexponential model accounting for both the

Table 6.2 Published ADC ($\times 10^{-3}$ mm^2/s) values for normal peripheral zone, normal central gland, and prostate cancer from selected studies

	b-values (s/mm^2)	Peripheral zone	Central gland	Prostate cancer
Reinsberg et al. 2007[29]	0, 300, 500, 800	1.51 ± 0.27	1.31 ± 0.20	1.03 ± 0.18
Sato et al. 2005[30]	0, 300, 600	1.68 ± 0.40		1.11 ± 0.41
Issa et al. 2002[28]	64, 144, 257, 401, 578, 786	1.82 ± 0.53	1.62 ± 0.41	1.38 ± 0.52
Hosseinzadeh et al. 2004[27]	0, 1000	1.61 ± 0.26		1.27 ± 0.37
Gibbs et al. 2001[26]	0–720 (8 values)	2.49 ± 1.30		2.73 ± 0.70
deSouza et al. 2007[25]	0, 300, 500, 800	1.71 ± 0.16	1.46 ± 0.14	1.30 ± 0.30
Gibbs et al. 2006 (3 T)[22]	0, 700	1.86 ± 0.47		1.33 ± 0.32
Van As et al. 2008[37]	0, 300, 500, 800	1.7 ± 0.29	1.5 ± 0.29	1.3 ± 0.20

perfusion and diffusion components[38]. As scan time is increased with each *b*-value utilized then it is advantageous to use the minimum number of *b*-values to yield the maximum information, and acquisition of data with *b*-values at 0, 100, and 800 s/mm^2 therefore allows separation of coefficients associated with perfusion and diffusion using simple monoexponential fitting over the two separate *b*-value ranges. Studies have also looked at biexponential intravoxel incoherent motion[39] modeling of prostate diffusion over an extended *b*-value range up to 3000 s/mm$^{2[24]}$. After removal of the perfusion component, these studies postulate there are two further distinct diffusion coefficients, one fast and one slow. The possible cause of the two components is not understood; in brain imaging it has been suggested that they may reflect intra- and extracellular water but the inferred length scales of the two compartments are not physiologically feasible. However, care must be taken to ensure that insufficient SNR at high *b*-values does not cause monoexponential signal decay to appear biexponential due to the presence of irregularly distributed noise in magnitude data[40].

Fractional anisotropy

Reports investigating anisotropy within the prostate have shown that diffusion in prostate tissue is anisotropic and consistent with the tissue architecture of the prostate fiber orientations namely predominantly in a superior–inferior direction for both the peripheral zone and central gland[41]. Increased fractional anisotropy has also been reported in regions of prostate cancer compared with non-cancer[42]. Figure 6.5 shows a tractography image of the prostate obtained with diffusion tensor imaging (DTI). However,

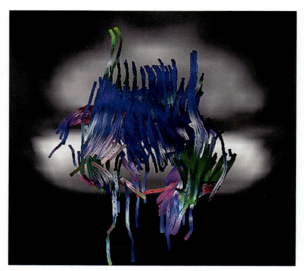

Figure 6.5 Tractography image of the prostate obtained with diffusion tensor imaging (DTI) using $b = 0$, 700 s/mm^2 and 32 directions. Blue indicates superior–inferior orientation of fiber structure within the gland; darker colors indicate increasing anisotropy. [Reproduced with permission from Gürses et al. 2008[41].]

simulation of various noise levels and investigation of fractional anisotropy vs. noise have shown a continuous increase in fractional anisotropy with decreasing SNR. Thus observed fractional anisotropy may well be due to the effects of system noise[43].

Utility of prostate DW-MRI in the clinic

Histological correlates

Studies defining tumors using T2-WI signal intensity and validating results against sextant biopsy or

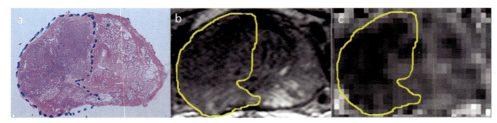

Figure 6.6 Patient with prostate cancer. (a) Hematoxylin-and-eosin stained histology section from a whole-mount prostatectomy specimen showing tumor outline (in blue). Axial T2-weighted image (b); this tumor outline has been warped to fit the T2-weighted image and then overlaid onto the ADC map (c). The tumor has lower ADC compared to the normal left peripheral zone.

step-section histology have reported ADC values of malignant prostate significantly lower than in non-malignant peripheral zone[25–30] (Table 6.2). Differences between normal peripheral zone and normal central gland tissue have been more variable[25,28,29] (Table 6.2). These studies automatically bias differences in ADC values of tumors away from normal tissue values by using T2-WI contrast or diffusion-weighted information to define the region of abnormality.

Determination of ADC values from histologically defined tumor and normal regions transposed onto the ADC maps by registering them with step-section histology revealed a smaller difference between tumor and non-tumor ADC values (1.45 ± 1.7 vs. $1.49 \pm 0.92 \times 10^{-3}$ mm^2/s) compared with previous studies[15]. Figure 6.6 shows a matching hematoxylin-and-eosin stained histology slide, T2-weighted image, and ADC map with the tumor region registered onto the ADC map for determination of histologically defined tumor and non-tumor ADC values. Differences between tumor and non-tumor ADCs were more marked if tumors of less than 1 cm^2 cross-section were excluded (1.38 ± 1.7 vs. $1.49 \pm 0.92 \times 10^{-3}$ mm^2/s) suggesting partial volume effects in the derivation of these values. Alternatively an inherent difference in diffusion in smaller tumors is possible.

Value in tumor detection

On conventional T2-WI, prostate cancer is mainly recognized as a focal low signal-intensity lesion within the peripheral zone (Fig 6.6). However, such change also may arise as a result of inflammatory process within the gland[44]. Furthermore, malignant lesions isointense with peripheral zone may not be distinguished as tumor. DW-MRI improves identification of tumor in these cases because of differences between tissue types[25,27,45]. The highly cellular regions encountered in prostate cancer result in restricted diffusion within reduced intracellular and interstitial spaces, compared with glandular normal prostate, and produces a substantial differential in ADC. With an experienced observer, one recent study showed that a combined T2-WI + DW-MRI approach over T2-WI alone improved sensitivity of prostate cancer detection from 46.5% to 71% on inclusion of the ADC maps in the evaluation[46]. Another study of 60 patients showed that the addition of DW-MRI to conventional T2-WI significantly improved tumor detectability[45]. This is reinforced by pre-clinical studies where improved prostate tumor detection in transgenic mice has been shown at 4.7 T using DW-MRI compared with T2 mapping[47]. The definitive role of DW-MRI in the detection of prostate cancer, however, remains to be established.

In the diagnosis of prostate cancer, subjective evaluation of ADC maps alongside corresponding T2-WI provides improved diagnostic performance[46]. ADC values derived from DW-MR images also can be used to separate nodules based on their cellularity. The ADC values of malignant prostate nodules appear significantly lower than in non-malignant prostate nodules[25,30]. This has particular implications for identifying the 30% of cancers that arise within the central gland. Malignant nodules are typically more cellular than the nodules of BPH, although there is significant heterogeneity in the latter where glandular BPH nodules, mixed BPH nodules, and stromal BPH nodules with different cellularity all coexist. It is this heterogeneity of DW-MRI within well-defined nodules in the central gland that identifies them as benign. Malignant central gland nodules are often more irregular and homogeneously low in signal intensity with mass effect. More recent data have shown anisotropy within BPH nodules, but not in tumor[48], indicating that eigenvalues may be a way of separating benign from malignant nodules in the central gland.

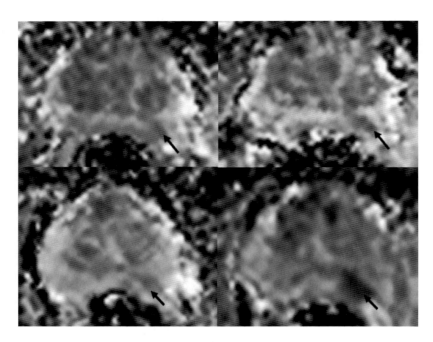

Figure 6.7 Top row: non-progressor to radical treatment showing tumor in the left midgland (arrow) at baseline (left) and after 24 months (right). No change in appearance between the two time-points is seen. Bottom row: progressor to radical treatment showing tumor in the left midgland (arrow) at baseline (left) and after 35 months (right). A change in appearance of the tumor on the ADC maps between the two time-points is evident. (See text for further details.)

Value as a prognostic biomarker

Active surveillance is an approach to the management of localized prostate cancer that aims to avoid over treatment of men with indolent cancers, while still providing treatment with radical intent within a window of curability for those who need it. Active surveillance programs rely on prostate-specific antigen (PSA) kinetics and repeat biopsies to risk stratify patients and guide decisions on who needs treatment and when. Risk stratification relies to an extent on information obtained from needle biopsy which is subject to potential sampling error.

DW-MRI is of major interest as a prognostic biomarker. It measures water movements within tissues which are substantially affected by cellular and structural changes (such as cell density, vascularity, viscosity of extracellular fluid, membrane permeability between intra- and extracellular compartments, active transport and flow, and directionality of tissue/cellular structures that impede water mobility) and thus offers potential for differentiating indolent from aggressive prostate cancers. A preliminary study on two cohorts of patients, one at low risk of disease progression and the other at high risk of disease progression, confirmed that ADC differences exist between low- and high-risk lesions. Figure 6.7 shows no change in tumor ADC between baseline and at 24 months follow-up in a patient who did not

progress to radical treatment, compared with a change in ADC between the two time-points in a patient who did progress to radical treatment[49]. Although ADC values are known to correlate with tissue structure this study used the National Comprehensive Cancer Network criteria to define risk groups rather than Gleason score in order to reduce the effects of biopsy sampling variability and reflect the fact that ADC values were averaged over the whole tumor region of interest (ROI).

The calculation of diffusion components weighted to low and high b-values can also be exploited when considering ADC as a prognostic biomarker. The slow diffusion component (associated with cell density[50]) shows differences between low- and high-risk groups may be due to highly cellular regions in high-risk patients. However, surprisingly, the fast diffusion component traditionally linked with capillary microcirculation is also diminished in high-risk patients[49]. It is possible that microcapillary perfusion is compromised in high-risk patients because of tumor hypoxia. This is supported by ex vivo findings of increased hypoxia in more aggressive tumor types[51].

Value in response assessment
Hormonotherapy

It is known that androgen ablation therapy shrinks the prostate and reduces the metabolite content. In a study of

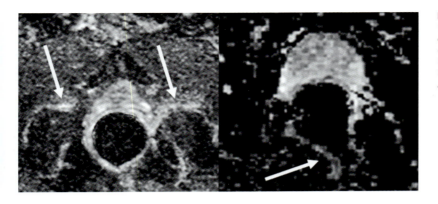

Figure 6.8 Axial ADC maps showing Nyquist ghosting (left) and diffusion gradient dependent geometric distortions (right) in the phase-encoding directions. Keeping the phase encoding direction left-to-right will prevent the artifacts from appearing within the prostate.

20 patients, the ADC of malignant tissue increased significantly after 3 months of androgen ablation therapy, whilst the ADC of central gland and peripheral zone ADC both reduced[52]. This indicates that there is a different effect of androgen deprivation on the tumor compared with the rest of the gland. The observed absolute changes in ADC of central gland and peripheral zone are likely to be caused by gross changes[53], which result in reduction of luminal space in normal tissue with hormone therapy[54]. The role of ADC in detecting disease recurrence in these treated glands remains to be evaluated.

Radiotherapy

There are limited reports of DW-MRI following radiation therapy (RT) in prostate cancer. A recent pilot study in nine patients showed that ADC values of prostate cancer showed a statistically significant increase after carbon-ion RT[55]. This was assumed to be due to a decrease in the size and number of neoplastic glands[56]. On the other hand, the ADC values of non-cancerous central gland and peripheral zone decreased after RT, but the changes were not significant. After radiotherapy, damage to vascular endothelial cells results in ischemia and leads to acinar distortion and atrophy. In addition, stromal fibrosis with granulation tissue formation arises in other areas of the prostate[56]. These structural changes are likely to account for the reduction in ADC in the non-cancerous gland. Inflammatory swelling of cells in association with radiotherapy causing a decrease in extracellular space may also be a contributory factor. In this pilot study, fractional anisotropy of prostate cancer and non-cancerous central gland and peripheral zone were low (range, 0.148–0.248), and showed no significant differences between before and after RT.

Minimally invasive therapy

There are very few data on the use of DW-MRI to monitor newer minimally invasive surgical techniques. Cryoablation and high-intensity focused ultrasound are increasingly popular in treating prostatic lesions. A recent study on canine prostate showed immediate reduction in ADC following cryoablation, which increased as the tissue recovered and regenerated[57] but studies establishing the relationship of ADC to subsequent tissue viability are lacking. High-intensity focused ultrasound provides very accurate destruction of tissue and under MR guidance provides opportunities for MR thermometry using T1-WI sequences. In this scenario, studies have largely been pre-clinical.

Artifacts and limitations

Most artifacts seen in prostate diffusion imaging are due to the use of the EPI sequence and are comparable to diffusion artifacts in other areas of the body such as the brain. EPI sequences will demonstrate Nyquist ghosting with the ghost image displaced by half the field of view (Figure 6.8). The bandwidth in the phase encoding direction of an EPI sequence is small and translates to a shift in fat/water signal of around 8 pixels at 1.5 T. This can be problematic because of periprostatic fat within the field of view.

The sensitivity of EPI sequences to phase incoherence means that eddy currents generated by the diffusion gradient will result in spatial encoding errors, causing diffusion gradient dependent geometric distortions in the phase-encode directions (Figure 6.8). This distortion can increase at higher b-values, and assessment of the distortion of the prostate at progressive b-values is important before calculating pixel-

81

by-pixel ADC values. To stop phase-encoding wrap in small field of view images, saturation bands can successfully be applied on either side of the field of view, reducing the need for oversampling and allowing the TE to be kept as short as possible.

Within the pelvis, the prostate exhibits periodic motion associated with peristalsis and respiration; peristalsis can be reduced with an intramuscular administration of hyoscine butyl bromide or glucagon. As respiratory motion occurs in the anterior–posterior direction, the phase-encoding direction should be right–left. Multishot EPI can be advantageous as it divides the acquisition into two, four, or eight segments which reduces the chemical shift and susceptibility artifacts due to increased bandwidth in the phase-encoding direction at the expense of increased scan time.

In a clinical setting, the overlap between ADC values of benign nodules within the central gland and tumor limits detection of central gland tumor. This excludes detection of ~30% of lesions which is a significant limitation of the technique.

Future directions

In order to improve the accuracy of diagnosis, staging, and prognosis, the future of prostate MRI is looking to multiparametric approaches. Several studies have used combinations of functional techniques to improve diagnostic accuracy. It has been suggested that a combination of ADC and MRS may have greater accuracy than sextant biopsy[58], and the combination has been found to be more accurate than either technique alone[29]. In one study histologically identified tumor regions larger than 1 cm^3 were mapped onto metabolite ratio and ADC maps and the investigators found significant increases in metabolite ratios and a decrease in ADC in tumor[59].

We have found a diagnostic advantage to using pairs of functional parameters (ADC, choline/citrate ratio, initial area under the gadolinium curve [IAUGC]) to improve the accuracy of prostate cancer detection[15]. Whilst no single functional parameter had a significantly greater area under the receiver operator curve for determining sensitivity and specificity, pairs of parameters did show increased diagnostic power. The combination of ADC and IAUGC improved detection over either parameter alone, whilst the inclusion of the choline/citrate ratio with either ADC or IAUGC improved detection over the

ADC and IAUGC but not the choline/citrate ratio alone. No further improvement in detection accuracy was found by combining all three functional parameters. The significantly increased power in separating tumor from non-tumor tissue with two functional techniques together suggests that information derived from the techniques is complementary. Because no pair of parameters gave a particular advantage, the choice of techniques can be based on time and cost restraints. As the easiest technique to implement and process is DW-MRI, it is suggested DW-MRI should be used in combination with either DCE-MRI or MRS, depending on the expertise of the imaging centre. As DCE-MRI has greater spatial resolution, combined DW-MRI and DCE-MRI may have greater potential for identifying smaller tumors in patients with biopsy results indicative of small tumors. Alternatively, patients with biopsy results suggesting the presence of tumor in the central gland region would benefit from the improved discrimination of MRS.

Summary and conclusions

DW-MRI of the prostate is proving of enormous interest. Its ease of implementation, relatively short scan times and readily analyzable datasets have resulted in its widespread use. However, detailed attention to methodology of data acquisition and analysis is crucial. Optimizing SNR by use of endorectal coils and higher field strengths, while reducing sequence artifacts is of paramount importance in achieving useful results. ADC maps have shown potential in detecting tumor when used in conjunction with T2 weighted images, although lesions in the central gland remain difficult to diagnose because of overlap of tumor ADC values with values in benign hyperplastic nodules.

Refinement of techniques such as measurement of fractional anisotropy may help in this regard. The value of ADC as a staging tool remains to be proven in large multicenter trials. It is likely that its performance in detecting seminal vesicle invasion in particular will improve staging accuracy. ADC values are also proving of interest as prognostic biomarkers. There is a crucial need to be able to differentiate those cancers that are likely to progress from those that will not in men managed on active surveillance programs. Development of threshold values in standardized protocols to differentiate aggressive disease is required. In these patients combination with other parameters such as tumor volume, contrast enhancement, and PSA velocity may be of benefit.

The utility of DW-MRI in response assessment, particularly to newer minimally invasive modalities, has not been proven, but given its value in other tumor sites, it is an area that demands further investigation. Unfortunately data are lacking on post-treatment values of ADC of the prostate so that its role in identifying recurrent disease remains to be established.

Acknowledgments

CRUK and EPSRC Cancer Imaging Centre in association with the MRC and Department of Health (England) Grant C1060/A10334.

NHS funding to the NIHR Biomedical Research Centre.

Sophie Riches is funded by a Personal Award Scheme Researcher Developer Award from the National Institute for Health Research.

References

1. CancerResearchUK. http://info.cancerresearchuk.org/cancerstats October 2009.

2. Reissigl A, Pointner J, Strasser H, *et al.* Frequency and clinical significance of transition zone cancer in prostate cancer screening. *Prostate* 1997;**30** (2):130–5.

3. Bill-Axelson A, Holmberg L, Ruutu M, *et al.* Radical prostatectomy versus watchful waiting in early prostate cancer. *N Engl J Med* 2005;**352** (19):1977–84.

4. Graser A, Heuck A, Sommer B, *et al.* Per-sextant localization and staging of prostate cancer: correlation of imaging findings with whole-mount step section histopathology. *Am J Roentgenol* 2007;**188** (1)84–90.

5. Kirkham AP, Emberton M, Allen C. How good is MRI at detecting and characterising cancer within the prostate? *Eur Urol* 2006;**50** (6)1163–74; discussion 1175.

6. Dhingsa R, Qayyum A, Coakley FV, *et al.* Prostate cancer localization with endorectal MR imaging and MR spectroscopic imaging: effect of clinical data on reader accuracy. *Radiology* 2004;**230** (1):215–20.

7. Futterer JJ, Scheenen TW, Heijmink SW, *et al.* Standardized threshold approach using three-dimensional proton magnetic resonance spectroscopic imaging in prostate cancer localization of the entire prostate. *Investig Radiol* 2007;**42** (2):116–22.

8. Wang L, Hricak H, Kattan MW, *et al.* Prediction of organ-confined prostate cancer: incremental value of MR imaging and MR spectroscopic imaging to staging nomograms. *Radiology* 2006;**238** (2):597–603.

9. Jackson AS, Parker CC, Norman AR, *et al.* Tumour staging using magnetic resonance imaging in clinically localised prostate cancer: relationship to biochemical outcome after neo-adjuvant androgen deprivation and radical radiotherapy. *Clin Oncol (R Coll Radiol)* 2005;**17** (3):167–71.

10. deSouza NM, Gilderdale DJ, Puni R, *et al.* A solid reusable endorectal receiver coil for magnetic resonance imaging of the prostate: design, use, and comparison with an inflatable endorectal coil. *J Magn Reson Imag* 1996;**6** (5):801–4.

11. Husband JE, Padhani AR, MacVicar AD, *et al.* Magnetic resonance imaging of prostate cancer: comparison of image quality using endorectal and pelvic phased array coils. *Clin Radiol* 1998;**53** (9): 673–81.

12. Futterer JJ, Engelbrecht MR, Jager GJ, *et al.* Prostate cancer: comparison of local staging accuracy of pelvic phased-array coil alone versus integrated endorectal-pelvic phased-array coils. Local staging accuracy of prostate cancer using endorectal coil MR imaging. *Eur Radiol* 2007;**17** (4):1055–65.

13. Rosen Y, Bloch BN, Lenkinski RE, *et al.* 3 T MR of the prostate: reducing susceptibility gradients by inflating the endorectal coil with a barium sulfate suspension. *Magn Reson Med* 2007;**57** (5):898–904.

14. Choi H, Ma J. Use of perfluorocarbon compound in the endorectal coil to improve MR spectroscopy of the prostate. *Am J Roentgenol* 2008;**190** (4):1055–9.

15. Riches SF, Payne GS, Morgan V, *et al.* MRI in the detection of prostate cancer: combined apparent diffusion coefficient, metabolite ratio, and vascular parameters. *Am J Roentgenol* 2009;**193** (6):1583–91.

16. Park BK, Kim B, Kim CK, *et al.* Comparison of phased-array 3.0-T and endorectal 1.5-T magnetic resonance imaging in the evaluation of local staging accuracy for prostate cancer. *J Comput Assist Tomogr* 2007;**31** (4):534–8.

17. Torricelli P, Cinquantini F, Ligabue G, *et al.* Comparative evaluation between external phased array coil at 3 T and endorectal coil at 1.5 T: preliminary results. *J Comput Assist Tomogr* 2006;**30** (3):355–61.

18. Heijmink SW, Futterer JJ, Hambrock T, *et al.* Prostate cancer: body-array versus endorectal coil MR imaging at 3 T: comparison of image quality, localization, and staging performance. *Radiology* 2007;**244** (1):184–95.

19. Miao H, Fukatsu H, Ishigaki T. Prostate cancer detection with 3-T MRI: comparison of diffusion-weighted and T2-weighted imaging. *Eur J Radiol* 2007;**61** (2):297–302.

20. Pickles MD, Gibbs P, Sreenivas M, *et al.* Diffusion-weighted imaging of normal and malignant prostate tissue at 3.0T. *J Magn Reson Imag* 2006;**23** (2):130–4.

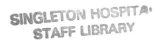

21. Gibbs P, Pickles MD, Turnbull LW. Repeatability of echo-planar-based diffusion measurements of the human prostate at 3 T. *Magn Reson Imag* 2007.

22. Gibbs P, Pickles MD, Turnbull LW. Diffusion imaging of the prostate at 3.0 tesla. *Investig Radiol* 2006;**41** (2): 185–8.

23. Kozlowski P, Chang SD, Goldenberg SL. Diffusion-weighted MRI in prostate cancer: comparison between single-shot fast spin echo and echo planar imaging sequences. *Magn Reson Imag* 2008;**26** (1):72–6.

24. Mulkern RV, Barnes AS, Haker SJ, *et al.* Biexponential characterization of prostate tissue water diffusion decay curves over an extended b-factor range. *Magn Reson Imag* 2006;**24** (5):563–8.

25. deSouza NM, Reinsberg SA, Scurr ED, *et al.* Magnetic resonance imaging in prostate cancer: the value of apparent diffusion coefficients for identifying malignant nodules. *Br J Radiol* 2007;**80** (950):90–5.

26. Gibbs P, Tozer DJ, Liney GP, *et al.* Comparison of quantitative T2 mapping and diffusion-weighted imaging in the normal and pathologic prostate. *Magn Reson Med* 2001;**46** (6);1054–8.

27. Hosseinzadeh K, Schwarz SD. Endorectal diffusion-weighted imaging in prostate cancer to differentiate malignant and benign peripheral zone tissue. *J Magn Reson Imag* 2004;**20** (4):654–61.

28. Issa B. In vivo measurement of the apparent diffusion coefficient in normal and malignant prostatic tissues using echo-planar imaging. *J Magn Reson Imag* 2002;**16** (2):196–200.

29. Reinsberg SA, Payne GS, Riches SF, *et al.* Combined use of diffusion-weighted MRI and 1H MR spectroscopy to increase accuracy in prostate cancer detection. *Am J Roentgenol* 2007;**188** (1):91–8.

30. Sato C, Naganawa S, Nakamura T, *et al.* Differentiation of noncancerous tissue and cancer lesions by apparent diffusion coefficient values in transition and peripheral zones of the prostate. *J Magn Reson Imag* 2005;**21** (3):258–62.

31. Hayashida Y, Hirai T, Morishita S, *et al.* Diffusion-weighted imaging of metastatic brain tumors: comparison with histologic type and tumor cellularity. *Am J Neuroradiol* 2006;**27** (7):1419–25.

32. Xing D, Papadakis NG, Huang CL, *et al.* Optimised diffusion-weighting for measurement of apparent diffusion coefficient (ADC) in human brain. *Magn Reson Imag* 1997;**15** (7):771–84.

33. Bito Y, Hirata S, Yamamoto E. Optimum gradient factors for apparent diffusion coefficient measurements. *Proc Int Soc Mag Reson Med* 1995; 913.

34. Kitajima K, Kaji Y, Kuroda K, *et al.* High b-value diffusion-weighted imaging in normal and malignant peripheral zone tissue of the prostate: effect of signal-to-noise ratio. *Magn Reson Med Sci* 2008; 7 (2):93–9.

35. Dietrich O, Heiland S, Sartor K. Noise correction for the exact determination of apparent diffusion coefficients at low SNR. *Magn Reson Med* 2001; **45** (3):448–53.

36. Walker-Samuel S, Orton M, McPhail LD, *et al.* Robust estimation of the apparent diffusion coefficient (ADC) in heterogeneous solid tumors. *Magn Reson Med* 2009;**62** (2):420–9.

37. Van As N, Charles-Edwards E, Jackson A, *et al.* Correlation of diffusion-weighted MRI with whole mount radical prostatectomy specimens. *Br J Radiol* 2008;**81** (966):456–62.

38. Riches SF, Hawtin K, Charles-Edwards EM, *et al.* Diffusion-weighted imaging of the prostate and rectal wall: comparison of biexponential and monoexponential modelled diffusion and associated perfusion coefficients. *NMR Biomed* 2008.

39. Le Bihan D, Breton E, Lallemand D, *et al.* Separation of diffusion and perfusion in intravoxel incoherent motion MR imaging. *Radiology* 1988;**168** (2):497–505.

40. Kristoffersen A. Optimal estimation of the diffusion coefficient from non-averaged and averaged noisy magnitude data. *J Magn Reson* 2007;**187** (2):293–305.

41. Gürses B, Kabakci N, Kovanlikaya A, *et al.* Diffusion tensor imaging of the normal prostate at 3 tesla. *Eur Radiol* 2008;**18** (4):716–21.

42. Tozer D, Gibbs P, Turnbull LS. Diffusion tensor imaging of the prostate. *Proc Int Soc Mag Reson Med* **2003**;460.

43. Reinsberg S, Brewster J, Payne GS, *et al.* Anisotropic diffusion in prostate cancer: fact or artefact? In *Proc 13th Annual Meeting International Society for Magnetic Resonance in Medicine*: Miami;. 2005.

44. Shukla-Dave A, Hricak H, Eberhardt SC, *et al.* Chronic prostatitis: MR imaging and 1H MR spectroscopic imaging findings – initial observations. *Radiology* 2004;**231** (3):717–24.

45. Shimofusa R, Fujimoto H, Akamata H, *et al.* Diffusion-weighted imaging of prostate cancer. *J Comput Assist Tomogr* 2005;**29** (2):149–53.

46. Morgan VA, Kyriazi S, Ashley SE, *et al.* Evaluation of the potential of diffusion-weighted imaging in prostate cancer detection. *Acta Radiol* 2007;**48** (6):695–703.

47. Song SK, Qu Z, Garabedian EM, *et al.* Improved magnetic resonance imaging detection of prostate cancer in a transgenic mouse model. *Cancer Res* 2002;**62** (5):1555–8.

48. Xu J, Humphrey P, Kibel A, *et al.* Magnetic resonance diffusion characteristics of histologically defined

prostate cancer in humans. In *Proc 16th Scientific Meeting International Society for Magnetic Resonance in Medicine*: Toronto; 2008.

49. deSouza NM, Riches SF, Vanas NJ, *et al.* Diffusion-weighted magnetic resonance imaging: a potential non-invasive marker of tumour aggressiveness in localized prostate cancer. *Clin Radiol* 2008;**63** (7):774–82.

50. Valonen PK, Lehtimaki KK, Vaisanen TH, *et al.* Water diffusion in a rat glioma during ganciclovir-thymidine kinase gene therapy-induced programmed cell death in vivo: correlation with cell density. *J Magn Reson Imag* 2004;**19** (4):389–96.

51. Zhao D, Ran S, Constantinescu A, *et al.* Tumor oxygen dynamics: correlation of in vivo MRI with histological findings. *Neoplasia* 2003;**5** (4):308–18.

52. Riches SF, Morgan V, Payne GS, Dearnaley D, deSouza N. Diffusion weighted imaging of androgen deprivation hormone therapy prostate cancer patients. *Proc Int Soc Mag Reson Med* 2007:793.

53. D'Amico AV, Halabi S, Tempany C, *et al.* Tumor volume changes on 1.5 tesla endorectal MRI during neoadjuvant androgen suppression therapy for higher-risk prostate cancer and recurrence in men treated using radiation therapy: results of the phase II

CALGB 9682 study. *Int J Radiat Oncol Biol Phys* 2008;**71** (1):9–15.

54. Cohen RJ, Fujiwara K, Holland JW, *et al.* Polyamines in prostatic epithelial cells and adenocarcinoma; the effects of androgen blockade. *Prostate* 2001;**49** (4):278–84.

55. Takayama Y, Kishimoto R, Hanaoka S, *et al.* ADC value and diffusion tensor imaging of prostate cancer: changes in carbon-ion radiotherapy. *J Magn Reson Imag* 2008;**27** (6):1331–5.

56. Petraki CD, Sfikas CP. Histopathological changes induced by therapies in the benign prostate and prostate adenocarcinoma. *Histol Histopathol* 2007;**22** (1):107–18.

57. Chen J, Daniel BL, Diederich CJ, *et al.* Monitoring prostate thermal therapy with diffusion-weighted MRI. *Magn Reson Med* 2008;**59** (6):1365–72.

58. Kumar V, Jagannathan NR, Kumar R, *et al.* Correlation between metabolite ratios and ADC values of prostate in men with increased PSA level. *Magn Reson Imag* 2006;**24** (5):541–8.

59. Mazaheri Y, Shukla-Dave A, Hricak H, *et al.* Prostate cancer: identification with combined diffusion-weighted MR imaging and 3D 1H MR spectroscopic imaging: correlation with pathologic findings. *Radiology* 2008;**246** (2):480–8.

Breast applications of diffusion-weighted MRI

Yong Guo

Abbreviations

ADC	apparent diffusion coefficient
BI-RADS	Breast Imaging Reporting and Data System
CHESS	chemical shift selective suppression
DCE-MRI	dynamic contrast-enhanced MRI
DWI	diffusion-weighted MRI
FOV	field of view
EPI	echo-planar imaging
MRS	magnetic resonance spectroscopy
NACT	neoadjuvant chemotherapy
NPV	negative prospective value
PET	positron emission tomography
ROI	region of interest
SENSE	sensitivity encoding
SNR	signal-to-noise ratio
SS EPI	single-shot EPI
STIR	short tau inversion recovery
T1-WI	T1-weighted imaging
T2-WI	T2-weighted imaging
TE	echo time
TR	repetition time

Introduction

The widespread use of mammography and ultrasound allows earlier detection of breast cancer and has been shown to improve survival of women with breast cancer[1–2]. Early detection of breast cancer allows also conservative surgery as an alternative to mastectomy[3–4]. However, breast lesions remain difficult to diagnose and characterize, especially in dense fibroglandular breasts. Magnetic resonance imaging (MRI) is emerging as the most sensitive available modality for the detection of primary or recurrent breast cancer[5–6]. MRI can help detect occult breast cancers, and this modality is playing an increasingly important role in the clinical setting, including a role in screening high-risk women[7–9]. It improves pre-operative local staging, which is useful for surgical planning[10–11], and for assessment of tumors' response to therapy. The most useful diagnostic criteria that are in use for differential diagnosis are based on lesion morphology (type of enhancement, mass shape and margins, distribution of non-mass-like enhancement, internal architecture)[12–13]. Enhancement pattern on dynamic contrast-enhanced (DCE) imaging provides information about a variety of parameters that reflect vascular changes, such as vascular permeability, interstitial pressure, and extracellular space[14–17]. Since the microvascular properties of cancers differ from those of benign lesions, enhancement patterns provide another useful diagnostic criterion for differentiation of benign and malignant lesions. On DCE-MRI, three different time–intensity curve shapes have been described: a persistent curve (continuous enhancement increasing with time), a "plateau" curve (after an initial peak enhancement, the signal intensity remains constant), and a washout curve defined as a decrease in signal intensity after an initial peak enhancement during the first 2–3 min after injection[18]. When these patterns are associated with analysis of lesion morphology, they can detect malignant lesions with good sensitivity (85–100%)[18–25]. The first edition of the MR BI-RADS lexicon[26] provides a sound basis for the reporting of a breast MR study and incorporates both morphologic and kinetic criteria.

Depiction of fine morphologic details of lesion margins is thought to be the most import feature for differentiating benign from malignant breast lesions and is best assessed during the early post-contrast phase, before the washout occurs in cancers and morphologic details are masked by adjacent enhancing fibroglandular tissue. In order to characterize the different enhancement patterns of breast lesions (especially for lesions with equivocal morphologic features), fast dynamic imaging is required. In breast MRI, however, acquisition speed and spatial resolution are diverging demands. Any increase in spatial resolution is associated with an increase in acquisition time. With state-of-the-art MR systems, these matrices are acquired fast enough to allow arterial phase imaging and to track the time course of enhancing lesions.

A 3D fast spoiled gradient recalled echo sequence with parallel imaging is generally used (we propose the following parameters: TR/TE 6/2 ms, flip angle 10°, slice thickness 2.2 mm, 350×350 matrix, with parallel imaging and an 8-channel breast array coil) for better depiction of lesion morphology. This sequence enables high-resolution imaging of both breasts with the same acquisition time used to image a single breast. Using breast MRI, negative prospective values (NPV) as high as 98% have been reported in single-center studies[11,27], which is the highest published NPV of all breast imaging modalities currently available, including positron emission tomography (PET) and scintimammography[28–30]. However, an overlap in appearance between benign and malignant lesions still exists and the specificity of the technique is relatively low, reported to vary between 40% and 80%[11,18,21,23,31–32]. The lack of specificity motivates the need to develop new MRI techniques, such as MR spectroscopy (MRS) and diffusion-weighted imaging (DWI). In 1997, a feasibility study by Englander et al.[33] showed that normal fibroglandular breast tissue had a different apparent diffusion coefficient (ADC) value from that of fatty breast tissue. In 1998, Lucas-Quesada et al.[34]

reported different ADC values of benign and malignant breast lesions. Subsequently, a series of reports on breast DWI were published, including a study tracking changes in ADC during the menstrual cycle,[35] assessment of DWI to characterize breast lesions;[36–37] and a correlation of tumor ADC with histopathologic degree of cellularity.[36] Preliminary studies that measured ADCs in both the normal breast and in breast lesions demonstrated that benign pathology and normal breast tissue have higher ADCs than those of malignant breast tumors. These findings suggest that the measurement of water diffusion may be an additional feature that could further increase the specificity of the classification of breast lesions. As cellularity and other tissue properties vary in normal tissue and malignant and benign breast lesions, ADC has also been suggested as a potential marker of tumor treatment response.

Breast diffusion acquisition and processing

Diffusion-weighted single-shot EPI (SS EPI) is the most often performed sequence for the diagnostic assessment of breast lesions, but despite its excellent contrast resolution, it suffers from susceptibility and chemical shift artifacts[38]. The combination of parallel imaging such as sensitivity encoding (SENSE) decreases distortion, susceptibility, and chemical shift artifacts caused by EPI[39–41]. Image distortion can be further reduced by increasing the field of view (FOV) and/or decreasing the image matrix. Image contrast in DWI varies greatly with the diffusion sensitizing factor b, which is a parameter that should be set carefully. The optimum b factor depends on target organs and available equipment. The optimum b factor should sufficiently suppress the background signal of the breast and should provide sufficient tumor signal to allow confident diagnosis. Both the background and tumor signal decrease as the b factor is increased. In our experience, using a b factor of 750 s/mm^2, tumor and normal breast tissue could be differentiated. At $b = 1000$ s/mm^2, the background signal decreased to near noise levels, whereas tumor signal remained visible. With a b factor at 1500 s/mm^2, the background signal decreases to noise levels in most cases; tumor signal is further reduced, but images were still diagnostic. When the b factor was increased to 2000 s/mm^2, both the background signal and tumor signal decreased to near noise levels, making image interpretation impossible[42].

We use the following parameters at our institution: repetition time (TR) 2500, echo time (TE) minimum, thickness/spacing 6/1 mm, FOV to cover bilateral breasts, matrix 128×128, two averages.

Values of ADC are affected by both the molecular diffusion of water and blood microcirculation in the capillary network (perfusion). Influence of perfusion is increased when diffusion images are acquired with small b-values (less than 400 s/mm^2),[43] especially for malignant lesions with higher microvessel counts than benign lesions, and could reduce the difference of ADCs between malignant and benign lesions. With a high b-value, ADC values would be less affected by perfusion, and the ADC discrepancy between malignant and benign lesions could be larger. Therefore, higher b-values are suggested for breast DWI. However, higher b-values would require a longer TE and would increase image distortion. Several studies have suggested that non-breath-hold diffusion images could be of acceptable image quality when the maximum b-value of 750–1000 s/mm^2 is used. The use of parallel imaging enables the use of high b-values of 1000–1500 s/mm^2 for breast diffusion[44].

High fat content in the breast makes fat saturation techniques necessary to identify lesions on diffusion. Two main fat-suppression techniques are available: chemical shift selective suppression (CHESS) and short tau inversion recovery (STIR). The STIR method used for diffusion-weighted whole-body imaging with background body signal suppression provides steady fat suppression, but its signal-to-noise ratio (SNR) is lower than that of CHESS. The CHESS method does not always provide uniform fat suppression, but its SNR is higher. Wenkel et al.[45] compared the two different fat-suppression sequences for breast DWI, and both methods appear to provide equivalent ADC quantification. However, CHESS EPI provided better lesion delineation compared to STIR EPI sequence. EPI CHESS demonstrated also a significantly lower standard deviation of ADC measurement. Due to better lesion delineation, better ADC quantification, and shorter acquisition time, EPI CHESS is preferred to EPI STIR sequence.

Accurate positioning of the region of interest (ROI) is essential for an accurate measure of ADC. Rubesova et al.[46] and Woodhams et al.[47] suggested placing the ROI using subtracted DCE images as

a reference. The easiest method is to copy and paste the ROI from contrast-enhanced images to ADC maps[45]. However, misregistration can happen between DCE and diffusion images due to EPI related distortion or patient movement, especially for small lesions.

Marini et al.[48] measured the ADC of malignant lesions with diameter greater than 3 cm, with the center and lesion edges well defined on ADC maps. The ADC values of central portion of tumors ($1.07 \pm 0.21 \times 10^{-3}$ mm^2/s) were significantly increased with respect to peripheral ADC values ($0.94 \pm 0.18 \times 10^{-3}$ mm/s)^2. In these cases, the histopathologic examination confirmed the presence of necrosis in the center of the lesion, due to the large dimension of the lesion and more cell-packed components at the edges of the lesion. Therefore, placement of ROIs in necrotic, cystic, or hemorrhagic components should be avoided by referring to other MR sequences.

DWI can be performed using breath-hold or free-breathing acquisitions. Regarding the acquisition plane, breast DWI can be performed in sagittal, transverse, or coronal plane. However, it is recommended to choose the same plane as used for DCE imaging.

Results of breast DWI
Lesion detection

Most breast lesions, especially malignant tumors, can be demonstrated on DWI. However, approximately 6% to 37.5% of malignant breast lesions are not visible on DWI, especially small lesions[49–51]. Detection and characterization of small breast lesions represent a difficulty not only with DWI but also with conventional sequences (using morphologic analysis and enhancement pattern)[52]. Small breast lesions, especially benign lesions, are difficult to localize on ADC maps because of limited spatial resolution and poor contrast with surrounding glandular tissue[46]. For example, we have reported three adenomas smaller than 1 cm in diameter that were not demonstrable on DWI[36]. Park et al.[49] reported eight daughter nodules of breast cancers ranging in size from 0.4 to 0.8 cm that were not detected on DWI. Wenkel et al.[45] reported three breast cancers with a maximum diameter of less than 1 cm that were not visible on DWI. To summarize, a lesion smaller than 1 cm in diameter may not be visualized on DWI. Rubesova et al.[46] suggested not to perform ADC

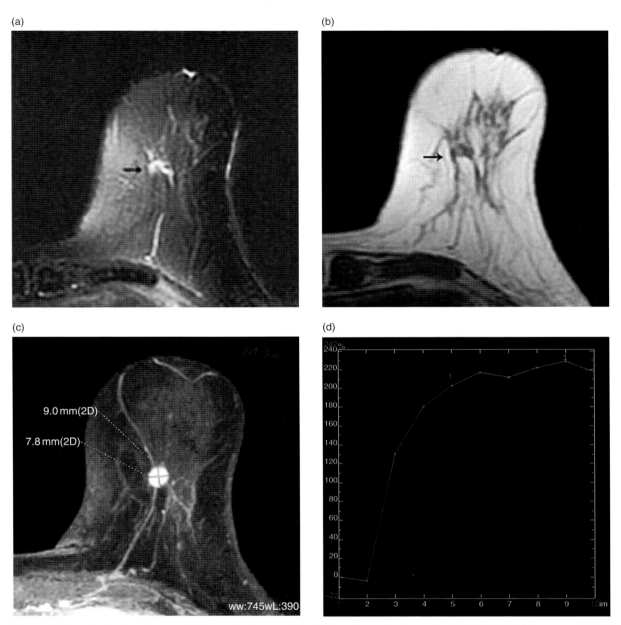

Figure 7.1 Invasive ductal carcinoma misdiagnosed with conventional MRI and correctly diagnosed with DWI. (a) Axial fat-suppressed T2-WI (TR/TE = 6260/90 ms), (b) axial T1-WI (TR/TE = 600/11.5 ms), (c) axial dynamic 3D fat-suppressed T1-WI contrast-enhanced image (TR/TE 4.8/2.3, TI = 16, NEX = 0.8, matrix 380 × 320, FOV 320 mm, dynamic acquisition time 60 s), (d) time–intensity curve, DWI (b = 1000), (e) SSPEI DWI (b = 1000). A 9-mm nodule in the inferior quadrant of left breast is present (arrow), demonstrating benign features on conventional sequences (round shape with smooth margins, homogeneous enhancement, and persistent time–signal intensity curve) compatible with BI-RADS category 2 (benign findings). However, the nodule demonstrated high signal on DWI, with low ADC (0.863 × 10^{-3} mm^2/s), which raised suspicion for malignancy. The nodule was confirmed to be an invasive ductal carcinoma.

measurements on lesions smaller than 0.7 cm in which the ROI contained an insufficient number of pixels and could not provide an accurate measure of ADC. However, visual assessment can still be of diagnostic value even in small lesions. For example, a small lesion in high signal on DWI which is also visible on subtracted images should raise the suspicion of malignancy (Fig. 7.1).

Lesion characterization

ADCs of malignant and benign breast lesions are listed in Table 7.1, which demonstrates a wide range of ADC values and proposed thresholds, related to differences in b-values[53–54] and differences in patient population and lesions assessed. Most prior studies,

(e)

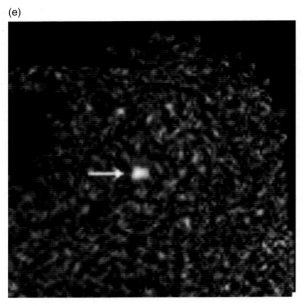

Figure 7.1 (*Cont.*)

except the study by Sinha et al.,[37] showed a statistical difference between ADCs of malignant and benign breast lesions,[36–37,47,49,51,55] with substantially lower ADC values in malignant lesions compared to benign lesions, with some degree of overlap, as shown in Fig. 7.2. In the study by Rubesova et al.,[46] a threshold ADC value between 1.08 and 1.19×10^{-3} mm^2/s provided sensitivity and specificity above 80%. This value is compared to a threshold ADC of 1.3×10^{-3} mm^2/s (using max $b = 1000$) in our experience.

In biological tissues, microscopic motion includes both the molecular diffusion of water and blood microcirculation in the capillary network. Both diffusion and perfusion thus affect the ADCs obtained from biological tissues. The pseudo-diffusion coefficient of capillary microcirculation is typically many times greater than the diffusion coefficient of pure water. However, the volume of blood flowing in the perfused capillaries is only a small percentage of the total water content in normal brain tissue[56]. In breast tumors, although higher microvessel counts were recorded for malignant than for benign pathology[57] and higher ADCs may be expected in cancers compared to benign conditions, they showed lower mean ADCs than did benign lesions. This suggests that molecular diffusion of water may overcome the opposite effect of perfusion in cancers and has a major impact on the ADCs in breast lesions.

Table 7.1 Mean ($\pm$ SD) ADCs ($\times 10^{-3}$ mm^2/s) of malignant and benign breast lesions and ADC cut-offs used for diagnosing malignant lesions reported in the literature

Reference	Number of lesions	Max. b-value	ADC malignant lesions	ADC benign lesions	Suggested ADC cut-off
Sinha et al.[37]	23	235	1.6 ± 0.36	2.01 ± 0.46	
Kinoshita et al.[51]	21	700	1.21 ± 0.18	1.49 ± 0.18	
Woodhams et al.[47]	76	750	1.12 ± 0.24		
Wenkel et al.[45]	56	800	0.90 ± 0.18	1.76 ± 0.42	1.44
Hatakenaka et al.[58]	136	1000	1.15 ± 0.26	1.66 ± 0.30	1.48
Guo et al.[36]	52	1000	0.97 ± 0.20	1.57 ± 0.23	1.30
Rubesova et al. [46]	78	1000	0.99	1.48	1.13
Marini et al.[48]	60	1000	0.95 ± 0.18	1.48 ± 0.37	1.1–1.31
Kuroki et al.[44]	60	1000	1.021 ± 0.23	1.44 ± 0.45	

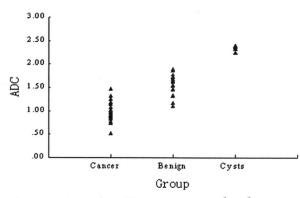

Figure 7.2 Scatterplots of the ADC values ($\times 10^{-3}$ mm²/s) obtained in benign and malignant breast lesions and cysts. An overlap is present between the ADCs of malignant and benign breast lesions.

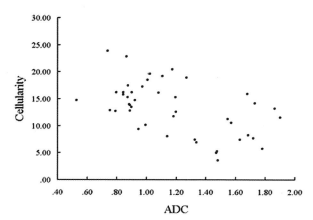

Figure 7.3 Correlation of tumor cellularity (44 lesions) with lesion ADC. There was a moderate significant correlation between cellularity and lesion ADC (r −0.542, $p < 0.01$) [From Guo et al. 2002[36].]

Water inside cells is known to have lower ADC values as compared to extracellular water, which is believed to be due to restrictive structural components inside the cell and higher viscosity from increased concentrations of macromolecules. Diffusion has been shown to decrease in tissues with high cellularity. It has been shown that ADC of breast tumors correlates significantly with tumor cellularity (Fig. 7.3)[36,58]. Malignant breast tumors had a higher cellularity and a lower ADC than benign breast tumors (Fig. 7.4, 7.5). Hence, a malignant tumor with low cellularity, such as in the case of squirrhous adenocarcinomas (Fig. 7.6), may demonstrate a high ADC and consequently be a potential false negative. Conversely, a benign tumor with high cellularity, such as in the case of papillomas (Fig. 7.7), may demonstrate a low ADC and be a potential false positive. Water diffusion is also influenced by the tissue structure such as mucous protein or necrosis[59]. Therefore, the ADCs of ductal ectasia with mucous protein may be decreased (Fig. 7.8), and the ADCs of invasive ductal carcinomas with central necrosis may be increased (Fig. 7.9). A small area of necrosis or cystic changes not detectable on DCE-MRI may also increase the ADC. Another factor that may influence ADC measurement is intratumoral hemorrhage[60], which may modify signal intensity on DWI and ADC value (Fig 7.10). To summarize, diffusion measurements can reflect differences in tissue cellularity, microstructure, and water compartmentalization. A low ADC value might indicate high cell density and dense mucus tissue.

Tumor staging

There is limited data on the use of DWI for local staging of breast cancer. For example, Woodhams et al.[47] have compared the spatial distribution of ADC values in tumors with histopathologic local tumor staging, and showed that tumor extension was accurate in 75% of cases and was overestimated in 20% of cases. The major reason for overestimation of local tumor invasion was the presence of benign proliferative lesions, which decreased ADC values. The low ADC value of benign proliferative lesions may be due to high cellularity, leukocytes, fibrosis, and inflammatory changes. The study by Woodhams et al. was limited by the lack of reference to dynamic contrast-enhanced MRI. Because of the limited spatial resolution of DWI, we do not suggest the use of DWI alone for assessment of tumor extension.

Comparison and combination with conventional sequences and mammography

Park et al.[49] evaluated tumor detection using DWI, and pre-contrast T1-WI and T2-WI in 41 patients with 65 enhancing lesions diagnosed on dynamic contrast-enhanced images. DWI, T1-WI, and T2-WI detected 86%, 62%, and 75% of lesions, respectively. DWI showed higher detection rate of breast tumors than T1-WI and T2-WI, but lower than that of DCE images. Therefore, DWI cannot replace

(a)

(b)

(c)

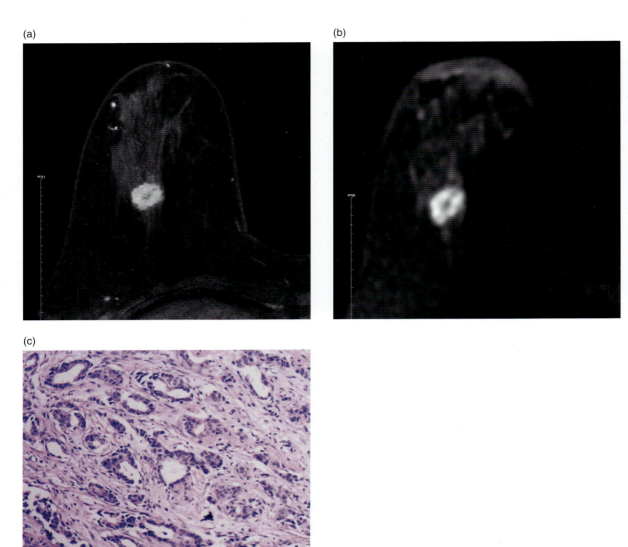

Figure 7.4 Invasive ductal carcinoma diagnosed with conventional MRI and DWI. (a) Early phase of an axial fat-suppressed contrast-enhanced image; an oval mass with irregular margin and heterogeneous enhancement is present. (b) DWI ($b = 1000$). The mass shows high signal intensity on DWI, with low ADC (0.83×10^{-3} mm^2/s). (c) Histological examination revealed invasive ductal carcinoma with high cellularity.

contrast-enhanced imaging, but DWI is a better method for tumor detection compared to T1-WI and T2-WI if contrast-enhanced imaging is contra-indicated. Yoshikawa et al.[50] examined 48 women with 53 breast cancers using DWI and mammography before surgery. Breast cancer detection rates by DWI and mammography were 94.3% and 84.9%, respectively, indicating a statistically significant difference.

The diagnosis of tumors was possible even in extremely dense breast tissue with DWI, compared to mammography. Thus, DWI may be useful for detecting breast cancer in a wide age group of women, including young women who have dense mammary glands, without exposing them to radiation. Therefore, DWI may be complementary to mammography. However, at present, there is no sufficient evidence to

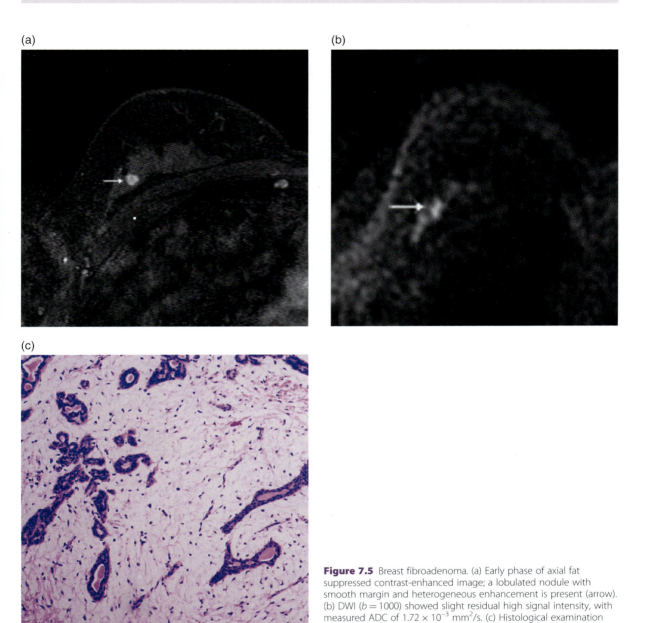

Figure 7.5 Breast fibroadenoma. (a) Early phase of axial fat suppressed contrast-enhanced image; a lobulated nodule with smooth margin and heterogeneous enhancement is present (arrow). (b) DWI ($b = 1000$) showed slight residual high signal intensity, with measured ADC of 1.72×10^{-3} mm^2/s. (c) Histological examination revealed fibroadenoma with low cellularity.

evaluate the effectiveness of using DWI for cancer screening, and future studies are warranted.

Treatment response

Neoadjuvant chemotherapy (NACT) provides the option of breast conservation surgery in patients with inoperable locally advanced breast cancer by reducing tumor size[61]. Moreover, it permits in vivo monitoring of tumor response. However, considering the high toxicity of chemotherapeutic drugs, early assessment of therapeutic response of the tumor is essential for patient management. Based on the treatment response, a second-line therapy or early surgery may be planned for non-responders, and prognosis and overall survival of patients can be predicted[62].

93

(a)

(b)

(c)

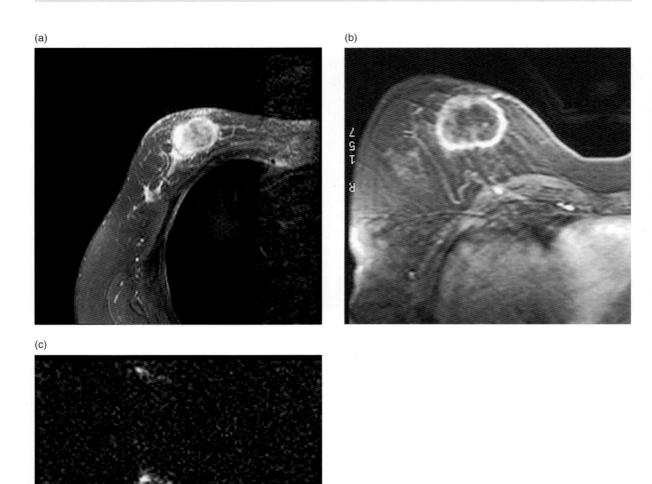

Figure 7.6 Squirrhous breast adenocarcinoma. (a) Axial fat-suppressed T2-WI (TR/TE = 6260/90 ms). (b) Axial fat-suppressed contrast-enhanced image at an early phase. (c) Sagittal DWI (b = 1000). There is a well-circumscribed oval mass in the upper inner quadrant of the right breast, with low signal in the lesion center on T2-WI, rim enhancement and rim in high signal with central low signal on DWI. ADC of the central portion was higher than the peripheral portion (1.48 vs. 1.12 × 10^{-3} mm^2/s), due to lower cellularity. The lesion was confirmed to be squirrhous adenocarcinomas.

The current purposes of imaging during and after NACT are to evaluate the extent of residual disease and try to predict the pathological response as early as possible after the initiation of treatment. Conventional imaging procedures such as mammography, ultrasound, conventional MRI sequences, and clinical examination evaluate the tumor response by measuring changes in tumor size. However, the major drawback of these methodologies is that they may not accurately provide early assessment of response because of slow changes in size. Thus, a technique that provides an early assessment of therapeutic response is essential in treatment planning and management of breast cancer. PET is such a technique and has an established role for the early assessment of response behaviour[63–67]. There is now increasing evidence that

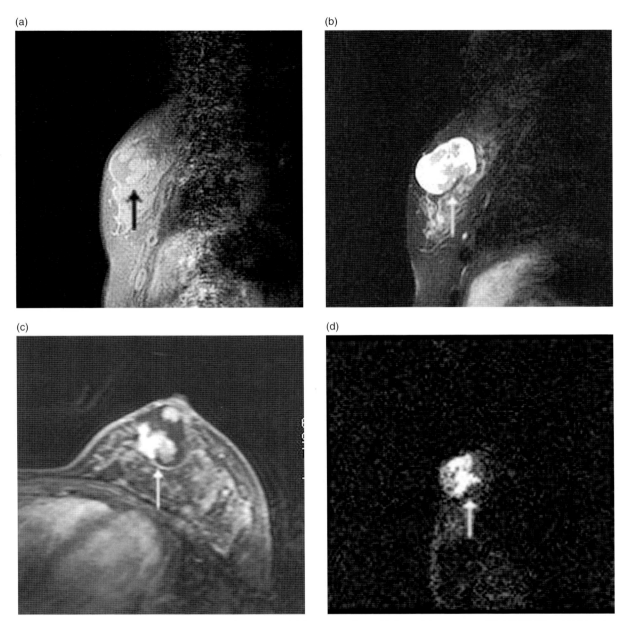

Figure 7.7 False positive of DWI in a 42-year-old female with left breast papilloma. (a) Sagittal fat-suppressed T1-WI (TR/TE = 600/30 ms). (b) Sagittal fat-suppressed T2-WI (TR/TE = 6260/90 ms). (c) Early phase of an axial fat-suppressed contrast-enhanced image. (d) Sagittal DWI (b = 1000). Ultrasound detected a mass with cystic and solid component. MRI demonstrated a well-circumscribed tumor in upper inner quadrant of left breast. The papillary nodule in a cyst showed isosignal intensity on T2-WI and T1-WI, enhancement with plateau time–signal intensity curve, and high signal on DWI, with low ADC (1.11×10^{-3} mm²/s), due to high cellularity. The mass was a surgically confirmed papilloma.

functional information may also be obtained by using DCE-MRI, MRS, and DWI. Using DCE imaging, a change of enhancement kinetics has been observed (slower wash-in rate, absence of a washout pattern – i.e., flattening of the enhancement curve), and preceded changes in tumor size and morphology by several weeks. Proton MRS of the breast is demonstrating great promise in the early evaluation of the effects of

95

(a)

(b)

(c)

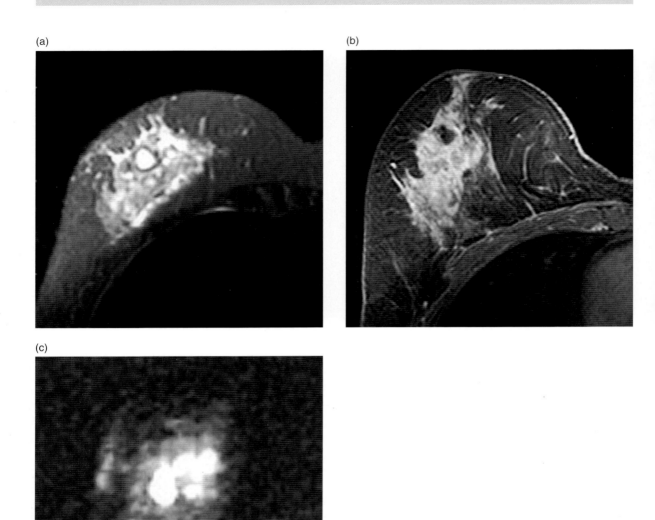

Figure 7.8 False positive of DWI in a 29-year-old female with surgically confirmed duct ectasia. (a) Axial fat-suppressed T2-WI (TR/TE = 6260/90 ms) (b) Axial fat-suppressed contrast-enhanced image. (c) Sagittal DWI (b = 1000). MRI demonstrated large patchy bright signal on T2-WI with multiple small cystic lesions in right breast, heterogeneous enhancement with plateau time–signal intensity curve. The multiple small cystic lesions showed high signal intensity on DWI, with low ADC of 0.77×10^{-3} mm^2/s, due to mucous protein contents.

chemotherapeutic agents. DWI can be used to detect changes in the ADC associated with changes in tissue structure. Galons *et al.*[68] reported an early increase in ADC in breast cancer responding to therapy. Sharma *et al.*[69] reported that the change in ADC after the first cycle of NACT was statistically significant compared with volume and diameter. After the third cycle, the

sensitivity for differentiating responders from non-responders was 89% for volume and diameter and 68% for ADC, and the respective specificities were 50%, 70%, and 100%. A sensitivity of 84% (specificity of 60% with an accuracy of 76%) was achieved when all three variables were taken together to predict the response. The results show that ADC is more useful

(a)

(b)

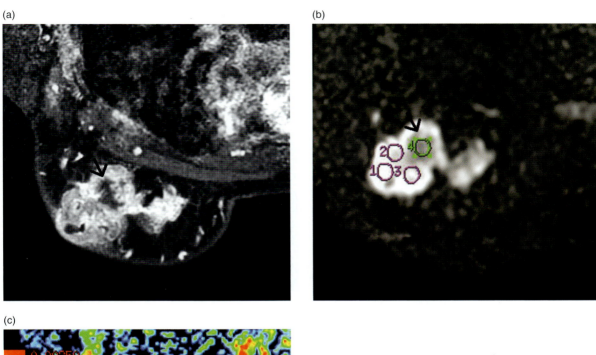

(c)

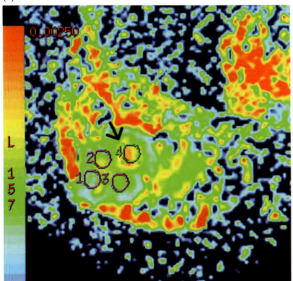

Figure 7.9 Necrotic invasive ductal carcinoma. (a) Axial fat-suppressed contrast-enhanced image. (b) Axial DWI ($b = 1000$). (c) ADC map. There is a large mass of the left breast, with central necrosis (arrow) identified on contrast-enhanced image, and increased ADC value (1.71×10^{-3} mm^2/s) compared to the peripheral cellular portion (0.86–1.22×10^{-3} mm^2/s) on ADC map.

for predicting early tumor response to chemotherapy than morphological changes. The early increase in ADC after treatment may be due to cell damage mediated by the therapeutic interventions. Moreover, the integrity of cell membranes is compromised, and the fractional volume of the interstitial space increases because of apoptosis or cell loss.[68] A decrease in cellularity of breast cancer after NACT compared with pre-therapy has also been documented[70]. It has been reported that NACT increases apoptosis within 24 h after its initiation in breast cancer[71]. In summary, DWI is showing great potential in assessing early response to NACT, and further clinical evaluation is needed.

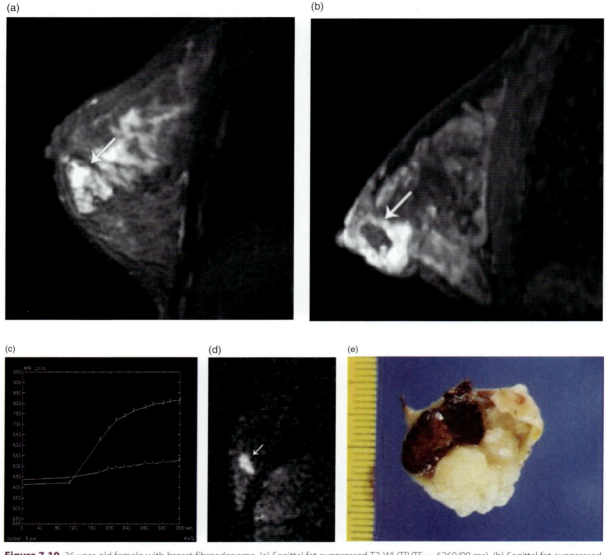

Figure 7.10 36-year-old female with breast fibroadenoma. (a) Sagittal fat-suppressed T2-WI (TR/TE = 6260/90 ms). (b) Sagittal fat-suppressed contrast-enhanced image. (c) Time–signal intensity curve. (d) Sagittal DWI. (e) Gross specimen. The tumor demonstrates heterogeneous signal on T2-WI, no enhancement in the central portion (labeled as curve 1 on the time–signal intensity curve), gradual enhancement in the peripheral portion (labeled as curve 2 on the time–signal intensity curve), and high signal on DWI, with ADC of 1.26–1.33 × 10^{-3} mm²/s. Gross tumor specimen reveals hemorrhagic changes in tumor.

Limitations of breast DWI

These include limited spatial resolution and the possibility of false negatives and false positives. Areas of high signal intensity on DWI do not always represent malignant lesions, and non-focal mass lesions as often seen in ductal carcinoma in situ (DCIS) may not be categorized correctly with DWI even with a small ROI due to diffuse tumor spread and partial volume effects. It is therefore suggested to combine DWI with other MR sequences.

Future directions

With continued improvement in image quality, DWI is expected to play an important role in breast cancer in the future. Its role in differentiating benign from malignant lesions and in improving the specificity of breast MR imaging may result in a decreased number of breast biopsies. DWI may be useful for detecting breast cancer in a wide age group of women, including young women who have dense breasts, for detecting mammographically and clinically occult breast carcinomas, even for screening breast cancer without DCE-MRI.

Moreover, in the setting of monitoring response to neoadjuvant chemotherapy, the results to date have been extremely promising. Large multicenter trials are needed and represent a vital step in the establishment of this technique in the clinical setting.

Conclusion

DWI is a non-contrast method, with short acquisition time and easy processing which may add useful information to conventional sequences, including lesion detection and characterization. Multiparametric imaging of the breast based on the combination of DCE-MRI, MRS, and DWI will likely improve specificity of morphology and kinetic data analysis. However, radiologists should be aware of limitations and pitfalls of DWI.

References

1. Senie RT, Lesser M, Kinne DW, Rosen PP. Method of tumor detection influences disease-free survival of women with breast carcinoma. *Cancer* 1994;**73** (6): 1666–72.

2. Margolin FR. Detecting early breast cancer: experience in a community hospital. *Cancer* 1989; **64** (12 Suppl):2702–5.

3. Thibault F, Nos C, Meunier M, *et al.* MRI for surgical planning in patients with breast cancer who undergo preoperative chemotherapy. *Am J Roentgenol* 2004; **183** (4):1159–68.

4. Esserman L, Hylton N, Yassa L, *et al.* Utility of magnetic resonance imaging in the management of breast cancer: evidence for improved preoperative staging. *J Clin Oncol* 1999;**17** (1): 110–19.

5. Kuhl C. The current status of breast MR imaging. I. Choice of technique, image interpretation, diagnostic accuracy, and transfer to clinical practice. *Radiology* 2007;**244** (2):356–78.

6. Kuhl CK. Current status of breast MR imaging. II. Clinical applications. *Radiology* 2007;**244** (3): 672–91.

7. Liberman L. Breast cancer screening with MRI: what are the data for patients at high risk? *N Engl J Med* 2004;**351** (5):497–500.

8. Robson ME, Offit K. Breast MRI for women with hereditary cancer risk. *JAMA* 2004;**292** (11): 1368–70.

9. Morris EA, Liberman L, Ballon DJ, *et al.* MRI of occult breast carcinoma in a high-risk population. *Am J Roentgenol* 2003;**181** (3):619–26.

10. Bedrosian I, Mick R, Orel SG, *et al.* Changes in the surgical management of patients with breast carcinoma based on preoperative magnetic resonance imaging. *Cancer* 2003;**98** (3):468–73.

11. Fischer U, Kopka L, Grabbe E. Breast carcinoma: effect of preoperative contrast-enhanced MR imaging on the therapeutic approach. *Radiology* 1999; **213** (3):881–8.

12. Hochman MG, Orel SG, Powell CM, *et al.* Fibroadenomas: MR imaging appearances with radiologic-histopathologic correlation. *Radiology* 1997; **204** (1):123–9.

13. Nunes LW, Schnall MD, Orel SG. Update of breast MR imaging architectural interpretation model. *Radiology* 2001;**219** (2):484–94.

14. Kaiser WA, Zeitler E. MR imaging of the breast: fast imaging sequences with and without Gd-DTPA – preliminary observations. *Radiology* 1989;**170** (3 Pt 1): 681–6.

15. Buadu LD, Murakami J, Murayama S, *et al.* Patterns of peripheral enhancement in breast masses: correlation of findings on contrast medium enhanced MRI with histologic features and tumor angiogenesis. *J Comput Assist Tomogr* 1997; **21** (3):421–30.

16. Su MY, Jao JC, Nalcioglu O. Measurement of vascular volume fraction and blood-tissue permeability constants with a pharmacokinetic model: studies in rat muscle tumors with dynamic Gd-DTPA enhanced MRI. *Magn Reson Med* 1994; **32** (6):714–24.

17. Stack JP, Redmond OM, Codd MB, Dervan PA, Ennis JT. Breast disease: tissue characterization with Gd-DTPA enhancement profiles. *Radiology* 1990; **174** (2):491–4.

18. Kuhl CK, Mielcareck P, Klaschik S, *et al.* Dynamic breast MR imaging: are signal intensity time course data useful for differential diagnosis of enhancing lesions? *Radiology* 1999;**211** (1):101–10.

19. Bluemke DA, Gatsonis CA, Chen MH, *et al.* Magnetic resonance imaging of the breast prior to biopsy. *JAMA* 2004;**292** (22):2735–42.

20. Wiener JI, Schilling KJ, Adami C, Obuchowski NA. Assessment of suspected breast cancer by MRI: a prospective clinical trial using a combined kinetic and morphologic analysis. *Am J Roentgenol* 2005; **184** (3):878–86.

21. Macura KJ, Ouwerkerk R, Jacobs MA, Bluemke DA. Patterns of enhancement on breast MR images: interpretation and imaging pitfalls. *Radiographics* 2006;**26** (6):1719–34.

22. Schnall MD, Blume J, Bluemke DA, *et al.* Diagnostic architectural and dynamic features at breast MR imaging: multicenter study. *Radiology* 2006; **238** (1):42–53.

23. Szabo BK, Aspelin P, Wiberg MK, Bone B. Dynamic MR imaging of the breast: analysis of kinetic and morphologic diagnostic criteria. *Acta Radiol* 2003; **44** (4):379–86.

24. Heywang-Kobrunner SH, Bick U, Bradley WG Jr, *et al.* International investigation of breast MRI: results of a multicentre study (11 sites) concerning diagnostic parameters for contrast-enhanced MRI based on 519 histopathologically correlated lesions. *Eur Radiol* 2001;**11** (4):531–46.

25. Kinkel K, Helbich TH, Esserman LJ, *et al.* Dynamic high-spatial-resolution MR imaging of suspicious breast lesions: diagnostic criteria and interobserver variability. *Am J Roentgenol* 2000; **175** (1):35–43.

26. ACR breast imaging reporting and data system (BIRADS). *Breast Imaging Atlas*. Reston, VA:American College of Radiology; 2003.

27. Kuhl CK, Schmutzler RK, Leutner CC, *et al.* Breast MR imaging screening in 192 women proved or suspected to be carriers of a breast cancer susceptibility gene: preliminary results. *Radiology* 2000;**215** (1):267–79.

28. Smyczek-Gargya B, Fersis N, Dittmann H, *et al.* PET with [^{18}F]fluorothymidine for imaging of primary breast cancer: a pilot study. *Eur J Nucl Med Mol Imag* 2004;**31** (5):720–4.

29. Samson DJ, Flamm CR, Pisano ED, Aronson N. Should FDG PET be used to decide whether a patient with an abnormal mammogram or breast finding at physical examination should undergo biopsy? *Acad Radiol* 2002;**9** (7):773–83.

30. Avril N, Rose CA, Schelling M, *et al.* Breast imaging with positron emission tomography and fluorine-18 fluorodeoxyglucose: use and limitations. *J Clin Oncol* 2000;**18** (20):3495–502.

31. Eliat PA, Dedieu V, Bertino C, *et al.* Magnetic resonance imaging contrast-enhanced relaxometry of breast tumors: an MRI multicenter investigation concerning 100 patients. *Magn Reson Imag* 2004;**22** (4):475–81.

32. Jacobs MA, Barker PB, Bluemke DA, *et al.* Benign and malignant breast lesions: diagnosis with multiparametric MR imaging. *Radiology* 2003; **229** (1):225–32.

33. Englander SA, Ulug AM, Brem R, Glickson JD, van Zijl PC. Diffusion imaging of human breast. *NMR Biomed* 1997;**10** (7):348–52.

34. Lucas-Quesada FA, Sinha S, DeBruhl N, Sinha U, Bassett LW. Estimation of diffusion coefficients for benign and malignant breast lesions using echo planar MRI. (Abstract.) *Radiology* 1998;**209**;468.

35. Partridge SC, McKinnon GC, Henry RG, Hylton NM. Menstrual cycle variation of apparent diffusion coefficients measured in the normal breast using MRI. *J Magn Reson Imag* 2001;**14** (4):433–8.

36. Guo Y, Cai YQ, Cai ZL, *et al.* Differentiation of clinically benign and malignant breast lesions using diffusion-weighted imaging. *J Magn Reson Imag* 2002;**16** (2):172–8.

37. Sinha S, Lucas-Quesada FA, Sinha U, DeBruhl N, Bassett LW. In vivo diffusion-weighted MRI of the breast: potential for lesion characterization. *J Magn Reson Imag* 2002;**15** (6):693–704.

38. Schmithorst VJ, Dardzinski BJ, Holland SK. Simultaneous correction of ghost and geometric distortion artifacts in EPI using a multiecho reference scan. *IEEE Trans Med Imag* 2001;**20** (6):535–9.

39. Kurihara Y, Yakushiji YK, Tani I, Nakajima Y, Van Cauteren M. Coil sensitivity encoding in MR imaging: advantages and disadvantages in clinical practice. *Am J Roentgenol* 2002;**178** (5):1087–91.

40. Lee RF, Westgate CR, Weiss RG, Bottomley PA. An analytical SMASH procedure (ASP) for sensitivity-encoded MRI. *Magn Reson Med* 2000; **43** (5):716–25.

41. Bammer R, Keeling SL, Augustin M, *et al.* Improved diffusion-weighted single-shot echo-planar imaging (EPI) in stroke using sensitivity encoding (SENSE). *Magn Reson Med* 2001;**46** (3):548–54.

42. Kuroki Y, Nasu K. Advances in breast MRI: diffusion-weighted imaging of the breast. *Breast Cancer* 2008; **15** (3):212–17.

43. Le Bihan D, Breton E, Lallemand D, *et al.* Separation of diffusion and perfusion in intravoxel incoherent motion MR imaging. *Radiology* 1988;**168** (2): 497–505.

44. Kuroki Y, Nasu K, Kuroki S, *et al.* Diffusion-weighted imaging of breast cancer with the sensitivity

encoding technique: analysis of the apparent diffusion coefficient value. *Magn Reson Med Sci* 2004; **3** (2):79–85.

45. Wenkel E, Geppert C, Schulz-Wendtland R, *et al.* Diffusion weighted imaging in breast MRI: comparison of two different pulse sequences. *Acad Radiol* 2007;**14** (9):1077–83.

46. Rubesova E, Grell AS, De Maertelaer V, *et al.* Quantitative diffusion imaging in breast cancer: a clinical prospective study. *J Magn Reson Imag* 2006; **24** (2):319–24.

47. Woodhams R, Matsunaga K, Iwabuchi K, *et al.* Diffusion-weighted imaging of malignant breast tumors: the usefulness of apparent diffusion coefficient (ADC) value and ADC map for the detection of malignant breast tumors and evaluation of cancer extension. *J Comput Assist Tomogr* 2005; **29** (5):644–9.

48. Marini C, Iacconi C, Giannelli M, *et al.* Quantitative diffusion-weighted MR imaging in the differential diagnosis of breast lesion. *Eur Radiol* 2007;**17** (10): 2646–55.

49. Park MJ, Cha ES, Kang BJ, Ihn YK, Baik JH. The role of diffusion-weighted imaging and the apparent diffusion coefficient (ADC) values for breast tumors. *Korean J Radiol* 2007;**8** (5):390–6.

50. Yoshikawa MI, Ohsumi S, Sugata S, *et al.* Comparison of breast cancer detection by diffusion-weighted magnetic resonance imaging and mammography. *Radiat Med* 2007;**25** (5):218–23.

51. Kinoshita T, Yashiro N, Ihara N, *et al.* Diffusion-weighted half-Fourier single-shot turbo spin echo imaging in breast tumors: differentiation of invasive ductal carcinoma from fibroadenoma. *J Comput Assist Tomogr* 2002;**26** (6):1042–6.

52. Langer SA, Horst KC, Ikeda DM, *et al.* Pathologic correlates of false positive breast magnetic resonance imaging findings: which lesions warrant biopsy? *Am J Surg* 2005;**190** (4):633–40.

53. Kim T, Murakami T, Takahashi S, *et al.* Diffusion-weighted single-shot echoplanar MR imaging for liver disease. *Am J Roentgenol* 1999; **173** (2):393–8.

54. Bammer R. Basic principles of diffusion-weighted imaging. *Eur J Radiol* 2003;**45** (3):169–84.

55. Woodhams R, Matsunaga K, Kan S, *et al.* ADC mapping of benign and malignant breast tumors. *Magn Reson Med Sci* 2005;**4** (1):35–42.

56. Le Bihan D, Breton E, Lallemand D, *et al.* MR imaging of intravoxel incoherent motions: application to diffusion and perfusion in neurologic disorders. *Radiology* 1986;**161** (2):401–7.

57. Buadu LD, Murakami J, Murayama S, *et al.* Breast lesions: correlation of contrast medium enhancement patterns on MR images with histopathologic findings and tumor angiogenesis. *Radiology* 1996;**200** (3):639–49.

58. Hatakenaka M, Soeda H, Yabuuchi H, *et al.* Apparent diffusion coefficients of breast tumors: clinical application. *Magn Reson Med Sci* 2008; **7** (1):23–9.

59. Yamashita Y, Tang Y, Takahashi M. Ultrafast MR imaging of the abdomen: echo planar imaging and diffusion-weighted imaging. *J Magn Reson Imag* 1998;**8** (2):367–74.

60. Kang BK, Na DG, Ryoo JW, *et al.* Diffusion-weighted MR imaging of intracerebral hemorrhage. *Korean J Radiol* 2001;**2** (4):183–91.

61. Buzdar AU, Singletary SE, Booser DJ, *et al.* Combined modality treatment of stage III and inflammatory breast cancer: M.D. Anderson Cancer Center experience. *Surg Oncol Clin N Am* 1995;**4** (4): 715–34.

62. Partridge SC, Gibbs JE, Lu Y, *et al.* MRI measurements of breast tumor volume predict response to neoadjuvant chemotherapy and recurrence-free survival. *Am J Roentgenol* 2005;**184** (6):1774–81.

63. Wahl RL, Zasadny K, Helvie M, *et al.* Metabolic monitoring of breast cancer chemohormonotherapy using positron emission tomography: initial evaluation. *J Clin Oncol* 1993;**11** (11): 2101–11.

64. Bassa P, Kim EE, Inoue T, *et al.* Evaluation of preoperative chemotherapy using PET with fluorine-18-fluorodeoxyglucose in breast cancer. *J Nucl Med* 1996;**37** (6):931–8.

65. Smith IC, Welch AE, Hutcheon AW, *et al.* Positron emission tomography using [(18)F]-fluorodeoxy-D-glucose to predict the pathologic response of breast cancer to primary chemotherapy. *J Clin Oncol* 2000;**18** (8):1676–88.

66. Schelling M, Avril N, Nahrig J, *et al.* Positron emission tomography using [(18)F]fluorodeoxyglucose for monitoring primary chemotherapy in breast cancer. *J Clin Oncol* 2000;**18** (8):1689–95.

67. Chen X, Moore MO, Lehman CD, *et al.* Combined use of MRI and PET to monitor response and assess residual disease for locally advanced breast cancer treated with neoadjuvant chemotherapy. *Acad Radiol* 2004;**11** (10):1115–24.

68. Galons JP, Altbach MI, Paine-Murrieta GD, Taylor CW, Gillies RJ. Early increases in breast tumor xenograft water mobility in response to

paclitaxel therapy detected by non-invasive diffusion magnetic resonance imaging. *Neoplasia* 1999;**1** (2):113–17.

69. Sharma U, Danishad KK, Seenu V, Jagannathan NR. Longitudinal study of the assessment by MRI and diffusion-weighted imaging of tumor response in patients with locally advanced breast cancer undergoing neoadjuvant chemotherapy. *NMR Biomed* 2009;**22** (1):104–13.

70. Rajan R, Poniecka A, Smith TL, *et al.* Change in tumor cellularity of breast carcinoma after neoadjuvant chemotherapy as a variable in the pathologic assessment of response. *Cancer* 2004; **100** (7):1365–73.

71. Archer CD, Parton M, Smith IE, *et al.* Early changes in apoptosis and proliferation following primary chemotherapy for breast cancer. *Br J Cancer* 2003; **89** (6):1035–41.

Diffusion-weighted MRI of lymph nodes

Taro Takahara and Thomas C. Kwee

Abbreviations

ADC	apparent diffusion coefficient
CT	computed tomography
DWI	diffusion-weighted MRI
DWIBS	diffusion-weighted whole-body imaging with background body signal suppression
EPI	echo-planar imaging
FDG	^{18}F-fluoro-2-deoxyglucose
FNAC	fine-needle aspiration cytology
IVIM	intravoxel incoherent motion
PET	positron emission tomography
ROI	region of interest
SNR	signal-to-noise ratio
STIR	short tau inversion recovery
SUV	standardized uptake value
TR	repetition time
USPIO	ultrasmall superparamagnetic iron oxide

Introduction
Importance of lymph node assessment in oncology

Cancer is a major public health problem in the United States and many other parts of the world. Currently, one in four deaths in the United States is due to cancer. A total of 1 479 350 new cancer cases and 562 340 deaths from cancer are projected to occur in the United States in 2009[1]. After a primary malignant tumor has been detected, it is important to accurately stage the tumor, because this allows appropriate treatment planning and determining prognosis. Asssessment of lymph node status plays a crucial role in the staging work-up of patients with cancer. Prostate cancer and breast cancer, the most frequent types of cancer in men and women, respectively,[1] are very suitable to illustrate the crucial role of nodal staging. In prostate cancer, the detection of a metastasis in a single lymph node can rule out curative treatment[2]. In addition, it has been reported that 10-year survival of patients without lymph node involvement is 57%, whereas that of patients with lymph node involvement is only 17%[3]. Furthermore, axillary lymph nodal status is the most important prognostic factor in the treatment evaluation of patients with newly diagnosed breast cancer[4]; reported 5-year survival for patients without lymph node involvement is 82.8% compared with 73% for 1–3 positive nodes, 45.7% for 4–12 positive nodes, and 28.4% for $\geq$13 positive nodes[5].

Another special patient group consists of those who present with symptomatic lymphadenopathy (i.e., one or more pathologically enlarged lymph nodes) or those in whom lymphadenopathy is incidentally discovered at imaging. Lymphadenopathy has a wide differential diagnosis, but is most frequently due to local or systemic infection. Although more rarely, it can also be caused by a malignant disease[6]. Most patients can be diagnosed on the basis of a careful history and physical examination. However, in case of unexplained lymphadenopathy, it is important to differentiate between benign and

Table 8.1 Results of selected studies correlating lymph node size to metastatic infiltration in several cancer types

Reference	Cancer type	Diameter of lymph nodes (mm)		Lymph nodes ≤10 mm in diameter (%)	
		Non-metastatic	Metastatic	Non-metastatic	Metastatic
Schröder et al.[15]	Esophageal cancer	5.1 ± 3.8	6.7 ± 4.2	89.5	10.5
Mönig et al.[16]	Gastric cancer	4.1 ± 2.7	6.0 ± 4.7	74.9	25.1
Mönig et al.[17]	Colon cancer	3.8 ± 2.3	5.9 ± 3.4	82	18
Prenzel et al.[18]	Lung cancer	7.1 ± 3.8	10.7 ± 4.7	91.6	8.4

malignant causes of lymphadenopathy and, in case of malignancy, to determine which histological classification is applicable, because all these entities have different additional diagnostic, therapeutic, and prognostic implications[6].

Crucial role of imaging

(Sentinel) lymph node biopsy or lymph node dissection, followed by histopathological examination, are considered the gold standard for the assessment of lymph nodes. However, surgical removal of lymph nodes is a costly and invasive procedure with associated complications. In prostate cancer, for example, pelvic lymph node dissection may result in the development of lymphocele, lower extremity edema, deep venous thrombosis/pulmonary embolism, pelvis abscess, ureteral injury, neurovascular injury, and/or ileus[7]. In patients with breast cancer, sentinel node biopsy is a good alternative to immediate axillary lymph node dissection. However, there remains a clinically relevant risk of lymphedema, pain, and impaired shoulder mobility following this procedure[8,9]. Another limitation of surgical lymph node mapping in general is that lymph nodes outside the surgical field are missed. Furthermore, although ultrasound-guided fine-needle aspiration cytology (FNAC) is gaining popularity in the assessment of lymph nodes, it is still an invasive and operator-dependent procedure with a high incidence of false-negative cases[10]. Cross-sectional imaging modalities, including computed tomography (CT), magnetic resonance imaging (MRI), and positron emission tomography (PET), provide a noninvasive approach to visualize and characterize lymph nodes, in the entire body[11]. As such, they may reduce the number of invasive procedures that are needed for lymph node assessment and increase the diagnostic yield of surgical lymph node mapping and FNAC alone. However, imaging has not yet reached the desired accuracy for characterizing lymph nodes[11]. Therefore, the development of more advanced techniques that will decrease the need for invasive lymph node diagnosis is of crucial importance.

From anatomical to functional lymph node imaging

The use of size criteria for determining nodal status by means of anatomical imaging (either ultrasound, CT, or MRI) was established by numerous studies that were published in the 1980s and 1990s[12–14]. Lymph nodes with a (short-axis) diameter larger than 10 mm are generally considered malignant. Since size data are a continuum, the use of a size criterion smaller than 10 mm will increase sensitivity at the expense of specificity and vice versa for a larger size criterion. Size measurements are still the only widely accepted method for discriminating metastatic from non-metastatic lymph nodes in routine clinical practice. However, size criteria are imperfect, because lymph nodes can enlarge as a result of benign inflammatory or infectious processes, and normal-sized lymph nodes may contain (micro)metastatic tumor cells. Morphometric studies of lymph node specimens obtained from patients with cancer have shown that although the mean diameter of non-metastatic lymph nodes is significantly lower than that of metastatic lymph nodes, there is a considerable overlap between both groups. In addition, a considerable proportion of lymph nodes with a diameter equal to or less than 10 mm still contains metastatic tumor cells[15–18]. The results of selected studies on this issue are summarized in Table 8.1. Thus, size criteria cannot be used a reliable indicator for lymph node metastasis.

On the other hand, it is assumable that lymph node pathology may result in altered lymph node function and physiology. Therefore, there is a need for new imaging modalities that go beyond anatomical lymph node assessment and are able to assess functional and physiological processes in the lymph nodes. In this respect, PET (combined with either CT or MRI to improve localization of abnormal radiotracer uptake) and new MRI techniques that offer both anatomical and functional lymph node information have been shown to outperform anatomical imaging alone[19–21]. One of the functional MRI techniques that may be of value in the assessment of lymph nodes is diffusion-weighted MRI (DWI). In this chapter, the rationale for the use of DWI for lymph node assessment, its development to a "volumetric" whole-body imaging modality, and its diagnostic opportunities and limitations in the evaluation of lymph nodes will be reviewed and illustrated. Furthermore, this chapter will discuss novel concepts regarding the use of DWI for the evaluation of lymph nodes.

DWI for lymph node evaluation in the entire body: opportunities and limitations

Rationale

DWI allows visualizing and quantifying diffusion in biological tissue without using any ionizing radiation and without administering any contrast agents or radiotracers, and can be performed in all modern MRI systems[22]. Furthermore, anatomical (T1- and T2-weighted) MRI sequences can be obtained during the same scan session, which may be useful to improve anatomic localization of lymph nodes that are detected at DWI. For these reasons, DWI is a patient- and operator-friendly technique for functional lymph node imaging that can easily be implemented in routine clinical practice. Lymph nodes have a relatively long T2 relaxation time[23,24] and an impeded diffusion due to their high cellularity[25]. Therefore, lymph nodes can generally easily be identified as high signal intensity structures at DWI. Furthermore, assessment of signal intensity at DWI or quantification of diffusion in lymph nodes by means of apparent diffusion coefficient (ADC) measurements may aid in the histological characterization of lymph nodes, because different pathologic processes may lead to differences in diffusion due to differences in cellularity, intracellular architecture, necrosis, and perfusion[22].

Development of "volumetric" whole-body DWI: diffusion-weighted whole-body imaging with background body signal suppression (DWIBS)

The development of high-performance magnetic field gradients and, most importantly, the introduction of parallel imaging, have made DWI feasible in any part of the body[26]. Until recently, breath-hold or respiratory-triggered acquisitions were still the most common approaches to performing DWI in the body, because bulk tissue motion (in particular respiratory motion) was thought to be a serious impediment when performing DWI of moving organs in the chest and (upper) abdomen. However, in a breath-hold acquisition it is impossible to apply a high number of excitations to compensate for the low signal-to-noise ratio (SNR) on high b-value images, due to the availability of only a limited scan time. Consequently, in order to maintain a sufficiently high SNR on high b-value images, thick slices (typically 7–9 mm) should be obtained. However, these thick slices are not suitable to create multiplanar reformats and 3D renderings (such as maximum intensity projections, surface shaded displays, and volume renderings). In addition, given the sizes of the metastatic lymph nodes that are shown in Table 8.1, a minimum slice thickness of 5 mm is recommended for DWI of lymph nodes in order to minimize the effect of partial volume averaging effects on ADC measurements (Figure 8.1). In a respiratory-triggered acquisition, SNR can be increased by applying multiple excitations, which allows obtaining thinner slices. This, in turn, may increase lesion conspicuity at DWI. However, actual scan time of a respiratory-triggered acquisition is approximately two to three times longer than its effective scan time. Therefore, although respiratory triggering is preferred for DWI of upper abdominal organs like the liver, it is not a clinically feasible approach to acquiring whole-body diffusion-weighted images for lymph node evaluation, which is, for example, necessary for staging malignant lymphoma. Furthermore, it should be realized that the repetition time (TR) in a respiratory-triggered acquisition is

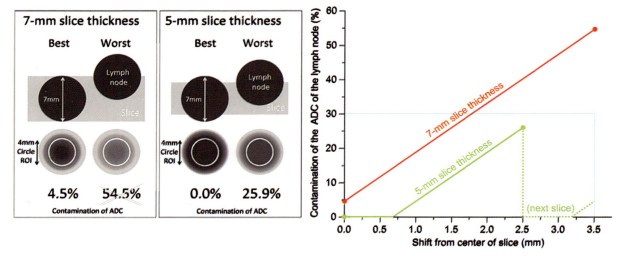

Figure 8.1 Panels and graph illustrating the importance of applying an appropriate (thin) slice thickness for DWI when aiming to obtain accurate ADC measurements of lymph nodes. In this example, it is assumed that the diameter of the lymph node of interest is 7 mm (which is a common size for both non-metastatic and metastatic lymph nodes, as can be seen in Table 8.1) and that a circular region of interest (ROI) with a conservative diameter of 4 mm is used to measure its ADC (in order to avoid contamination of the ADC from surrounding structures that may occur in the peripheral area of the lymph node). Note that the shape of the lymph node in this example is assumed to be spherical, which is a simplification of reality because normal lymph nodes usually tend to have an oval or cigar shape with a central hilum. The best (i.e., most accurate) ADC measurement can be obtained when the lymph node is in the center of the slice. However, when the lymph node shifts outside the center of the slice, ADC measurements will become increasingly inaccurate due to partial volume averaging effects with the surrounding tissue. If the lymph node is exactly at the center of two different slices, the worst (i.e., most inaccurate measurement) will be obtained. When using of a slice thickness of 7 mm, the most accurate ADC measurement will still have a contamination from surrounding tissue of approximately 4.5% and the most inaccurate ADC measurement will have a contamination of approximately 54.5%, which can be considered as unacceptable. On the other hand, when using a slice thickness of 5 mm, ADC measurements will be more accurate, with less than 30% contamination from surrounding tissue, ranging between (approximately) 0% and 25.9%. As we can learn from this simulation, it is necessary to obtain even thinner slices (less than 5 mm) to obtain reasonably accurate ADC measurements of lymph nodes of even smaller size (i.e. less than 7 mm). It should also be realized that non-metastatic lymph nodes are frequently of smaller size than metastatic lymph nodes (Table 8.1), which implies that ADC measurements of the former are generally less accurate than those of the latter.

equal to the respiratory cycle of the patient. If the respiratory cycle and the TR become shorter than four or five times the T1 relaxation time of tissue, recovery of longitudinal magnetization will be incomplete, resulting in less longitudinal magnetization at the time of the next excitation pulse; this will lead to anomalous ADCs[27]. Moreover, the use of a short TR will lead to relatively more signal decrease in metastatic lymph nodes (i.e., decreased visibility) than in normal lymph nodes because malignant tissue, including metastatic lymph nodes, generally has both a long T1 and a long T2 relaxation time.

The limitations of breath-hold and respiratory-triggered acquisitions in the body have relatively recently been overcome by the demonstration of the feasibility of DWI under free breathing, which is also known as the concept of diffusion-weighted whole-body imaging with background body signal suppression (DWIBS)[28]. The feasibility of a free-breathing acquisition can be explained by the fact that

respiratory motion can be considered as *coherent* intravoxel motion during the short period in which the diffusion-sensitizing gradients are applied, and as such, does not result in signal loss at intravoxel *incoherent* motion imaging[29]. Moreover, although DWI is performed under free breathing, there are many relatively motionless periods during image acquisition, for example at the end of expiration. The advantage of DWIBS is the possibility to obtain thin slices with multiple excitations without prolonging scan time (although at the expense of slight image blurring), making it a suitable method to acquire near volumetric whole-body diffusion-weighted images. Furthermore, in DWIBS, high b-values (on the order of 1000 s/mm²) and a long TR (>3000 ms) are applied. Using these parameters, structures with a relatively long T2 relaxation time and impeded diffusion, including (relatively small-sized) lymph nodes, are highlighted, while signal of the majority of surrounding structures (including muscles, vascular structures, and bowel) are

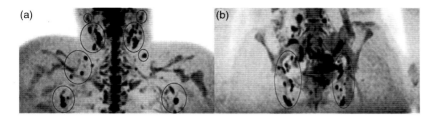

Figure 8.2 DWI in a 23-year-old healthy female. Coronal maximum intensity projection gray-scale inverted diffusion-weighted images (acquired using the concept of diffusion-weighted whole-body imaging with background body signal suppression (DWIBS) and by applying a single-shot spin-echo echo-planar imaging sequence with a b-value of 1000 s/mm^2) of the neck (a) and pelvis (b) highlight normal cervical, supraclavicular, infraclavicular, axillary, pelvic, and inguinal lymph nodes (encircled).

suppressed[28]. Thus, the concept of DWIBS is a very attractive method for the evaluation of lymph nodes throughout the entire body (Figure 8.2).

Lymph node detection

Contrast-to-noise ratio of lymph nodes at DWI is high thanks to the suppression of signals from surrounding normal structures, especially at high b-value. In fact, lymph node-to-background contrast at DWI is superior to that at CT and other MRI sequences. Furthermore, DWI is potentially more useful for the detection of lymph nodes than PET, because attainable spatial resolution of the former is considerably higher than that of the latter. Of note, in a study by Nakai et al.,[30] in 18 patients with uterine cancer who underwent pelvic lymph node dissection, it was shown that only 136 (40%) of 340 dissected lymph nodes were identified on T2-weighted images, whereas 249 (73%) of 340 dissected lymph nodes were identified on diffusion-weighted images in addition to T2-weighted images. Thus, DWI is a good technique to visualize lymph nodes, irrespective of their histological composition. As such, it may provide a map of lymph nodes and draw the attention of the reader to suspicious lymph nodes that may require further characterization by means of ADC measurements or other methods such as ultrasmall superparamagnetic iron oxide (USPIO)-enhanced high-resolution T2*-weighted imaging[31,32] or PET (given the anticipated advent of combined PET/MRI systems)[33]. However, although lymph node detectability is generally good at DWI (especially in the head, neck, axillary, pelvic, and inguinal regions), lymph nodes close to the heart (e.g., mediastinal and hilar lymph nodes) are less well depicted because cardiac motion causes intravoxel incoherent motion (IVIM) and consequent signal loss of adjacent structures.

Diagnosis of lymphadenopathy

Several studies[34–42] have investigated the value of DWI with ADC measurements for the differentiation between various causes of lymphadenopathy, with all but two[38,42] being performed in patients with cervical lymphadenopathy. The results of these studies[34–42] are summarized in Table 8.2. Importantly, it should be realized that the results of these studies are only applicable to pathologically enlarged lymph nodes, because most of the analyzed lymph nodes were larger than 10 mm in the short-axis diameter. A consistent finding in several studies[34,35,39,40] was that ADCs of malignant lymphomas were significantly lower than those of metastatic and benign lymphadenopathies (Figure 8.3). This can be explained by the fact that malignant lymphomas mostly consist of densely packed cellular tissue with very little extracellular space[25], which considerably impedes the diffusivity of water molecules. It can be speculated that ADCs of metastatic and benign lymphadenopathy are higher because of relatively lower cellularity, lower nucleus-to-cytoplasm ratios, more (micro)necrosis, and/or a higher perfusion due to hypervascularity[25]. Several studies[34–36,38,39,41,42] also showed a significant difference in ADCs between metastatic and benign lymphadenopathy. Interestingly, however, the direction of this difference was variable; two studies[34,35] reported that ADCs of benign lymphadenopathy were lower than those of metastatic lymphadenopathy, whereas five other studies[36,38,39,41,42] reported the opposite. One possible explanation for this discrepancy is the inclusion or exclusion of necrotic areas in the ADC measurements. Another interesting observation is that reported ADCs within the groups metastatic lymphadenopathy (range, [0.410–1.423] $\times$ 10^{-3} mm^2/s), benign lymphadenopathy ([0.302–1.64] $\times$ 10^{-3} mm^2/s),

Table 8.2 ADCs of different types of lymphadenopathies (i.e., pathologically enlarged lymph nodes)

Reference	b-values (s/mm^2)	Method of ADC measurement	Type of lymphadenopathy (n)	Mean ADC ± SD (× 10^{-3} mm^2/s)	Pairwise comparisons
Sumi et al.[34]	500, 1000	Average of one to four lymph node sections	1. Metastatic (25)[a] 2. Benign (25) 3. Lymphoma (5)[b]	0.410 ± 0.105 0.302 ± 0.062 0.223 ± 0.056	1 vs. 2; $p < 0.01$ 1 vs. 3; $p < 0.01$ 2 vs. 3; $p < 0.05$
Sumi et al.[35]	500, 1000	All lymph node sections	1. Metastatic (24)[a] 2. Benign (35) 3. Lymphoma (14)[c]	1.167 ± 0.447 0.652 ± 0.101 0.601 ± 0.427	1 vs. 2; $p < 0.001$ 1 vs. 3; $p < 0.001$ 2 vs. 3; $p < 0.01$
Abdel Razek et al.[36]	0, 1000	Single lymph node section	1. Metastatic (51)[a] 2. Benign (15) 3. Lymphoma (21)[c]	1.09 ± 0.11 1.64 ± 0.16 0.97 ± 0.27	1 vs. 2; $p < 0.04$ 1 vs. 3; NS 2 vs. 3; $p < 0.04$
King et al.[37]	0, 100, 200, 300, 400, 500	All lymph node sections	1. Metastatic (18)[a] 2. Metastatic (17)[d] 3. Lymphoma (8)[c]	1.163 ± 0.228 0.845 ± 0.109 0.739 ± 0.107	1 vs. 2; $p < 0.001$ 1 vs. 3; $p < 0.001$ 2 vs. 3; $p = 0.171$
		Single lymph node section, no necrotic areas	1. Metastatic (18)[a] 2. Metastatic (17)[d] 3. Lymphoma (8)[c]	1.057 ± 0.169 0.802 ± 0.128 0.664 ± 0.071	1 vs. 2; $p < 0.001$ 1 vs. 3; $p < 0.001$ 2 vs. 3; $p = 0.04$
Akduman et al.[38]	0, 600	NR	1. Metastatic (16)[e] 2. Benign (40)	1.84 ± 0.37 2.38 ± 0.29	1 vs. 2; $p < 0.0005$
Holzapfel et al.[39]	0, 500, 1000	Single lymph node section, no necrotic areas	1. Metastatic (25)[a] 2. Benign (24) 3. Lymphoma (6)[b]	0.78 ± 0.09 1.24 ± 0.16 0.64 ± 0.09	1 vs. 2; $p < 0.05$ 1 vs. 3; $p < 0.05$ 2 vs. 3; $p < 0.05$
Sumi & Nakamura[40]	500, 1000	All lymph node sections	1. Metastatic (88)[a] 2. Lymphoma (79)[c]	1.092 ± 0.436 0.587 ± 0.334	1 vs. 2; $p < 0.001$
			1. Metastatic without focal necrosis (18)[a] 2. Lymphoma without focal necrosis (62)[c]	0.960 ± 0.310 0.449 ± 0.096	1 vs. 2; $p < 0.001$
			1. Metastatic with focal necrosis (63)[a] 2. Lymphoma with focal necrosis (17)[c]	1.423 ± 0.529 1.091 ± 0.405	1 vs. 2; $p = 0.057$
			1. Focal necrotic defects in metastasis (63)[a] 2. Focal necrotic defects in lymphoma (17)[c]	1.905 ± 0.6401 1.091 ± 0.405	1 vs. 2; $p < 0.001$
Koşucu et al.[41]	50, 400	NR	1. Metastatic (19)[f] 2. Benign (72)	1.012 ± 0.025 1.511 ± 0.075	1 vs. 2; $p < 0.0005$
Perrone et al.[42]	0, 500, 1000	All lymph node sections, no necrotic areas	1. Metastatic or lymphoma (14)[c,g] 2. Benign (17)	0.85 ± NR 1.448 ± NR	1 vs. 2; $p < 0.01$

Notes: [a]Metastatic lymph nodes from primary squamous cell carcinoma in the head and neck region.
[b]Non-Hodgkin lymphoma.
[c]Non-Hodgkin lymphoma and Hodgkin disease.
[d]Metastatic lymph nodes from nasopharyngeal carcinoma.
[e]Metastatic lymph nodes in patients with various abdominal malignancies or lung cancer.
[f]Metastatic lymph nodes from non-small cell or small cell lung cancer.
[g]Metastatic lymph nodes from squamous cell carcinoma or rhabdomyosarcoma.
NR, not reported; NS, not significant.

(a)

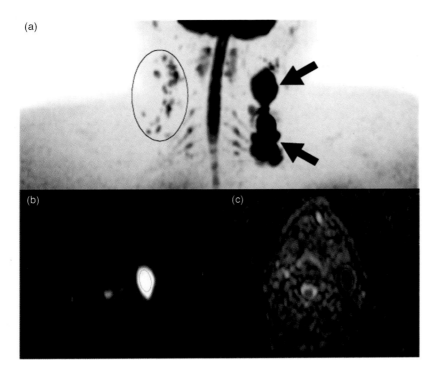

(b)

(c)

Figure 8.3 DWI in a 56-year-old male who presented with cervical lymphadenopathy. Coronal maximum intensity projection gray-scale inverted diffusion-weighted image (acquired using the concept of diffusion-weighted whole-body imaging with background body signal suppression (DWIBS) and by applying a single-shot spin-echo echo-planar imaging sequence with a b-value of 1000 s/mm^2) (a) shows a large left-cervical/infraclavicular mass (arrows). Note several normal-sized contralateral cervical lymph nodes (encircled). Axial source diffusion-weighted image (b) and corresponding ADC map (created using b-values of 0 and 1000 s/mm^2 (c) with region of interest in the pathologically enlarged cervical lymph node revealed a relatively low ADC of $(0.54 \pm 0.07) \times 10^{-3}$ mm^2/s, suggestive of malignant lymphoma. Subsequent excisional biopsy and histopathological analysis of the cervical lymph node established the diagnosis of mantle cell lymphoma.

and lymphomatous lymphadenopathy (range, $[0.223–1.091] \times 10^{-3}$ mm^2/s) vary widely (Table 8.2)[34–42]. These observations can be attributed to several causes. First, different b-values were used; the use of a relatively low minimum b-value (e.g., <150 s/mm^2) for the calculation of the ADC includes perfusion effects and results in an ADC that is an overestimation of the true diffusion coefficient[22]. Second, as mentioned previously, the method of ADC measurement varied; above all, the inclusion of necrotic areas can lead to considerably higher ADCs[40]. Third, different histological subtypes were included, which may all have different ADCs due to differences in tissue architecture. Fourth, ADC measurements may vary due to imperfect inter- and intra-observer reproducibility. Fifth, a number of instrumental factors can give rise to random or systematic errors in estimates of the ADC. Random errors can arise from image noise and motion artifacts. Systematic errors can arise from incorrect values used for the diffusion gradient amplitudes, the presence of imaging, susceptibility, or eddy current gradient cross-terms unaccounted for in the b-value calculation, errors in the b-value calculation, image noise, and gradient calibration inaccuracy[43]. Because of these issues, no cut-off ADC values can currently

be recommended to differentiate the different causes of lymphadenopathy. For the same reason, and because studies determined their cut-off ADC values by applying post-hoc analyses of their data (which may have lead to an inflated accuracy of ADC measurements),[34–37,39,40,42] it is currently difficult to provide a general statement on the performance of ADC measurements in diagnosing lymphadenopathy in terms of sensitivity and specificity.

Nodal staging

As mentioned previously, DWI is an excellent method for lymph node detection. Although imperfect,[15–18] classical size criteria may be used for discriminating metastatic from non-metastatic lymph nodes that are detected at DWI. However, because of the lack of an anatomical reference, size measurements of lymph nodes at DWI are highly dependent on the applied window level and window width. In addition, there are no published studies comparing nodal measurements at DWI with those at conventional imaging (either CT or T1- and T2-weighted images). Thus, at present, it is recommended that sizes of lymph nodes that are suspicious for malignancy at DWI are

Table 8.3 ADCs in nodal staging (i.e., lymph node characterization in patients with primary cancer)

Reference	b-values (s/mm²)	Method of ADC measurement	Lymph node status (n)	Mean ADC ± SD (× 10^{-3} mm²/s)	Pairwise comparisons
De Bondt et al.[21]	0, 1000	All lymph node sections, no necrotic areas	1. Metastatic (26)[a] 2. Non-metastatic (191)[b]	0.85 ± 0.19 1.2 ± 0.24	1 vs. 2; $p < 0.05$
Nakai et al.[30]	0, 800	NR	1. Metastatic (7)[c] 2. Non-metastatic (134)[d]	1.4 ± 0.4 1.3 ± 0.24	1 vs. 2; $p = 0.28$
Lin et al.[44]	0, 1000	Single lymph node section	1. Metastatic (12)[c] 2. Non-metastatic (71)[d]	0.83 ± 0.15 0.75 ± 0.19	1 vs. 2; $p = 0.639$
Kim et al.[45]	0, 1000	Single lymph node section	1. Metastatic (30)[c] 2. Non-metastatic (220)[d]	0.7651 ± 0.1137 1.0021 ± 0.1859	1 vs. 2; $p < 0.001$
Park et al.[46]	0, 1000	Single lymph node section	1. Metastatic (29)[c] 2. Non-metastatic (226)[d]	0.748 ± 0.160 0.996 ± 0.196	1 vs. 2; $p < 0.01$
Vandecaveye et al.[47]	0, 1000	All lymph node sections, no necrotic areas	1. Metastatic (74)[a] 2. Non-metastatic (227)[b]	0.85 ± 0.27 1.19 ± 0.22	1 vs. 2; $p < 0.001$
Sakurada et al.[48]	0, 1000	Single lymph node section	1. Metastatic (NR)[e] 2. Non-metastatic (NR)[f]	1.46 ± 0.35 1.15 ± 0.25	1 vs. 2; $p < 0.001$
Yasui et al.[49]	0, 800	NR	1. Metastatic (76)[g] 2. Non-metastatic (87)[h]	1.36 ± 0.42 1.85 ± 0.53	1 vs. 2; $p = 0.001$

Notes: [a]Metastatic lymph nodes from primary squamous cell carcinoma in the head and neck region.
[b]Non-metastatic lymph nodes in patients with primary squamous cell carcinoma in the head and neck region.
[c]Metastatic lymph nodes from cervical or uterine cancer.
[d]Non-malignant lymph nodes (not further specified) in patients with cervical or uterine cancer
[e]Metastatic lymph nodes from esophageal cancer.
[f]Non-metastatic lymph nodes in patients with esophageal cancer.
[g]Metastatic lymph nodes from colorectal cancer.
[h]Non-metastatic lymph nodes in patients with colorectal cancer.
NS, not significant; NR, not reported.

measured on conventional T1-weighted or T2-weighted images for verification.

Several studies[21,30,44–49] have investigated the value of DWI with ADC measurements for nodal staging. It is expected that malignant tissue, including metastatic lymph nodes, generally exhibits hypercellularity, increased nucleus-to-cytoplasm ratios, and an increased amount of macromolecular proteins[25], resulting in decreased diffusion in the extra- and intracellular compartments compared to normal lymph nodes[22]. However, it is important to pay attention to the difference between the detection of metastases in lymph nodes and the detection of primary tumors or metastases in other tissues. In contrast to other organs like the liver, kidneys, or lungs, normal lymph nodes already have a relatively long T2 relaxation time and an impeded diffusion due

to their high cellularity. Thus, it should be realized that it is generally more difficult to detect metastases in lymph nodes than detecting cancerous lesions in other tissues. Results of studies investigating the value of ADC measurements for nodal staging are summarized in Table 8.3. Importantly, the majority of analyzed lymph nodes in these studies were of normal size (i.e., they measured less than 10 mm in the short-axis diameter); these lymph nodes are, in contrast to pathologically enlarged lymph nodes, the ones that pose the most diagnostic difficulties in nodal staging. Six studies[21,45–49] found a significant difference in ADCs between metastatic and non-metastatic lymph nodes, indicating that ADC measurements may increase the diagnostic performance of size measurements alone. In five of six studies,[21,45–47,49] ADCs of metastatic lymph nodes were significantly lower than those of non-metastatic lymph nodes. This can be explained by the fact that malignant tissue generally exhibits hypercellularity, increased nucleus-to-cytoplasm ratios, and an increased amount of macro-molecular proteins,[25] resulting in an decreased diffusion in the extra- and intracellular compartments[22]. However, one study in patients with esophageal cancer (mainly squamous cell carcinoma type)[48] reported the ADCs of metastatic lymph nodes to be significantly higher than those of non-metastatic lymph nodes. On the other hand, two studies[30,44] reported that ADCs of metastatic and non-metastatic lymph nodes were not significantly different. As mentioned previously, because of the use of different b-values, different methods of ADC measurement, inter- and intra-observer reproducibility issues in ADC measurements, the inclusion of different histological subtypes, the possible effect of instrumental factors in the different studies, and the post-hoc determination of cut-off values by the different studies,[21,44–49] no general cut-off ADC value can currently be recommended that would yield a certain sensitivity and specificity for the differentiation between metastatic and non-metastatic lymph nodes.

Comparative studies with other imaging modalities are still largely lacking. However, one study[50] compared minimum ADC measurements to (modified) standardized uptake value (SUV) measurements from ^{18}F-fluoro-2-deoxyglucose (FDG)-PET for nodal staging in 88 patients with non-small cell lung cancer. A minimum ADC value of 1.6×10^{-3} mm^2/s proved to be the best cut-off value for discriminating metastatic from non-metastatic lymph nodes, with metastatic lymph nodes having minimum ADCs below this cut-off value. Diagnostic accuracy of DWI with minimum ADC measurements for nodal staging was 89% (78/88), whereas that of FDG-PET/CT with (modified) SUV measurements was 78% (69/88); this difference was statistically significant ($p = 0.012$). In addition, specificity of DWI for nodal staging was significantly higher ($p = 0.002$) than that of FDG-PET/CT. Thus, this study indicates that DWI may be a potential alternative to FDG-PET/CT for nodal staging in non-small cell lung cancer, with fewer false-positive results[50]. However, a significant limitation of Nomori *et al.*'s study[50] is that only lymph nodes with a long-axis diameter of more than 10 mm were analyzed.

An important issue is the reproducibility of ADC measurements of lymph nodes; especially normal-sized lymph nodes may be less reliable to measure due the combination of image distortions (especially adjacent to air-containing organs), insufficient spatial resolution, and partial volume averaging effects (Figure 8.1). One study[51] performed an inter- and intra-observer reproducibility analysis regarding ADC measurements of normal-sized lymph nodes. In this study[51] that used a standard protocol for (whole-body) DWI, mean ADC difference $\pm$ limits of agreement (in 10^{-3} mm^2/s) for inter-observer agreement were as high as 0.02 ± 0.31. In addition, mean ADC difference $\pm$ limits of agreement (in 10^{-3} mm^2/s) for intra-observer agreement were as high as 0.04 ± 0.32. Given these relatively large limits of agreement, inter- and intra-observer reproducibility of ADC measurements of normal-sized lymph nodes can be considered as rather poor. It can be argued that the use of improved echo-planar imaging (EPI) technology, dedicated coils, and dedicated sequence optimization may improve spatial resolution and reduce susceptibility and motion artifacts, as a result of which reliability and reproducibility of ADC measurements may improve. However, another important issue is that although tissue diffusivity may differ between metastatic and non-metastatic lymph nodes, there is a considerable overlap (Table 8.3 and Figure 8.4), as various conditions such as ischemia and inflammation also reduce ADC. In addition, false-negative ADC measurements may occur in case of a low intranodal metastatic volume, because this is

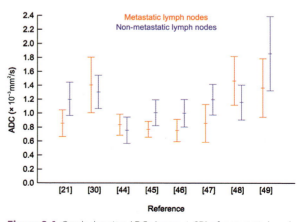

Figure 8.4 Graph showing ADCs (mean $\pm$ SD) of metastatic lymph nodes compared to those of non-metastatic lymph nodes per study. Although ADCs generally differ between both groups, there is considerable overlap.

less likely to form sufficient tissue boundaries to impede water diffusion. Therefore, clinical utility of ADC measurements in the assessment of lymph nodes is still questionable.

Whole-body DWI for staging malignant lymphoma

One of the most promising applications of whole-body DWI (using the concept of DWIBS) lies in the evaluation of patients with malignant lymphoma. Unlike CT and FDG-PET/CT, MRI does not use any ionizing radiation or iodinated contrast agents, which may cause secondary cancers and induce allergic reactions, respectively[52,53]. Malignant lymphomas are characterized by a relatively long T2 relaxation time and a considerably impeded diffusion[34–37,39,40,42]. Therefore, malignant lymphomas exhibit a very high signal intensity at DWI. The high lesion-to-background contrast of DWI is expected to improve staging performance of conventional (T1- and T2-weighted) whole-body MRI alone. One study[54] compared a combination of conventional whole-body MRI (T1-weighted and short tau inversion recovery [STIR] sequences) and whole-body DWI to CT for the staging of 28 patients with newly diagnosed malignant lymphoma. Lymphomatous lesions were diagnosed at MRI based on size criteria and signal abnormalities. Staging results of combined conventional whole-body MRI and whole-body DWI were equal to those of CT in 75% (21/28), higher in 25% (7/28), and lower in 0% (0/28) of patients, with correct/incorrect overstaging relative to CT in 6 and 1 patient(s), respectively. Interestingly, the combination of conventional whole-body MRI with whole-body DWI correctly upstaged 4 of 28 patients compared to conventional whole-body MRI alone, which well reflects the potential additional diagnostic value of DWI[54]. Nevertheless, although these initial results appear very promising, more studies with larger sample sizes are needed, and whole-body DWI should also be compared to FDG-PET(/CT). Furthermore, attempts should be made to develop ADC criteria for discriminating normal lymph nodes from lymphomatous lymph nodes in the staging work-up of patients with malignant lymphoma; this would especially be helpful in the assessment of borderline lymph nodes. Figure 8.5 shows an example of whole-body DWI in a patient with malignant lymphoma.

Challenges and future considerations
Normalization of ADC

ADC measurements have an inherent limitation with regard to the general application of a certain threshold due to variances in acquisition protocols, method of ADC measurements, and the possible effect of instrumental errors. For this reason, it can be argued that each center should develop its own ADC criteria for each MRI system. To overcome this limitation, and to allow future meta-analyses and comparisons of results of different studies, it has been proposed to normalize the ADC[44,46]. In this context, Lin et al.[44] proposed to calculate a relative ADC by subtracting the mean ADC of the lymph node from the mean ADC of the primary tumor; this approach is based on the hypothesis that metastatic lymph nodes exhibit a cellularity and/or microarchitecture similar to that of the primary tumor, and that their ADCs are similar. In their study in 50 patients with cervical or uterine cancers, Lin et al.[44] indeed showed that the relative ADC of metastatic lymph nodes ($[0.06 \pm 0.03] \times 10^{-3}$ mm^2/s) was significantly lower ($p < 0.001$) than that of non-metastatic lymph nodes ($[0.21 \pm 0.18] \times 10^{-3}$ mm^2/s), whereas the conventional ADC was not significantly different between the groups. Park et al.[46] investigated which anatomical reference site (spleen, liver, renal cortex, lumbar spine, lumbar spinal cord, or gluteus maximus) would be most suitable for normalizing the ADC of lymph nodes in 50 patients with uterine cervical cancer. The renal cortex proved to be the most suitable reference site in terms of inter- and intra-observer reproducibility of ADC measurements. The relative ADC (defined as ADC lymph node/ADC renal cortex) of metastatic lymph nodes (0.3832 ± 0.080) was significantly lower ($p < 0.01$) than that of non-metastatic lymph nodes (0.538 ± 0.111). In addition, although the conventional ADC was also different between the groups, area under the receiver operating characteristic curve was significantly higher ($p = 0.007$) for the relative ADC (0.914) than for the normal ADC (0.872). However, although a normalized ADC may be more generally applicable and even more accurate than a conventional ADC,[44,46] it still does not solve the diagnostic difficulties related to the overlap in ADCs between metastatic and non-metastatic lymph nodes. Another method for the assessment of lymph nodes at DWI that can generally be applied consists of dividing the

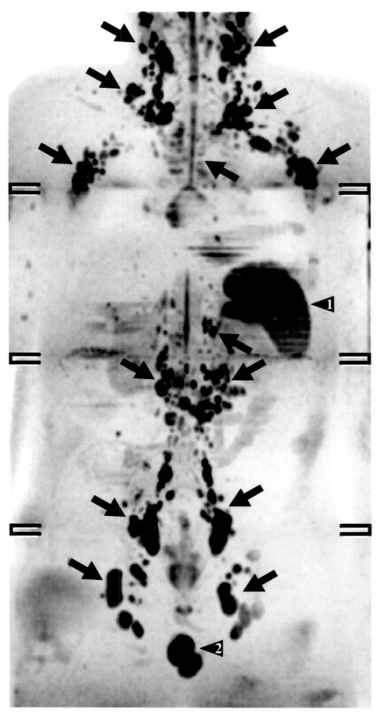

Figure 8.5 Whole-body DWI in a 47-year-old male with Ann Arbor stage III follicular lymphoma. Coronal maximum intensity projection gray-scale inverted diffusion-weighted image (acquired using the concept of diffusion-weighted whole-body imaging with background body signal suppression (DWIBS) and by applying a single-shot sp n-echo EPI sequence with a b-value of 1000 s/mm^2) shows widespread supra- and infradiaphragmatic lymph node involvement (arrows). Also note normal high signal intensity of the spleen (arrowhead 1) and testis (arrowhead 2).

signal intensity of the lymph node of interest by the signal intensity of a reference organ (e.g., the spinal cord) on native diffusion-weighted images. The advantage of such semi-quantitative measurements on native diffusion-weighted images over ADC-based measurements is that it takes into account both diffusion and T2 relaxation time (which is often prolonged in malignant tissue)[55]. Furthermore, unlike ADC measurements, such an approach does not suffer from measurement errors due to misregistration of images with different b-values. Nevertheless, the exact value of this method still has to be established.

Ultrasmall superparamagnetic iron oxide-enhanced DWI

DWI is an excellent method for the detection of lymph nodes, but its diagnostic performance may be limited due to overlap in ADCs between metastatic and non-metastatic lymph nodes, as was outlined in previous sections. Therefore, there is a need for improved imaging techniques. USPIO-enhanced MRI was introduced in the beginning of the 1990s as a promising method for nodal staging, irrespective of size[31]. USPIO particles are taken up by macrophages in the reticuloendothelial system, predominantly within the lymph nodes. Normal homogeneous uptake of USPIO particles in non-metastatic lymph nodes shortens the T2 and T2* relaxation times, turning these lymph nodes hypointense on T2- and T2*-weighted images, whereas malignant lymph nodes lack uptake and remain hyperintense[31]. Will et al.[32] performed a meta-analysis of 38 studies that investigated the diagnostic performance of USPIO-enhanced MRI for nodal staging in various tumors, and reported that overall (lymph node-based) sensitivity and specificity of USPIO-enhanced MRI (88% and 96%, respectively) were higher than those of unenhanced MRI (63% and 93%, respectively). However, because of the low lymph node-to-background contrast at conventional (T1-, T2, and T2*-weighted) MRI sequences, detectability of lymph nodes is relatively low at conventional USPIO-enhanced MRI. Consequently, image interpretation can be very time-consuming, and malignant lymph nodes of small size may be missed. Similar to T2*-weighted imaging, diffusion-weighted EPI is very susceptible to magnetic field inhomogeneities that are caused by the USPIO particles. Performing DWI after USPIO

administration may overcome disadvantages of DWI and conventional USPIO-enhanced MRI alone. Theoretically, in USPIO-enhanced DWI only malignant lymph nodes are highlighted; the high metastatic lymph node-to-background contrast will reduce image interpretation time and may increase sensitivity for the detection of small metastatic lymph nodes. The feasibility of this new concept has recently been proven in a study involving 28 patients with urinary bladder and prostate cancer[56]. In this study,[56] (patient-based and pelvis side-based) diagnostic accuracies for the detection of lymph node metastasis were comparable between USPIO-enhanced DWI and conventional USPIO-enhanced MRI (both 90%), but interpretation time of the former (median, 13 min; range, 5–90 min) was significantly shorter ($p < 0.0001$) than that of the latter (median, 80 min; range, 45–180 min). Although a very promising method, attention should be paid to possible over-suppression by USPIO contrast agents, as a result of which micrometastases may be missed. Thus, studies investigating the most appropriate dose of USPIO contrast agents and optimization of the DWI sequence (in terms of sensitivity to susceptibility effects) are necessary to fully exploit this new concept. Another, perhaps more important, issue is that the availability of USPIO contrast agents is currently limited, and currently still not FDA approved in the United States. Nevertheless, USPIO-enhanced DWI has great potential and may become a very important method for nodal staging in the near future.

Short inversion time inversion recovery and single-axis DWI

Given the (considerable) overlap in ADCs between metastatic and non-metastatic lymph nodes and the very promising results of USPIO-enhanced MRI in nodal staging[32], it is likely that the main role of DWI will shift towards lymph node detection rather than lymph node characterization. Diffusion-weighted images are most frequently acquired by using spectral fat saturation and by applying diffusion-sensitizing gradients in three orthogonal directions, which yields a trace (isotropic) image. However, a STIR pre-pulse provides superior fat suppression over an extended field of view compared to spectral fat saturation[57]. Furthermore, STIR may also be useful for suppressing bowel signal, which often has a short T1 relaxation time[28]. Thus, the use of STIR may improve lymph

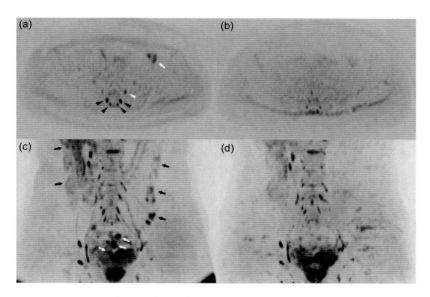

Figure 8.6 Trace DWI (acquired by applying pairs of diffusion-sensitizing gradients in three orthogonal directions) with spectral fat saturation compared to single-axis DWI (acquired by applying only one pair of diffusion-sensitizing gradients in the superior–inferior direction) with STIR in a 28-year-old healthy male. All images were acquired using the concept of diffusion-weighted whole-body imaging with background body signal suppression (DWIBS) and by applying a single-shot spin-echo echo-planar imaging sequence with a b-value of 1000 s/mm². Axial gray-scale inverted trace diffusion-weighted image obtained with spectral fat saturation (a) shows sacral nerves and ganglia as high signal intensity structures (black arrowheads), one of them mimicking a lymph node (white arrowhead). Also note high signal intensity of the bowel, making the image "crowded." Corresponding coronal maximum intensity projection gray-scale inverted trace diffusion-weighted image obtained with spectral fat saturation (c) shows high signal intensity of the bowel system (black arrows), which may obscure lymph nodes. Note that some of the bowel signal looks very similar to lymph nodes (white arrows). Axial (b) and coronal maximum intensity projection (d) gray-scale inverted single-axis diffusion-weighted image obtained with STIR suffers considerably less from unwanted signals that may mimic, overlap, or obscure lymph nodes. This is because the application of only one pair of diffusion-sensitizing gradients in the superior–inferior direction suppresses the nerves of the lumbosacral plexus, and STIR suppresses bowel signal because it often has a short T1 relaxation time.

node conspicuity at DWI, especially in the abdomen and pelvis. Other structures that are frequently highlighted at DWI are the peripheral nerves, because of their relatively long T2 relaxation time and impeded diffusivity[58]. Peripheral nerves may mimic (on axial images), overlap, or obscure (on coronal maximum intensity projection images) lymph nodes at DWI, especially in the brachial plexus (neck) and lumbosacral plexus (pelvic) regions. It is well known that diffusion in the human nervous system is anisotropic[59]. In other words, diffusion is more impeded perpendicular to the course of the nerves, while the highest diffusivity can be expected parallel to the course of the nerves. Since the nerves of the brachial and lumbosacral plexus mainly course in a superior–inferior direction, these nerves can theoretically be suppressed by applying only one pair of diffusion-sensitizing gradients in the superior–inferior direction. Note that an opposite approach (e.g., applying one pair of diffusion-sensitizing gradients in the anterior–posterior direction) will offer the highest signal of the nerves[60]. Thus, similar to the use of STIR, a single-axis DWI approach may improve lymph node detectability. Figure 8.6 shows an example of trace DWI with spectral fat saturation compared to single-axis DWI with STIR.

Conclusion

DWI is a non-invasive method for functional lymph node assessment. It is particularly useful for the detection of lymph nodes and may, to a certain extent, aid in the diagnosis of lymphadenopathy and in discriminating metastatic from non-metastatic lymph nodes. However, DWI may have some diagnostic difficulties in the characterization of lymph nodes, because diffusion properties of different nodal pathologies and normal lymph nodes overlap, and because of the limited spatial resolution of DWI. Thus, it is likely that the main role of DWI will shift towards lymph

115

node detection rather than lymph node characterization. Combining DWI with USPIO contrast agents has great potential and may become a very important method for nodal staging in the near future.

References

1. Jemal A, Siegel R, Ward E, *et al*. Cancer statistics, 2009. *CA Cancer J Clin* 2009;**59**:225–49.

2. Damber JE, Aus G. Prostate cancer. *Lancet* 2008;**371**:1710–21.

3. Gervasi LA, Mata J, Easley JD, *et al*. Prognostic significance of lymph nodal metastases in prostate cancer. *J Urol* 1989;**142**:332–6.

4. Banerjee M, George J, Song EY, Roy A, Hryniuk W. Tree-based model for breast cancer prognostication. *J Clin Oncol* 2004;**22**:2567–75.

5. Fisher B, Bauer M, Wickerham DL, and other NASAAB P investigators. Relation of number of positive axillary nodes to the prognosis of patients with primary breast cancer: an NSABP update. *Cancer* 1983;**52**:1551–7.

6. Ferrer R. Lymphadenopathy: differential diagnosis and evaluation. *Am Fam Physician* 1998;**58**:1313–20.

7. Allaf ME, Partin AW, Carter HB. The importance of pelvic lymph node dissection in men with clinically localized prostate cancer. *Rev Urol* 2006;**8**:112–19.

8. McLaughlin SA, Wright MJ, Morris KT, *et al*. Prevalence of lymphedema in women with breast cancer 5 years after sentinel lymph node biopsy or axillary dissection: objective measurements. *J Clin Oncol* 2008;**26**:5213–19.

9. Del Bianco P, Zavagno G, Burelli P, *et al*. Morbidity comparison of sentinel lymph node biopsy versus conventional axillary lymph node dissection for breast cancer patients: results of the sentinella-GIVOM Italian randomised clinical trial. *Eur J Surg Oncol* 2008;**34**:508–13.

10. Castelijns JA, van den Brekel MW. Imaging of lymphadenopathy in the neck. *Eur Radiol* 2002;**12**:727–38.

11. Torabi M, Aquino SL, Harisinghani MG. Current concepts in lymph node imaging. *J Nucl Med* 2004;**45**:1509–18.

12. Glazer GM, Gross BH, Quint LE, *et al*. Normal mediastinal lymph nodes: number and size according to American Thoracic Society mapping. *Am J Roentgenol* 1985;**144**:261–5.

13. Van den Brekel MW, Stel HV, Castelijns JA, *et al*. Cervical lymph node metastasis: assessment of radiologic criteria. *Radiology* 1990;**177**:379–84.

14. Dorfman RE, Alpern MB, Gross BH, Sandler MA. Upper abdominal lymph nodes: criteria for normal size determined with CT. *Radiology* 1991;**180**:319–22.

15. Schröder W, Baldus SE, Mönig SP, *et al*. Lymph node staging of esophageal squamous cell carcinoma in patients with and without neoadjuvant radiochemotherapy: histomorphologic analysis. *World J Surg* 2002;**26**:584–7.

16. Mönig SP, Zirbes TK, Schröder W, *et al*. Staging of gastric cancer: correlation of lymph node size and metastatic infiltration. *Am J Roentgenol* 1999;**173**:365–7.

17. Mönig SP, Baldus SE, Zirbes TK, *et al*. Lymph node size and metastatic infiltration in colon cancer. *Ann Surg Oncol* 1999;**6**:579–81.

18. Prenzel KL, Mönig SP, Sinning JM, *et al*. Lymph node size and metastatic infiltration in non-small cell lung cancer. *Chest* 2003;**123**:463–7.

19. Kyzas PA, Evangelou E, Denaxa-Kyza D, Ioannidis JP. ^{18}F-fluorodeoxyglucose positron emission tomography to evaluate cervical node metastases in patients with head and neck squamous cell carcinoma: a meta-analysis. *J Natl Cancer Inst* 2008;**100**:712–20.

20. Will O, Purkayastha S, Chan C, *et al*. Diagnostic precision of nanoparticle-enhanced MRI for lymph-node metastases: a meta-analysis. *Lancet Oncol* 2006;**7**:52–60.

21. De Bondt RB, Hoeberigs MC, Nelemans PJ, *et al*. Diagnostic accuracy and additional value of diffusion-weighted imaging for discrimination of malignant cervical lymph nodes in head and neck squamous cell carcinoma. *Neuroradiology* 2009;**51**:183–92.

22. Padhani AR, Liu G, Koh DM, *et al*. Diffusion-weighted magnetic resonance imaging as a cancer biomarker: consensus and recommendations. *Neoplasia* 2009;**11**:102–25.

23. Glazer GM, Orringer MB, Chenevert TL, *et al*. Mediastinal lymph nodes: relaxation time/pathologic correlation and implications in staging of lung cancer with MR imaging. *Radiology* 1988;**168**:429–31.

24. Ranade SS, Trivedi PN, Bamane VS. Mediastinal lymph nodes: relaxation time/pathologic correlation and implications in staging of lung cancer with MR imaging. *Radiology* 1990;**174**:284–5.

25. Ioachim HL, Medeiros LJ. *Ioachim's Lymph Node Pathology*. Philadelphia, PA: Lippincott Williams and Wilkins; 2009.

26. Koh DM, Collins DJ. Diffusion-weighted MRI in the body: applications and challenges in oncology. *Am J Roentgenol* 2007;**188**:1622–35.

27. Shiehmorteza M, Sirlin CB, Wolfson T, *et al*. Effect of shot number on the calculated apparent diffusion

coefficient in phantoms and in human liver in diffusion-weighted echo-planar imaging. *J Magn Reson Imag* 2009;**30**:547–53.

28. Takahara T, Imai Y, Yamashita T, *et al.* Diffusion weighted whole body imaging with background body signal suppression (DWIBS): technical improvement using free breathing, STIR and high resolution 3D display. *Radiat Med* 2004;**22**:275–82.

29. Le Bihan D, Breton E, Lallemand D, *et al.* MR imaging of intravoxel incoherent motions: application to diffusion and perfusion in neurologic disorders. *Radiology* 1986;**161**:401–7.

30. Nakai G, Matsuki M, Inada Y, *et al.* Detection and evaluation of pelvic lymph nodes in patients with gynecologic malignancies using body diffusion-weighted magnetic resonance imaging. *J Comput Assist Tomogr* 2008;**32**:764–8.

31. Weissleder R, Elizondo G, Wittenberg J, *et al.* Ultrasmall superparamagnetic iron oxide: an intravenous contrast agent for assessing lymph nodes with MR imaging. *Radiology* 1990;**175**:494–8.

32. Will O, Purkayastha S, Chan C, *et al.* Diagnostic precision of nanoparticle-enhanced MRI for lymph-node metastases: a meta-analysis. *Lancet Oncol* 2006;**7**:52–60.

33. Antoch G, Bockisch A. Combined PET/MRI: a new dimension in whole-body oncology imaging? *Eur J Nucl Med Mol Imag* 2009;**36** (Suppl 1):S113–20.

34. Sumi M, Sakihama N, Sumi T, *et al.* Discrimination of metastatic cervical lymph nodes with diffusion-weighted MR imaging in patients with head and neck cancer. *Am J Neuroradiol* 2003;**24**:1627–34.

35. Sumi M, Van Cauteren M, Nakamura T. MR microimaging of benign and malignant nodes in the neck. *Am J Roentgenol* 2006;**186**:749–57.

36. Abdel Razek AA, Soliman NY, Elkhamary S, Alsharaway MK, Tawfik A. Role of diffusion-weighted MR imaging in cervical lymphadenopathy. *Eur Radiol* 2006;**16**:1468–77.

37. King AD, Ahuja AT, Yeung DK, *et al.* Malignant cervical lymphadenopathy: diagnostic accuracy of diffusion-weighted MR imaging. *Radiology* 2007;**245**:806–13.

38. Akduman EI, Momtahen AJ, Balci NC, *et al.* Comparison between malignant and benign abdominal lymph nodes on diffusion-weighted imaging. *Acad Radiol* 2008;**15**:641–6.

39. Holzapfel K, Duetsch S, Fauser C, *et al.* Value of diffusion-weighted MR imaging in the differentiation between benign and malignant cervical lymph nodes. *Eur J Radiol* 2009;**72**:381–7.

40. Sumi M, Nakamura T. Diagnostic importance of focal defects in the apparent diffusion coefficient-based differentiation between lymphoma and squamous cell carcinoma nodes in the neck. *Eur Radiol* 2009;**19**:975–81.

41. Koşucu P, Tekinbaş C, Erol M, *et al.* Mediastinal lymph nodes: assessment with diffusion-weighted MR imaging. *J Magn Reson Imag* 2009;**30**:292–7.

42. Perrone A, Guerrisi P, Izzo L, *et al.* Diffusion-weighted MRI in cervical lymph nodes: differentiation between benign and malignant lesions. *Eur J Radiol* 2009; doi: 10.1016/j.ejrad.2009.07.039.

43. Tofts PS, Lloyd D, Clark CA, *et al.* Test liquids for quantitative MRI measurements of self-diffusion coefficient in vivo. *Magn Reson Med* 2000;**43**:368–74.

44. Lin G, Ho KC, Wang JJ, *et al.* Detection of lymph node metastasis in cervical and uterine cancers by diffusion-weighted magnetic resonance imaging at 3 T. *J Magn Reson Imag* 2008;**28**:128–35.

45. Kim JK, Kim KA, Park BW, Kim N, Cho KS. Feasibility of diffusion-weighted imaging in the differentiation of metastatic from nonmetastatic lymph nodes: early experience. *J Magn Reson Imag* 2008;**28**:714–19.

46. Park SO, Kim JK, Kim KA, *et al.* Relative apparent diffusion coefficient: determination of reference site and validation of benefit for detecting metastatic lymph nodes in uterine cervical cancer. *J Magn Reson Imag* 2009;**29**:383–90.

47. Vandecaveye V, De Keyzer F, Vander Poorten V, *et al.* Head and neck squamous cell carcinoma: value of diffusion-weighted MR imaging for nodal staging. *Radiology* 2009;**251**:134–46.

48. Sakurada A, Takahara T, Kwee TC, *et al.* Diagnostic performance of diffusion-weighted magnetic resonance imaging in esophageal cancer. *Eur Radiol* 2009;**19**:1461–9.

49. Yasui O, Sato M, Kamada A. Diffusion-weighted imaging in the detection of lymph node metastasis in colorectal cancer. *Tohoku J Exp Med* 2009;**218**:177–83.

50. Nomori H, Mori T, Ikeda K, *et al.* Diffusion-weighted magnetic resonance imaging can be used in place of positron emission tomography for N staging of non-small cell lung cancer with fewer false-positive results. *J Thorac Cardiovasc Surg* 2008;**135**:816–22.

51. Kwee TC, Takahara T, Luijten PR, Nievelstein RA. ADC measurements of lymph nodes: inter- and intra-observer reproducibility study and an overview of the literature. *Eur J Radiol* 2009; doi: 10.1016/j.ejrad.2009.03.026.

52. Brenner DJ, Hall EJ. Computed tomography: an increasing source of radiation exposure. *N Engl J Med* 2007;**357**:2277–84.

53. Namasivayam S, Kalra MK, Torres WE, Small WC. Adverse reactions to intravenous iodinated contrast media: a primer for radiologists. *Emerg Radiol* 2006;**12**:210–15.

54. Kwee TC, Quarles van Ufford HM, Beek FJ, *et al.* Whole-body MRI, including diffusion-weighted imaging, for the initial staging of malignant lymphoma: comparison to computed tomography. *Investig Radiol* 2009;**44**:683–90.

55. Uto T, Takehara Y, Nakamura Y, *et al.* Higher sensitivity and specificity for diffusion-weighted imaging of malignant lung lesions without apparent diffusion coefficient quantification. *Radiology* 2009;**252**:247–54.

56. Thoeny HC, Triantafyllou M, Birkhaeuser FD, *et al.* Combined ultrasmall superparamagnetic particles of iron oxide-enhanced and diffusion-weighted magnetic resonance imaging reliably detect pelvic lymph node metastases in normal-sized nodes of bladder and prostate cancer patients. *Eur Urol* 2009;**55**:761–9.

57. Delfaut EM, Beltran J, Johnson G, *et al.* Fat suppression in MR imaging: techniques and pitfalls. *Radiographics* 1999;**19**:373–82.

58. Takahara T, Hendrikse J, Yamashita T, *et al.* Diffusion-weighted MR neurography of the brachial plexus: feasibility study. *Radiology* 2008;**249**:653–60.

59. Beaulieu C. The basis of anisotropic water diffusion in the nervous system: a technical review. *NMR Biomed* 2002;**15**:435–55.

60. Takahara T, Hendrikse J, Kwee TC, *et al.* Diffusion-weighted MR neurography of the sacral plexus with unidirectional motion probing gradients. *Eur Radiol* 2009; doi: 10.1007/s00330-009-1665-2.

Diffusion-weighted MRI of female pelvic tumors

Hela Sbano and Anwar R. Padhani

Introduction

Magnetic resonance imaging (MRI) plays essential roles at every stage in the management of patients with gynecological cancer, from initial diagnosis and lesion characterization, to assessments of treatment effectiveness as well as for the determination of the activity of residual disease and the detection of recurrent active cancer. The limitations of morphological MRI assessments are well documented. For example, the detection of malignant lesions can be difficult particularly when disease burden is small or when disease is intermixed with normal or benign disease processes (e.g., detecting a small endometrial cancer in an endometrial polyp). Similarly, diagnostic accuracy of myometrial invasion by endometrial cancer is impaired particularly in patients with distortions of the endometrial cavity due to congenital abnormalities or fibroids or when there is scarring due to prior surgery. Coincident adenomyosis or a thinned/indistinct junctional zone can also impair assessments of depth of tumor invasion. Lesion characterization can be equally problematic, for example differentiating uterine sarcoma from degenerating leiomyomas or determining the nature of an adnexal mass. Detection and assessment of the activity of residual disease is also problematic for morphology-based imaging; for example, subtle serosal disease due to ovarian carcinoma is easily overlooked[1]. Finally, determining relapsed disease in areas of therapy-induced scarring can be problematic requiring careful comparisons to be made with prior examinations (e.g., it is often difficult to differentiate tumor recurrence from post-surgical/post-radiotherapy fibrosis following pelvic surgery).

These limitations of morphological-based imaging assessments have prompted a growing interest in the roles that functional imaging techniques such as diffusion-weighted (DW) MRI and dynamic contrast-enhanced (DCE) MRI could play in the management of patients with gynecological malignancies. Recent advances in MR technology such as high-performance gradient coils, parallel imaging techniques, and novel sequence designs have made the acquisition of DW-MR images feasible in the pelvis thus enabling everyday clinical use[2]. The greatest advantage of DW-MRI in the pelvis is its ability to delineate pathological lesions against generally suppressed background signals with excellent contrast resolution. This aids in the improved detection of small primary tumors including peritoneal metastases from gynecological malignancies[3]. Calculations of diffusivity (ADC: apparent diffusion coefficient) derived from DW-MRI also show promise for aiding in the discrimination of benign and malignant disease, as well as for monitoring therapeutic response, for example after uterine artery embolization (UAE), chemotherapy, and/or radiotherapy[4,5]. Additionally, by being able to assess tumor cellularity and tumor differentiation[6], DW-MRI may also aid in lesion characterization.

Diffusion tensor imaging (DTI) is an extension of DW-MRI wherein the degree of anisotropic diffusions of water molecules in tissues can be also determined. DTI yields higher quality diffusion weighted images and ADC maps with improved signal-to-noise ratio (SNR) with fewer distortions. DTI is feasible in the pelvis in vivo. Weiss et al.[7] have recently shown that DTI can enable the intrinsic fiber architecture of the uterus of non-pregnant patients to be determined in vitro. The clinical usefulness of DTI is yet to be established but appears to provide complementary information to high b-value DW-MRI.

Extra-Cranial Applications of Diffusion-Weighted MRI, ed. Bachir Taouli. Published by Cambridge University Press.
© Cambridge University Press 2011.

Table 9.1 Strategies for combating low SNR on pelvic DW-MRI

Strategy	Comments
Minimize TE (<100 ms)	Increase bandwidth – max about 1500; if too high ghosting increases Use parallel imaging (max × 2) Use bipolar gradient scheme if possible Use 3-scan approach (3 small gradients applied simultaneously = large net gradient achieved in much less time)
Image at 3 T	SNR scales with field strength
Multiple averages/NEX	Time penalties; max 6 averages (suggest trace approach instead)
Coarse matrix	128^2 at 1.5 T and 256^2 at 3 T (interpolate as needed) Also enables lower-amplitude imaging gradients to be used resulting in a smaller effect on changing the magnitude of low b-value diffusion gradients
Larger field of view	Maximum compatible with diagnosis; pelvis 22–24 cm Lower-amplitude imaging gradients have a smaller effect on changing the magnitude of low b-value diffusion gradients
Increase slice thickness	No less than 5–6 mm to match anatomical images
Trace approaches; i.e., diffusion gradients applied in 3 directions consecutively and then averaged	Adding signal from each image per direction is constructive but adding noise is destructive; therefore better SNR Blurring of ADC maps can occur due to distortions in x- and z-axes images

In this chapter, we assume that readers are already familiar with DW-MRI principles which are covered elsewhere in this book. We start by discussing strategies for improving SNR and provide a working protocol for the female pelvis. We will also discuss fusion imaging principles, provide interpretation guidelines, and illustrate potential pitfalls as well as illustrate clinical applications of DW-MRI in women with gynecological malignancies.

Clinical protocol

All DW-MRI regardless of anatomical site is impeded by poor SNR of high b-value images and is prone to artifacts, particularly image distortion. The strategies adopted by us to optimize SNR of pelvic DW-MRI are given in Table 9.1. These strategies have allowed us to develop a working pelvic tumor protocol that incorporates DW-MRI for use in daily clinical practice (Table 9.2). Our DW-MRI protocol has been developed for a Siemens 1.5-T Symphony scanner and should be adapted by readers for their own machines using the strategies outlined in Table 9.1. Single-shot, fat-suppressed T2-weighted echo-planar imaging (EPI) sequence with diffusion- weighting and parallel imaging acceleration is universally used. A bipolar (balanced) gradient scheme with the simultaneous application of multidirectional motion probing gradients (resulting in a larger overall gradient) should be used where possible (so-called three-scan trace/gradient overplus gradient schemes). This gradient scheme aids in reducing echo times (TEs) and helps reduce the effect of eddy current induced image distortions. Free-breathing techniques are preferred with a bowel relaxant where possible and an empty bladder.

Our practice is to undertake two DW-MRI data acquisitions which have distinct uses. The whole pelvis survey is undertaken initially; this is helpful for nodal mapping and for the detection of disease against a suppressed background. We find this sequence useful for detecting sites of disease which may be otherwise hidden. This sequence is quick and easy to perform, uses larger fields of view, inversion recovery for fat suppression, thicker slices, and few but very high b-values (≥ 1000 s/mm^2). This survey sequence can help the subsequent placement of high-resolution morphological T2-weighted images. The second DW-MRI sequence is required for detailed examination of a tumor or organ (thin slices, smaller field of view, and shorter z-axis resolution) and uses multiple b-values for the accurate calculation of ADC values. Generally b-values do not exceed 800 s/mm^2 in order to retain good SNR so as to reduce the error of calculated ADC values.

Table 9.2 Suggested protocol for DW-MRI in the pelvis at 1.5 T

	Whole pelvis survey	Tumor
Field of view (cm)[a]	260	260
Matrix size (x, y)[a]	160 × 256i (interpolated)	112 × 256i
Repetition time (ms)	>3500	4500
Echo time (ms)	Minimum	Minimum
Fat suppression	STIR	SPAIR
EPI factor	114	139
Parallel imaging	2	2
Signal averages	6	6
Section thickness (mm)/gap/slices	6/1/90–100	3–5/0/20
Directions of motion probing gradients	Phase + frequency + slice	Phase + frequency + slice
b-values (mm²/s)	0, 1100, 1400	0, 100, 500, 800
Pixel bandwidth (Hz)	1000–1500	1000–1500
Acquisition time (min)	3.11	4.48

Note: [a]Rectangular to fit body size and shape.
STIR, short tau inversion recovery; SPAIR, spectral presaturation attenuated by inversion recovery; EPI, echo-planar-imaging.

Image display

There are a number of ways of displaying high b-value images (where fat and background suppression is maximal). Inverted gray or arbitrary color scales (so called false-color maps) are often used to visualize the data as axial slices, multiplanar reconstructions, and maximal intensity projection (MIP) displays. It is also possible to fuse high b-value images with anatomical images using advanced software algorithms.

When fusion imaging is undertaken, it is recommended that one uses high b-value images that have good SNR, good background suppression, and minimal distortions; this means that in practice image fusion is undertaken using b-values greater than 500 s/mm² (Figure 9.1). Modern 3D fusion imaging visualization software works in three steps: (1) Super-imposition of datasets; datasets do not need to be acquired in the same plane, or to have identical field of views or even the same matrix sizes. (2) Alignment algorithms working with multiple degrees of freedom based on anatomical landmarks with the ability to work automatically with manual overrides if necessary. (3) Visualization blending of gray-scale anatomical images with pseudo-color high b-value images with adjustable balance between the two superimposed datasets. Readers should note that although no color scales are especially suited for the display of high b-value magnitude images, inverted gray-scale is often used. It is also important to remember that internal organ motion in the time interval between data acquisitions may require additional volume registrations/image warping to be performed. 3D fusion imaging software has a number of uses including detection, localization, and estimating extent of lesions. Fusion imaging can also be used for data presentation to clinicians, for analyses prior to reporting DW-MRI, and for guiding biopsy to variable tumor cell sites and therapy planning.

It is often stated that regions of interest (ROIs) should be drawn on high b-value images (>800–1000 s/mm²) as the estimated regional ADC values represent "viable tumor" (because the detrimental effects of necrosis are ameliorated by using high b-value images). Although a good idea, this method for defining ROIs is occasionally prone to error. For example, if the intrinsic T2-relaxation rates of background tissues are high (T2 shine-through) then tumor may not be seen; this is occasionally a problem when evaluating a nodule in a cystic adnexal mass. Furthermore, occasionally viscous water can demonstrate high signal intensity on very high b-value images (for example, in an obstructed endometrial cavity, Figure 9.2). It is also important to remember that well-differentiated tumors may not be seen on high b-value images and that there are other non-cancer causes of high signal intensity on high b-value pelvic images including normal lymph nodes, normal endometrium, and bowel mucosa. These observations mean that one needs to be cautious about using high b-value images exclusively for ROI definitions; these should always take into account findings on ADC maps and on corresponding anatomical images.

Image interpretation guidelines

Visual inspection of DW-MRI and co-registered anatomical images should always be undertaken together. Images at $b = 0$ s/mm² are fat suppressed with water

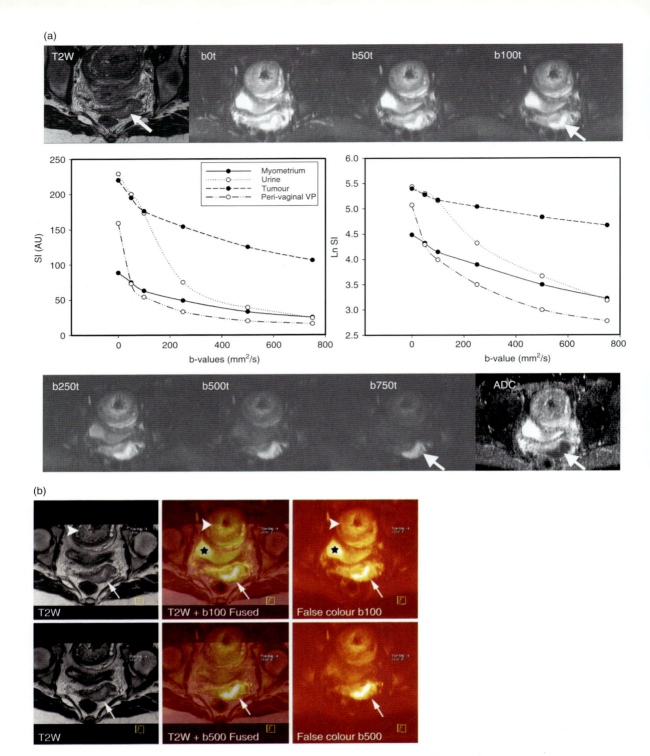

Figure 9.1 (a) Signal intensity changes with increasing *b*-values (t, trace image). Moderately differentiated squamous carcinoma of the vagina in a 29-year-old post-partum (arrow). Changes in signal intensity (left graph) and log$_n$ signal intensity (right graph) are show. Note the biexponential signal decay (most pronounced in the peri-vaginal venous plexus (VP). The signal decay of urine is more erratic because of turbulent urinary flow. For fusion imaging, it is necessary to ensure that background signals are adequately suppressed whilst maintaining good SNR. (b) Image selection for fusion imaging. Fusion of T2-W images with the *b* = 100 images demonstrates the tumor; however, the high signal intensity from the bladder (asterisk) is still visible. Fusion of the T2-W images with the *b* = 500 image provides better background and urinary water suppression and thus enables better tumor visualization. The uterus has been marked with an arrowhead.

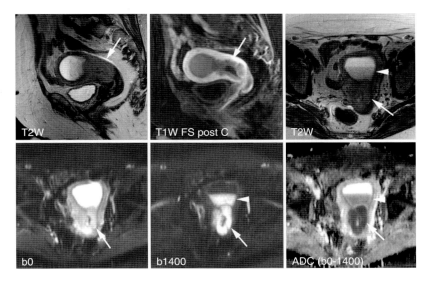

Figure 9.2 Viscous fluid with low ADC values. Large adenocarcinoma of the endometrium in the lower uterine segment with cervical invasion (arrow). There is extensive myometrial invasion by the tumor with right-sided parametrial extension. The tumor causes obstruction of the endometrial cavity. The inspissated, layered fluid within the endometrial cavity demonstrates low signal intensity on the ADC map with marked hyperintensity on the $b = 1400$ images (arrow head). T1-W fat-suppressed post contrast (T1-W FS post C).

appearing bright. It is on the higher b-value images that an initial idea of tissue cellularity and structure is obtained. From the outset, it is important for readers to remember that signal intensity on high b-value images is dependent on biophysical tissue properties including intrinsic proton density, tissue T2-relaxation rate, and ADC values as well as on sequence parameters. So as a first approximation one can say that areas retaining high signal intensity on $b = 800–1000$ s/mm^2 images usually indicate highly cellular tissues, whereas low signal intensity regions are seen in most normal tissues, glandular formation, cystic spaces, necrosis, or fibrosis. However, high signal intensities on $b = 800–1000$ s/mm^2 images are not always reliable indicators of increased cellularity. As we have already noted, occasionally fluid/edema remain high signal intensity because of high proton density; this observation is called T2 shine-through, and corresponding ADC maps should always be inspected and interpreted according to the guidance given in Table 9.3. This is illustrated in Figure 9.3, where T2 shine-through is demonstrated in a benign cervical polyp. T2 shine-through is also demonstrated in Figure 9.4b.

It is also important to remember that some normal pelvic tissues such as the normal lymph nodes, nerves, normal endometrium, and bowel mucosa can all have high signal intensity on high b-value images. It is essential not to interpret ADC maps or high b-value images in isolation and correlation with anatomical images is vital if errors are to be avoided.

Table 9.3 Scheme for the interpretation of DW-MRI images with reference to the signal intensity (represented by arrows) on T2-weighted and high b-value source images and on ADC maps

T2-W	High b-value source images (>800 s/mm^2)	ADC maps	Interpretation
↔	↑	↓	Generally, high cellularity tumor; rarely coagulative necrosis, highly viscous fluid or abscess
↑	↑	↑	T2 shine-through; often proteinaceous fluid
↓ ↔	↓	↓	Fibrous tissue with low water content with/without viable tumor cells
↑	↓	↑	Fluid; liquefactive necrosis; lower cellularity; gland formation

There is no unique cut-off ADC value that distinguishes cancer from non-cancer/normal tissues in gynecological assessments. There are a number of reasons for this including the fact that ADC values are dependent on the range of b-values used for calculations. This occurs principally because of the

123

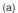

(a)

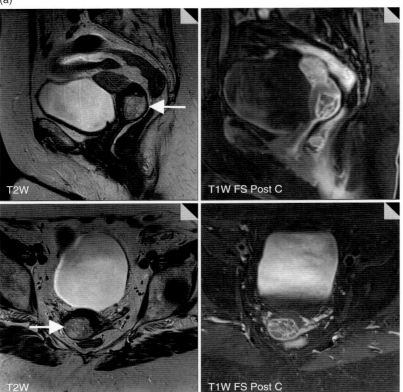

T2W

T1W FS Post C

T2W

T1W FS Post C

Figure 9.3 (a, b) T2 shine-through. A large mass at the external cervical os in an 80-year-old woman. The lesion has highly vascularised septae. T2 shine-through is demonstrated with high signal intensity on the high *b*-value images and ADC map. Histology confirmed a benign endocervical polyp composed of dilated glands with flattened epithelium in a fibrous stroma. This is reflected in the isotropic diffusion demonstrated on the fractional anisotropy (FA) map.

(b)

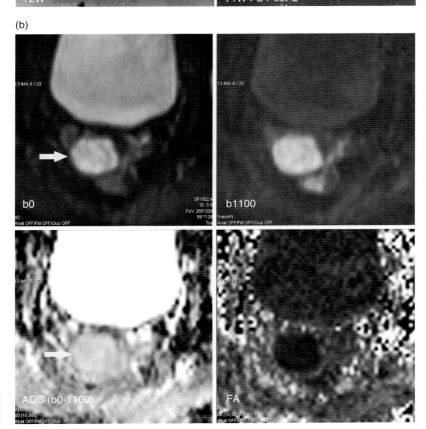

b0

b1100

ADC (b0-1100)

FA

(a)

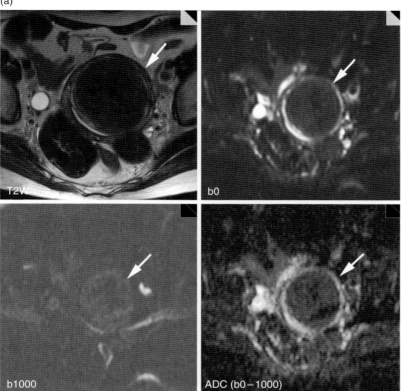

T2W

b0

b1000

ADC (b0 – 1000)

(b)

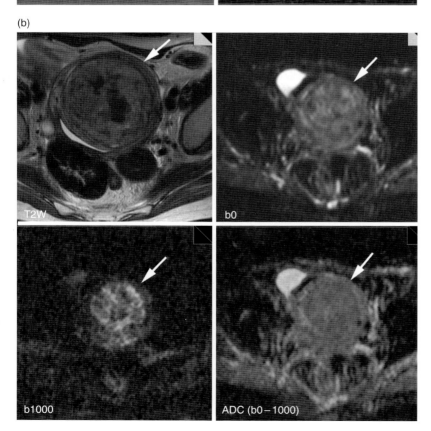

T2W

b0

b1000

ADC (b0 – 1000)

Figure 9.4 (a) A large uterine leiomyoma (arrow) with low signal intensity on T2-W, high *b*-value images and ADC map. (b) Following chemoradiation for associated cervical cancer (not shown), there is an increase in the size and signal intensity of the leiomyoma on the T2-W sequence and high *b*-value images in keeping with infarction of the leiomyoma (arrow). T2 shine-through is demonstrated in the infarcted tissue with high signal intensity on the high *b*-value images and the ADC map.

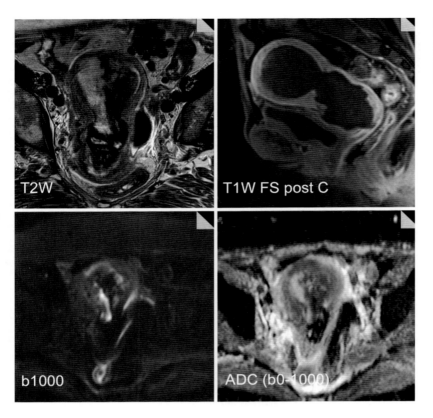

Figure 9.5 A large infarcted, poorly differentiated endometrial cancer with myometrial and cervical stromal invasion in a 72-year-old woman. The extent of this tumor is underestimated on the $b = 1000$ s/mm^2 image.

inclusion of $b0$ in ADC calculations which results in increased sensitivity to perfusion effects. Inclusion of $b0$ when calculating ADC maps may lead to errors in ADC calculation particularly for tissues with high blood flow. Other important points to recall include the fact that both well differentiated tumors and necrotic poorly differentiated tumors can have over-lapping high ADC values because DW-MRI does not distinguish between water movements in cystic structures and in areas of necrosis. Figure 9.5 is a large infarcted, poorly differentiated endometrial cancer with cervical stromal invasion. The extent of this tumor is underestimated on the $b = 1000$ s/mm^2 image and on the ADC map.

As already noted, the combination of hyperintensity on high b-value images with corresponding low ADC values is typically due to high cellular density within tumors (with exceptions in normal tissue as described above). However, such appearances can occasionally also be seen in patients with hydrosalpinx, some ovarian cysts, peritoneal collections including inspissated abscesses, and occasionally within an obstructed endometrial cavity (Figure 9.2).

These observations further emphasize the need for diagnostic characterization to integrate appearances from morphology, high b-value DW images, and ADC maps.

Appearance of the normal female pelvis

The global muscle and collagen fiber orientation in the human uterine myometrium has been analyzed extensively by microscopic techniques[7]. DTI has been successfully applied to the analysis and depiction of neuronal fibers in the living human brain and more recently qualitative agreements between the main diffusion directions and the fiber orientation in myocardium and skeletal muscle has been observed[7,8,9]. Recently, Weiss *et al.* showed marked anisotropy of the uterus by ex-vivo DTI measurements on five uteri from non-pregnant women[7]. Two systems of fibers were found running circularly along within the myometrium of the uterine body that merged caudally so building a closely fitting envelope of circular layers around the uterine cavity (Figure 9.6). In the

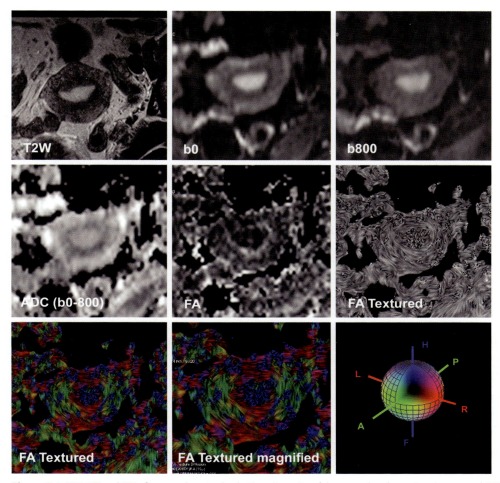

Figure 9.6 DW-MRI and DTI of a normal uterine body. Hyperintensity of the normal endometrium is seen on $b800$ image. Note the reduced ADC value of the inner myometrial layer with increased fractional anisotropy (FA). Fiber orientation is well shown on the black-and-white and colored textured FA maps which demonstrate the circular myometrial fibers around the uterine cavity. The direction of these fibers is color coded: head to foot (blue), left to right (red), and anterior–posterior (green).

cervix, circular fibers were observed in the outer part with mostly longitudinal fibers in the inner part[7] (Figure 9.7).

Figures 9.6 and 9.7 are typical DW images of the normal uterine body and cervix, respectively. Normal endometrium in women of reproductive age is composed of endometrial glands and stromal cells of high cellular density with abundance of cytoplasm, and will have high signal intensity on high b-value images (Figure 9.6)[6,4]. Tamai et al. demonstrated the ADC_{0-1000} values for histologically confirmed normal endometrium in 12 women to be $1.53 \pm 0.1 \times 10^{-3} \, mm^2/s$[6]. There are, however, no published ADC values of the normal endometrium during different stages of the menstrual cycle.

ADC_{0-1000} values for the normal myometrium appear to vary by study; Tamai et al. quote $1.62 \pm 0.11 \, (SD) \times 10^{-3} \, mm^2/s$[10], and Anstee et al. $1.15 \times 10^{-3} \, mm^2/s$ (interquartile range of 1.13–1.41 $\times 10^{-3} \, mm^2/s$, $n = 15$)[11]. Further studies are required to establish the entire range of ADC values for the normal myometrium.

It is difficult to comment very meaningfully about the normal ADC values of the cervix because most studies do not attempt to distinguish between cervix mucosa and stroma (Figure 9.7). One study report that normal cervical mucosa had higher ADC_{0-1000} values $(1.27 \times 10^{-3} \, mm^2/s)$ compared to stroma $0.58 \times 10^{-3} \, mm^2/s$ (interquartile range = 0.38–0.92, $n = 12$)[11]. Naganawa et al. found ADC_{0-600} values

127

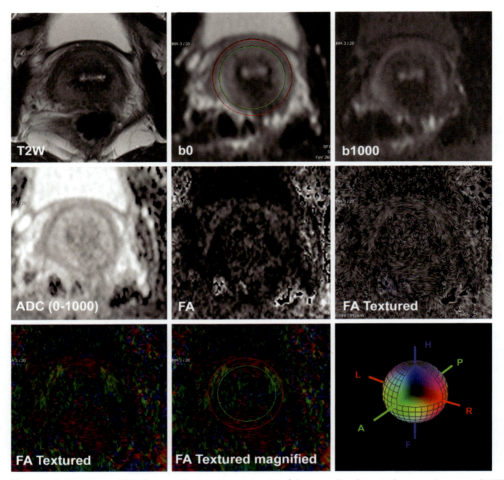

Figure 9.7 DW-MRI and DTI of a normal cervix. Hyperintensity of the normal endocervical mucosa is seen on *b*1000 image. Fiber orientation is well shown on the black-and-white and colored textured FA maps. Circular fibers are observed in the outer part of the cervix (between the green and red rings) with mostly longitudinal fibers in the inner part. The direction of these fibers is color coded: head to foot (blue), left to right (red), and anterior–posterior (green).

for the normal cervix to be $1.79 \pm 0.24 \times 10^{-3}$ mm^2/s $(n = 10)$[12]. Normal cervical ADC$_{0-600}$ values of $2.09 \pm 0.46 \times 10^{-3}$ mm^2/s were demonstrated by McVeigh *et al.* $(n = 26)$[2]. Once again further studies are required to establish the entire range of ADC values for the normal cervix.

Clinical applications of DW-MRI
Tumor cellularity and grade
With increasing tumor cellularity and architectural distortion, any increase in the tortuosity of the extra-cellular space will additionally contribute to decreased ADC values. It would, therefore, be expected that ADC values would correlate with tumor cellularity and grade[13]. High-grade adenocarcinoma lesions are typically of high cellular density with a high nuclear-to-cytoplasm ratio, so they would be expected to have lower ADC values; as a caveat necrosis which is often found in high-grade lesion will paradoxically increase ADC values thus potentially reducing the correlations between ADC values and tumor grade[13]. This may explain the trend for lower ADC values in higher-grade endometrial cancers noted by Tamai *et al.*[6], which did not achieve statistical significance. Hence, correlations between ADC value and cellularity are best done when ROIs are drawn on high *b*-value images which effectively removes the confounding effects of necrosis and cyst formation.

Tumor detection and characterization

As noted above the basic premise for using DW-MRI for tumor detection relates to the fact that malignant tissues are generally more cellular than normal tissues or benign processes. Unfortunately, no unique ADC cut-off value predicts for the presence of malignancy in the pelvis, as shown in Table 9.4; however, as a first approximation one can say that if a tumor is of very low ADC values then it is likely to have highly packed cells and therefore is more likely to be of higher grade.

Endometrial tumors

Endometrial cancer is the most common gynecological malignancy in developed countries[6,14]. The prognosis of endometrial cancer is determined by histological subtype and grade; tumor stage at diagnosis (including the depth of myometrial invasion); and the presence of lymph node and distant metastasis[6,15]. In endometrial cancer, the predominant histological subtype is endometrioid adenocarcinoma, which histologically is further classified into three grades based on architectural features.

MRI is a well-established modality for evaluating local stage including myometrial invasion and cervical involvement[6]. Conventional MRI does not always clearly demonstrate the tumor, particularly if small, since the signal intensity of the endometrial cancer can be variable, making cancer sometimes indistinguishable from normal endometrium or myometrium (Figure 9.8). Similarly, diagnostic detection may be reduced when the disease is intermixed with benign processes such as polyps or when there are endometrial cavity distortions such as those caused by fibroids, septae, and scars[6,16]. The reported diagnostic accuracy of lesion detection on T2-weighted imaging is 58–77% which can be improved by administering contrast medium (85–93%)[16–18]. Unfortunately, post-contrast-enhanced images can become degraded because of bladder filling towards the end of a long examination period. DW-MRI can also be helpful for detecting endometrial cancers in patients in whom contrast medium cannot be administered, for example because of impaired renal function.

Differences in the water diffusion profile between normal myometrium and tumor enable the detection of even small tumors on DW-MRI on high b-value images. Tamai et al. demonstrated lower mean ADC values of endometrial cancer compared to normal endometrium (Table 9.4). Anstee et al. demonstrated

similar results with endometrial carcinomas with median ADC_{0-1000} value of $0.74 \times 10^{-3}\,mm^2/s$ which was also found to be significantly lower than that of normal endometrium[11]. These findings were also confirmed by Inada et al.[19]

In addition, DW-MRI and ADC measurements can help in differentiating malignant from benign uterine endometrial cavity lesions[1]. There are a number of differentials for endometrial cavity lesions including; endometrial polyps, submucosal leiomyomas, endometrial carcinomas, carcinosarcomas (malignant mixed mullerian tumors), trophoblastic tumors, and retained products of conception. Most diseases of the endometrial cavity can be diagnosed via endometrial cytology or curettage; however, some can be difficult to detect and imaging findings are helpful in making diagnoses[1]. Fujii et al. found that malignant lesions such as endometrial carcinoma and carcinosarcoma had lower ADC values than benign lesions including submucosal leiomyomas (Figure 9.9) and endometrial polyps[21]. Endometrial polyps consist of endometrial glands and stroma of focally or diffusely dense fibrous or smooth muscle tissue[1,20]. Cystic glandular hyperplasia commonly occurs within the polyp. These tissue characteristics allow increased movement of water molecules, resulting in lower signal on high b-value images and increased ADC values[21]. Carcinosarcomas have poor prognosis in comparison with endometrial carcinomas. In dynamic contrast enhanced studies, most carcinosarcomas demonstrate early and persistent marked enhancement similar to that of myometrium which may be useful in differentiating carcinosarcoma from endometrial carcinoma[21,22]. ADC values of both endometrial carcinomas and carcinosarcomas have been shown to be relatively low (Figure 9.10), thus the distinction between high-grade endometrial cancer and carcinosarcoma cannot be made with ADC values.

Cervical tumors

DW-MRI has been shown to be useful for the evaluation of cervix tumors because ADC values of cancers are lower than the normal cervix with very little overlap (Table 9.4). In general, tumor detection of cervix tumors is not problematic and can be done by visual inspection of the ectocervix. However, occasionally after a knife-core biopsy histological margins can remain positive and DW-MRI can be useful for delineating the extent of remaining disease

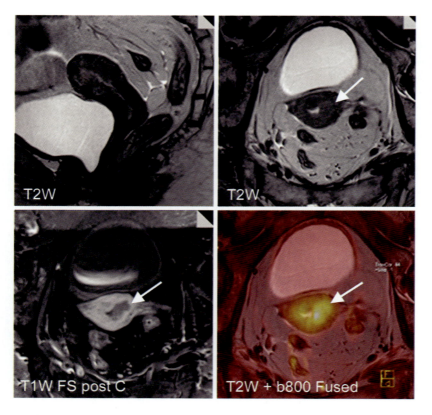

T2W

T2W

T1W FS post C

T2W + b800 Fused

Figure 9.8 Small well-differentiated endometrial carcinoma extending into the left cornua. There is inner myometrial invasion which was confirmed on histology. The tumor (arrow) is isointense with the surrounding myometrium on the T2-W sequence thus making it difficult to detect. Tumor position is well shown on both DW-MRI and contrast-enhanced images.

(Figure 9.11). Cervical inflammation after excision biopsy in the absence of active tumor shows minimal high signal on high b-value images compared to high signal on high b-value images (and lower ADC values) of residual cancer. Occasionally, cervical cancers which are largely ulcerative can destroy the cervix; in these cases we have found that DW-MRI can be less useful for tumor delineation. Endocervical adenocarcinomas can also be problematic to delineate on DW-MRI particularly when they are of low grade due to the abundance of glandular structures.

Myometrial tumors

Leiomyomas are the commonest benign uterine tumors. The diffusion MRI appearances of leiomyomas are variable thus reflecting the complex histological findings[23]. The common appearance of low signal intensity of leiomyomas on high b-value DW images can be explained by a low proton density which is also responsible for hypointensity on T2-weighted images[10,24,25] (Figure 9.12). These appearances are a reflection of histopathologic features

(accumulated clusters of uniform smooth muscle cells with intervening collagen)[21] which contributed to relatively high fractional anisotropy (FA) values. The relatively large standard deviation of ADC values of ordinary leiomyomas, which was also found by Shimada et al.[26], may reflect the known variety of their histological features[10]. Leiomyomas are associated with degenerative features such as hyalinization and edema, which occur in more than 50% of leiomyomas[21,27]. Hyalinization involves the presence of homogenous eosinophilic bands or plaques in the extracellular space, which causes a narrowing of the extracellular space[21], and is suggested to cause decreased ADC values. Edema, however, leads to increased ADC values because of increased extracellular water.

Malignant tumors of the myometrium consist of leiomyosarcoma, which is the most common, followed by endometrial stromal sarcoma[10,28]. Endometrial stromal sarcomas originate from endometrial stroma; they usually show extensive myometrial involvement and are frequently misdiagnosed as

Table 9.4 DW-MRI studies with ADC values in uterine and ovarian diseases

Authors	Site of lesions	Tumor and tissue (no. of subjects)	b-values	ADC (10^{-3} mm^2/s)	p-value
Naganawa et al.[12]	Cervical	Cervical cancer (12) Normal cervix (10)	0, 300, 600	1.09 ± 0.20 1.79 ± 0.24	<0.001
McVeigh et al.[2]	Cervical	Cervical cancer (47) Normal cervix (26)	0, 600	1.09 ± 0.20 2.09 ± 0.46	<0.0001
Tamai et al.[6]	Endometrial	Endometrial cancer (18) Normal endometrium (12)	0, 500, 1000	0.88 ± 0.16 1.53 ± 0.10	< 0.01
Fujii et al.[21]	Endometrial	Endometrial cancer (11) Carcinosarcoma (2) Submucosal leiomyoma (8) Endometrial polyp (4)	0, 1000	0.98 ± 0.21 0.97 ± 0.02 1.37 ± 0.28 1.58 ± 0.45	<0.01
Shen et al.[37]	Endometrial	Endometrial cancer (11) Endometrial polyp or hyperplasia (7)	0, 1000	1.86 ± 0.31 1.27 ± 0.22	<0.01
Inada et al.[19]	Endometrial	Endometrial cancer (22)		0.97 ± 0.19	<0.05
Anstee et al.[11]	Endometrial	Cervical mucosa (12) Cervical stroma (12) Myometrium (15) Endometrioid adenocarcinoma (21) Grade 1 (9) Grade 2 (7) Grade 3 (5)	0, 50, 150, 500, 1000	1.27 (median) 0.58 (median) 1.15 (median) 0.79 (median) 0.84 ± 0.04 0.73 ± 0.05 0.64 ± 0.06	<0.02
Tamai et al.[10]	Myometrial	Uterine sarcoma (7) Leiomyoma (51) Normal myometrium	0, 500, 1000	1.17 ± 0.15 0.88 ± 0.27 1.62 ± 0.11	<0.01
Moteki et al.[34]	Ovarian	Endometrial cyst (33) Serous cystadenoma (4) Mucinous cystadenoma (4) Malignant cystic tumor (12)	2, 188	1.00–1.09 ± 0.57–0.60 2.74 ± 0.37 1.59–1.88 ± 0.89–0.99 1.55–2.00 ± 0.59–1.01	<0.03
Katayama et al.[33]	Ovarian	Endometrial cyst (18) Mature cystic teratoma (29) Serous cystadenoma (2) Mucinous cystadenoma (7) Malignant cystic tumors (10)	200, 400, 600	1.24 ± 0.46 1.27 ± 0.66 1.64 ± 0.14 1.61 ± 0.61 1.64 ± 0.48	
Nakayama et al.[31]	Ovarian	Endometrial cyst (35) Mature cystic teratoma (54) Benign cystadenoma (14) Malignant cystic tumors (24)	0, 500, 1000	1.37 ± 0.66 0.89 ± 0.55 2.52 ± 0.32 2.28 ± 0.71	<0.01

Source: Adapted from Namimoto et al., Eur Radiol 2009; **19**(3) 745–60[5].

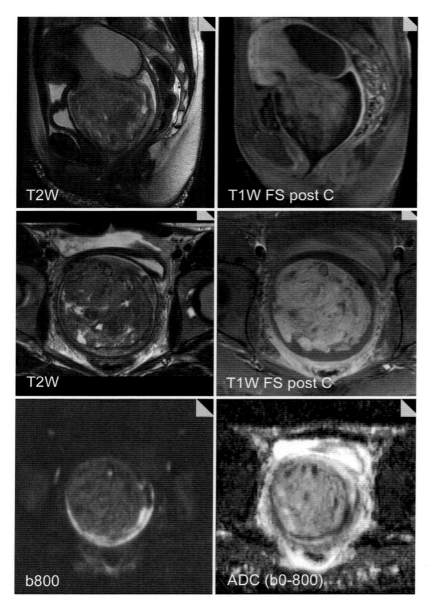

Figure 9.9 Large benign prolapsed submucosal leiomyoma with cavitary obstruction. Low signal intensity on high *b*-value DW image and high ADC values is in keeping with benign pathology.

benign leiomyomas[10,29]. Endometrial biopsy may not be helpful for the definitive diagnosis of uterine sarcoma; MRI plays an essential role for the diagnosis of these tumors and determining appropriate management. On MRI, uterine sarcomas are often large infiltrating masses of intermediate to high signal intensity on T2-weighted images[10,30]. In contradistinction, MRI usually allows specific diagnosis of benign leiomyomas, which as we have noted often

present as low signal intensity on T1- and T2-weighted imaging. However, the common occurrence of degenerating leiomyomas and cellular histological subtypes makes differentiation between benign degenerative and malignant myometrial tumors difficult on both morphological and contrast-enhanced sequences[10].

Tamai *et al.* found that uterine sarcomas show a high signal intensity on high *b*-value DW images[10].

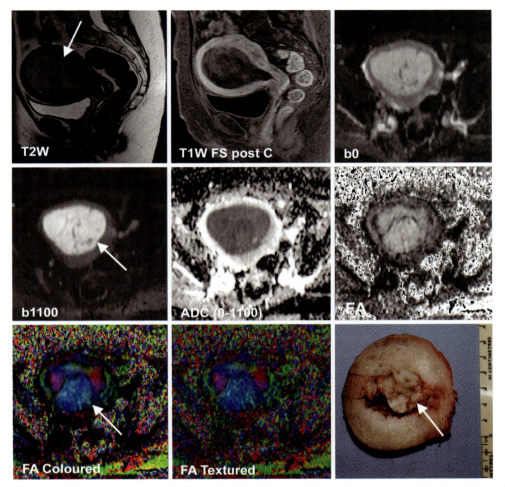

Figure 9.10 Large carcinosarcoma (malignant mixed mullerian tumor) occupying the endometrial cavity with superficial myometrial invasion posteriorly. The tumor (arrow) demonstrates restriction on diffusion imaging. This lesion is atypical in that it does not demonstrate enhancement post contrast. There is marked anisotropic diffusion within the tumor shown on the black-and-white and colored textured FA maps. The stalk of this polypoidal tumor shows marked water directionality which is color coded: head to foot (blue), left to right (red) and anterior–posterior (green).

In addition, the ADC value of sarcomas was lower than those of the normal myometrium and degenerating leiomyomas without any overlap[10]. However, uterine sarcomas demonstrated overlap in ADC values with ordinary leiomyomas and cellular leiomyomas[10]. Thus, cellular leiomyomas may not be distinguishable from sarcomas based on signal intensity on DW images and ADC values; however, cellular leiomyomas tend to be smaller and more homogeneous compared to sarcomas which are often large and degenerate. Degenerating leiomyomas tended to exhibit low signal intensity on DW images and higher ADC values in comparison to sarcomas.

Accordingly, DW images and ADC measurements can aid in the differentiation between degenerating leiomyoma and pelvic sarcomas.

Adnexal tumors

There have been a number of studies investigating the use of DW-MRI for characterizing cystic ovarian masses with inconsistent results. Nakayama *et al.* studied 131 patients with cystic ovarian masses, and demonstrated that mature cystic teratomas tended to show higher signal intensity on high *b*-value DW images and corresponding lower ADC values than endometrial cysts and other benign and malignant

133

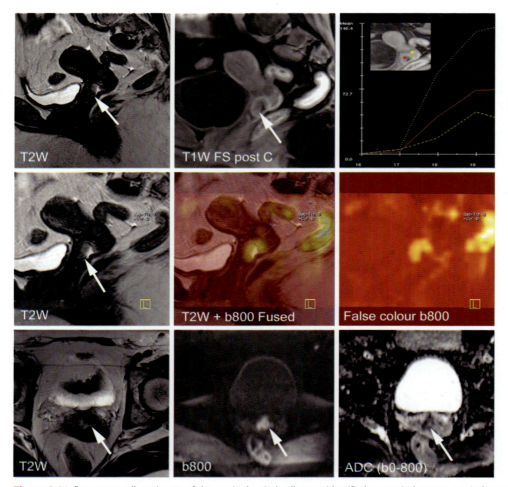

Figure 9.11 Squamous cell carcinoma of the cervix. Atypical cells were identified on cervical smears, cervical cancer was finally only diagnosed after cone biopsy. No mass was visible on the ectocervix. The extent of the mass is well shown on the DW-MRI. The mass is centrally hypovascular as shown on the dynamic contrast-enhanced image. Signal intensity versus time curves are shown for three regions of interest; the center of the tumor (red), tumor edge (green), and normal cervix (yellow).

neoplasm ($p < 0.005$)[31]. They ascribed these findings to the keratinoid substance within tumor cysts. Differences between endometriomas and ovarian neoplasms whether malignant or benign, were also significant ($p < 0.001$). This was thought to be due to T1 shortening secondary to blood products and hemosiderin within endometriomas[31]. However, when mature cystic teratomas and endometriomas were excluded from evaluation, the ADC of the benign lesions showed no statistically significant difference from that of malignant lesions[31]. These findings are similar to those made by Fujii *et al.* in their study of 123 ovarian lesions in 119 patients, who concluded neither signal intensity on high *b*-value

images nor ADC values of the solid component were useful for differentiating benign from malignant ovarian lesions[32]. Similarly, Katayama *et al.* evaluated 31 women with 61 cystic components of ovarian tumors and concluded that ADC values were not useful in discriminating benign from malignant lesions[33]. Only Moteki *et al.* have demonstrated significantly lower ADC values in malignant cystic ovarian tumors compared to benign ovarian cysts and serous cystadenomas[34] (Figure 9.13). Overall therefore DW-MRI and ADC values may add some useful information regarding differential diagnosis (mature cystic teratomas and endometriomas); however, undue reliance should not be placed on

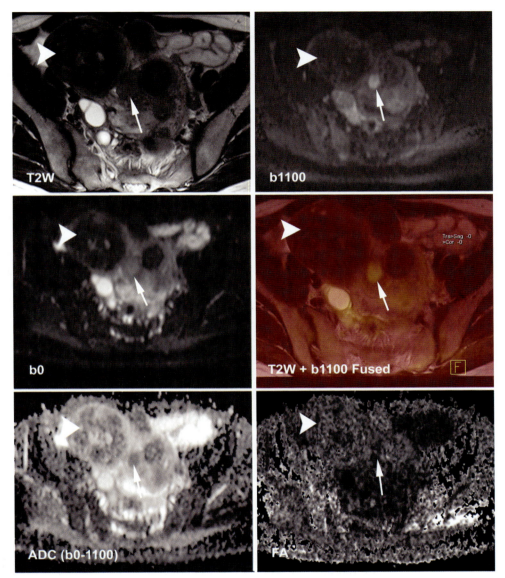

Figure 9.12 Multiple intramural and subserosal leiomyomas at varying degrees of degeneration in a 45-year-old woman. The large leiomyoma (arrowhead) has the common appearance of low signal intensity on high *b*-value DW images indicating low proton density with relatively high fractional anisotropy. Hypercellularity is demonstrated in one of the small leiomyomas (arrow).

DW-MRI alone in the differential diagnosis of the indeterminate adnexal mass. Correlation with morphological and contrast-enhanced MRI should always be sought for making this determination[35].

Depth of tumor invasion

In patients with endometrial cancer, DW-MRI can be a useful tool for determining depth of invasion, particularly in patients with distortions of the endometrial cavity due to congenital abnormalities, fibroids, or scars, in addition to those with adenomyosis or when a thinned or indistinct junctional zone is present. Since tumors of high cellularity appear very bright on high *b*-value images, fusion imaging with anatomical T2-weighted sequences can improve the visualization of the depth of tumor invasion into the myometrium (Figure 9.8). Currently, contrast

135

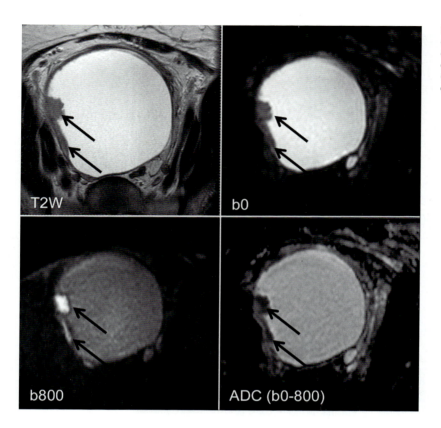

Figure 9.13 Serous cystadenocarcinoma of the ovary. Large complex cystic mass of the ovary with malignant nodules demonstrating restricted diffusion (arrows), with extension through the capsule (T3C).

medium enhancement using dynamic sequences is used which relies on the observation that the majority of endometrial tumors are hypovascular compared to the normal myometrium[36]. However, significant numbers of tumors are isovascular compared to myometrium impairing this assessment (occasional hypervascularization is also seen). DW-MRI is complementary to contrast enhancement for determining the depth of invasion[4,37,38]. Additionally post-contrast-enhanced images can be degraded by artifacts arising from concentrated contrast medium in the filling bladder and DW-MRI can be helpful in this regard. There are also instances in which renal impairment impedes the administration of contrast medium where DW-MRI can make a helpful contribution to tumor staging (Figure 9.14).

In a recent study of 48 women with histologically confirmed endometrial cancer, Lin *et al.* found that the addition of fused T2-weighted and DW-MRI to dynamic contrast-enhanced or dynamic contrast-enhanced and T2-weighted imaging was significantly better at assessing myometrial invasion compared

with dynamic contrast-enhanced imaging alone ($p < 0.001$) or dynamic contrast-enhanced and T2-weighted ($p = 0.001$) imaging[38]. Regarding assessment of deep myometrial invasion, they found that dynamic contrast-enhanced imaging and fused T2-weighted and DW-MRI yielded a comparable performance, with a sensitivity of 1.00 and 0.86 and a specificity of 0.93 and 1.00, respectively. Reader agreement was found to be excellent for fused T2-weighted and DW images (weighted kappa = 0.79), with a significant pathologic correlation regarding the depth of myometrial invasion ($r = 0.94$, $p = 0.0001$)[38].

Detection of peritoneal tumor

The peritoneal cavity is a common site of metastatic spread from gynecological malignancy especially ovarian cancer. Pre-operative imaging plays a number of roles including detection, assessment of tumor bulk, and assessment of suitability for surgical debulking. The detection of peritoneal dissemination by tumor can present difficulties due to poor contrast

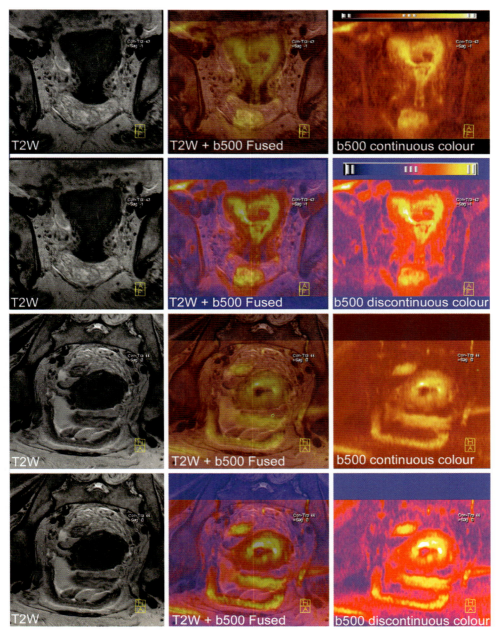

Figure 9.14 Large endometrial adenocarcinoma. The patient had renal failure and therefore intravenous gadolinium contrast was not administered. The complete loss of zonal morphology of the uterine body makes it difficult to assess the depth of myometrial invasion on morphological images. Diffusion images, however, demonstrate deep myometrial invasion which reaches the serosal surface in some areas. No cervical invasion demonstrated. Fusion images with both continuous and discontinuous color scale are shown; discontinuous scales are often better at demonstrating depth of invasion. Note hyperintensity on high *b*-value images of small bowel loops.

resolution compared to the surrounding organs and fat particularly on computed tomography (CT) scans and sometimes on MRI also. Recent studies have reported sensitivity and specificity to be 85–93% and 78–96% respectively on contrast-enhanced CT[3,39], and 95% and 80% respectively on contrast-enhanced MRI[3,40]. DW-MRI can help detect peritoneal tumor both in the abdomen and pelvis. Fujii *et al.* reported

137

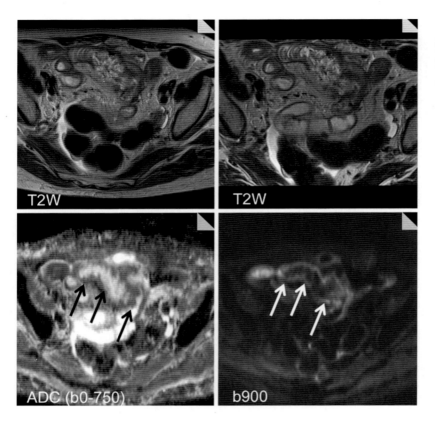

Figure 9.15 Endometrial carcinoma and peritoneal carcinomatosis in a 76-year-old woman. There is extensive serosal disease affecting several small and large bowel loops, better demonstrated on high *b*-value and ADC images (arrows).

DW-MRI sensitivity and specificity of 90% and 95.5% respectively for detection of peritoneal dissemination[3]. In this study, the majority of instances of peritoneal dissemination were demonstrated as moderate or strong high signal intensity on high *b*-value DW-MRI. The minimum size of peritoneal nodules detected was 5 mm. When making this determination it should be remembered that the mucosa of collapsed bowel can be quite hyperintense but is in general uniform and smooth unlike malignant serosal disease which is often irregularly thick (Figure 9.15).

Nodal assessment

Size alone to determine the presence of metastatic lymphadenopathy has been shown to be a poor discriminator in the pelvis[41]. MR sensitivity for distinguishing metastatic from benign nodes ranges from 24% to 73%[5,42–45]. This limited sensitivity is primarily related to the inaccurate detection of small metastatic lymph nodes. Even ^{18}F-fluoro-2-deoxyglucose

(FDG)-PET is unsatisfactory when metastatic lymph nodes are small[46–48]. The advantage of DW-MRI is that it is relatively independent of lesion size. In a recent study, Kim *et al.* demonstrated that DW-MRI is capable of differentiating metastatic from non-metastatic lymph nodes in patients with cervical cancer. In their study of 125 patients who underwent lymph node dissection, the ADC values were significantly lower in the metastatic lymph nodes (0.7651×10^{-3} mm^2/s ± 0.1137) than in the non-metastatic nodes (1.0021×10^{-3} mm^2/s ± 0.1859; $p = 0.001$). The sensitivity of ADC for differentiating metastatic from non-metastatic lymph nodes was 87%, with a specificity of 80%[48].

In our experience normal, benigns and metastatic lymph nodes can all appear bright on high *b*-value images with corresponding low ADC values. As a result, we are cautious about suggesting that lymph nodes are involved with cancer unless ADC values are very low. Our criterion for indicating that a lymph node might be suspicious on DW-MRI also takes into account the relative signal intensity (on very high

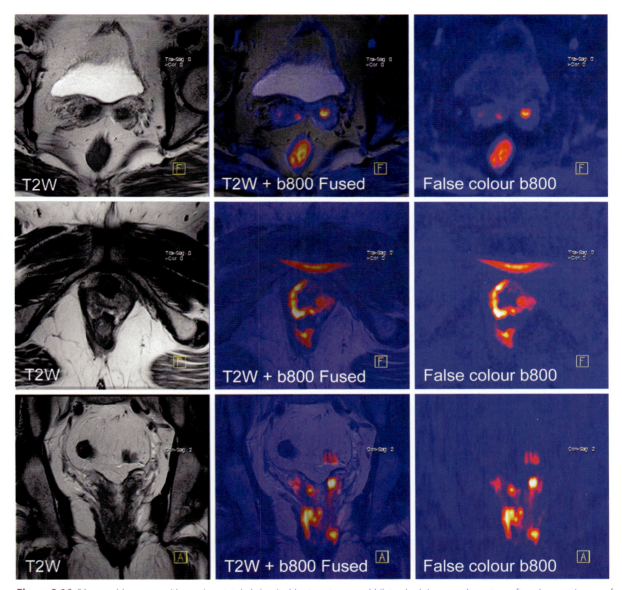

Figure 9.16 56-year-old woman with previous total abdominal hysterectomy and bilateral salpingo-oophorectomy for adenocarcinoma of the endometrium. There are multiple areas of recurrent tumor along the entire vagina from the vaginal vault to the level of the introitus. The extent of the tumor is well demonstrated on diffusion images.

b-value images >1000 s/mm²) compared to nodes that we "know" are benign (such as groin nodes in patients with endometrial or cervix cancer). Another approach is to compare the signal intensity of a lymph node to the primary tumor.

An interesting new approach to circumvent false-positive results (normal and benign reactive nodes appearing bright on high *b*-value images) has been described by Thoeny *et al.* (but in patients with prostate cancer)[49]. They made the critical observation that normal/benign nodes would take up the contrast agent Ferumoxatran-10 (an ultrasmall super-paramagnetic iron oxide particulate –[USPIO]) and thus eliminate the high signal intensity from normal/benign nodes. Using this approach they were able to detect micrometastasis as small as 3 mm using DW-MRI. This innovative approach looks promising and needs to be explored more fully.

Assessement of treatment response

Assessment of tumor response following chemotherapy and radiotherapy

The measurement of size change in response to therapy is the standard method of evaluation of treatment response. It is well known, however, that it has a number of shortcomings. Novel targeted molecular therapies can have clinical benefits without necessarily reducing tumor size and response rates are therefore underestimated. Initial reports have demonstrated the clinical potential for DW-MRI in assessment of tumor response in women with pelvic malignancies. A number of studies have demonstrated increases in the ADC following successful therapy[50–52] the biological basis for which is cell death resulting in increased water diffusion distances in tissues. The success of therapy can be assessed both quantitatively with ADC measurements and qualitatively by inspecting signal intensity changes on high b-value images[4].

Naganawa *et al.* found significant increases in lesion ADC values in patients with cervical cancer treated with combination chemotherapy and radiation therapy. In the partial responders, the differences in the ADC values were found to be relatively small with only a slight increase demonstrated[12]. In fact, changes in water diffusion might be seen before changes in tumor volume and, thus, DW-MRI can potentially act as an early biomarker of therapy[13].

Assessment of uterine fibroid therapy response

Jacob *et al.* examined 14 patients with uterine fibroids who underwent MRI-guided focused ultrasound treatment[53]. They demonstrated increased signal intensity on DW images within the area of ablated fibroid tissue with reduction of ADC values. The mean baseline ADC value in fibroids was 1.5×10^{-3} mm^2/s and post-treatment ADC values (1.08×10^{-3} mm^2/s). A significant difference between ADC values for treated (1.9×10^{-3} mm/sec) and non-treated (1.43×10^{-3} mm^2/s) fibroid tissue at 6-month follow-up was also observed[53]. This observation of an initial ADC decrease and later increase in the ADC probably reflects on the time course as the tissue undergoes transformation from a state of infarction to edema. It is suggested that this change may provide a measure by which to gauge the effectiveness of

treatment[53]. Liapi *et al.* also suggested that DW-MRI and ADC maps may serve as imaging tools for assessing treatment response after uterine fibroid embolization (UFE)[54]. They evaluated 32 fibroids in 11 patients treated with UFE. Treated lesions had low ADC values (1.22×10^{-3} mm^2/s) compared to untreated lesions (1.74×10^{-3} mm^2/s). Changes observed in an infarcted fibroid following chemoradiotherapy for cervix cancer are shown in Figure 9.4.

Assessment of disease recurrence

Diffusion MRI can be very helpful in detecting tumor recurrence particularly for high-grade lesions (Figure 9.16). It can be particularly useful in determining relapsed disease in areas of therapy-induced scarring or where there is very small volume of disease recurrence. It is important to be aware, however, that DW-MRI can underestimate disease recurrence in cases of poorly differentiated tumors or necrotic tumors as discussed earlier.

Conclusions

DW-MRI is a useful adjunct to conventional MR imaging for the evaluation of the female pelvis, providing additional information and improving radiologists' confidence in image interpretation without significant impact on total imaging time[5]. Differences in the water diffusion profile between normal structures and tumor enables improved tumor detection, staging, assessment of treatment response, and determination of the presence of disease recurrence. Furthermore, it has been shown to be helpful in assessing tumor cellularity and histological grade. Although DW-MRI is helpful in lesion characterization, there are no unique values of ADC that enable reliable distinction of malignancy from benign pelvic pathology particularly for ovarian masses and for pelvic nodal evaluations. For accurate reporting of DW-MRI, it is important to be aware of the potential pitfalls such as T2 shine-through, restriction in normal structures, and tumors of low cellular density. Readers must be aware of the benign causes of low ADC with hyperintensity on high b-value images such as abscesses, coagulative necrosis, and inspissated mucus. High b-value and ADC images should always be interpreted in association with morphological findings. Software fusion of high b-value DW images with anatomical images is useful in image interpretation and data presentation, and for therapy planning.

References

1. Inada Y, Matsuki M, Nakai G, *et al.* Body diffusion-weighted MR imaging of uterine endometrial cancer: is it helpful in the detection of cancer in nonenhanced MR imaging? *Eur J Radiol* 2009;**70** (1): 122–7.

2. McVeigh PZ, Syed AM, Milosevic M, Fyles A, Haider MA. Diffusion weighted MRI in cervical cancer. *Eur Radiol* 2008; **18**(5):1058–64.

3. Fujii S, Matsuse E, Kanasaki Y, *et al.* Detection of peritoneal dissemination in gynecological malignancy: evaluation by diffusion-weighted MR imaging. *Eur Radiol* 2008;**18**:18

4. Whittaker CS, Coady C, Culver L, *et al.* Diffusion-weighted MR imaging of female pelvic tumors: a pictorial review. *Radiographics* 2009;**29**:759–74.

5. Namimoto T, Awai K, Nakaura T, *et al.* Role of diffusion-weighted imaging in the diagnosis of gynecological diseases. *Eur Radiol* 2009;**19**(3):745–60.

6. Tamai K, Koyama T, Saga T *et al.* Diffusion-weighted MR imaging of uterine endometrial cancer. *J Magn Reson Imag* 2007;**26**:682–7.

7. Weiss S, Jaermann T, Schmid P, *et al.* Three dimensional fiber architecture of the non pregnant human uterus determined ex vivo using magnetic resonance diffusion tensor imaging. *Anat Rec A* 2006;**228**:84–90.

8. Schmid P, Jaermann T, Boesiger P, *et al.* Ventricular myocardial architecture as visualised in postmortem swine hearts using magnetic resonance diffusion tensor imaging. *Eur J Cardiothorac Surg* 2005;**27**:468–72.

9. Napadow VJ, Chen Q, Mai V, So P T C, Gilbert RJ. Quantitative analysis of three-dimensional-resolved fiber architecture in heterogeneous skeletal muscle tissue using NMR and optical imaging methods. *Biophys J* 2001;**80**:2968–75.

10. Tamai K, Koyama T, Saga T, *et al.* The utility of diffusion-weighted MR imaging for differentiating uterine sarcomas from benign leiomyomas. *Eur Radiol* 2007;**18**:723–30.

11. Anstee A, Scott F, Culver L, *et al.* Diffusion weighted MRI: correlation with tumor grade and stage in endometrial cancer and normal tissue. *Cancer Imag* 2006;**6**:158–62.

12. Naganawa S, Sato C, Kumada H, *et al.* Apparent diffusion coefficient in cervical cancer of the uterus: comparison with the normal uterine cervix. *EurRadiol* 2005;**15**(1):71–8.

13. Koh DM, Collins DJ. Diffusion-weighted MRI in the body: applications and challenges in oncology. *Am J Roentgenol* 2007;**188**(6):1622–35.

14. Jemal A, Murray T, Ward E, *et al.* Cancer statistics, 2005. *CA Cancer J Clin* 2005;**55**:10–30.

15. Klinkel K, Kaji Y, Yuk K, *et al.* Radiological staging in patients with endometrial cancer: a meta-analysis. *Radiology* 1999;**212**:711–18.

16. Manfredi R, Gui B, Maresca G, Fanfani F, Bonomo L. Endometrial cancer: magnetic resonance imaging. *Abdom Imag* 2005;**30**:626–36.

17. Yamashita Y, Harada M, Sawada T, *et al.* Normal uterus and FIGO stage 1 endometiral carcinoma: dynamic gadolinium-enhanced MR imaging. *Radiology* 1993; **186**:495–501.

18. Takahashi S, Murakami T, Narumi Y, *et al.* Preoperative staging of endometrial carcinoma: diagnostic effect of T2-weighted fast spin-echo MR imaging. *Radiology* 1998;**206**:539–47.

19. Inada Y, Matsuki M, Nakai G, *et al.* Body diffusion-weighted MR imaging of uterine endometrial cancer: is it helpful in the detection of cancer in nonenhanced MR imaging? *Eur J Radiol* 2009;**70** (1):122–7.

20. Silverberg SG, Kurman RJ. Tumors of the uterine corpus and gestational trophoblastic disease. In: Rosai J, Aovin I, eds. *Atlas of Tumor Pathology*, vol 3. Washington, DC: Armed Forces Institution of Pathology; 2002, 113–51.

21. Fujii S, Matsusue E, Kigawa J, *et al.* Diagnostic accuracy of the apparent diffusion coefficient in differentiating benign from malignant uterine endometrial cavity lesions: initial results. *Eur Radiol* 2008;**18**:384–9.

22. Ohguri T, Aoki T, Watanabe H, *et al.* MRI findings including gadolinium-enhanced dynamic studies of malignant, mixed, mesodermal tumors of the uterus: differentiation from endometrial carcinoma. *Eur Radiol* 2002;**12**:2737–42.

23. Ueda H, Togashi K, Konishi I, *et al.* Unusual appearances of uterine leiomyomas: MR imaging findings and their histopathologic backgrounds. *Radiographics* 1999;**19**:131–45.

24. Maldjian JA, Listerud J, Moonis G, Siddiqi F. Computing diffusion rates in T2-dark haematomas and areas of low T2 signal. *Am J Neuroradiol* 2001;**22**:112–18.

25. Hitwatashi A, Kinoshita T, Moritani T, *et al.* Hypointensity on diffusion-weighted MRI of brain related to T2 shortening and susceptibility effects. *Am J Roentgenol* 2003;**181**:1705–9.

26. Shimada K, Ohashi I, Kasahara I, *et al.* Differentiation between completely hyalinised uterine leiomyomas: three phase dynamic magnetic resonance imaging (MRI) vs. diffusion weighted MRI with very small b-factors. *J Magn Reson Imag* 2004; **20**:97–104.

27. Ueda H, Togashi K, Konishi I, *et al.* Unusual appearances of uterine leiomyomas: MR imaging findings and their histopathologic backgrounds. *Radiographics* 1999;**19**:131–45.

28. Kahanpaa KV, Wahlstrom T, Grohn P, *et al.* Sarcomas of the uterus: a clinicopathologic study of 119 patients. *Obstet Gynecol* 1986;**67**:417–24.

29. Zaloudek C, Hendrickson MR. Mesenchymal tumors of the uterus. In: Kurman RJ, ed. *Blaustein's Pathology of the Female Genital Tract.* 5th edn. New York: Springer; 2002, 561–616.

30. Sahdev A, Sohaib SA, Jacobs I, *et al.* MR imaging of uterine sarcoma. *Am J Roentgenol* 2001;**177**:1307–11.

31. Nakayama T, Yoshimitsu K, Irie H, *et al.* Diffusion weighted echo-planar MR imaging and ADC mapping in the differential diagnosis of ovarian cystic masses: usefulness of detecting keratinoid substancesin mature cystic teratomas. *J Magn Reson Imag* 2005;**22**:271–8.

32. Fujii S, Kakite S, Nishihara K, *et al.* Diagnostic accuracy of diffusion-weighted imaging in differentiating benign from malignant ovarian lesions. *J Magn Reson Imag* 2008;**28**:1149–56.

33. Katayama M, Masui T, Kobayashi S, *et al.* Diffusion-weighted echo planar imaging of ovarian tumors: is it useful to measure apparent diffusion coefficients? *J Comput Assist Tomogr* 2002;**26**:250–6.

34. Moteki T, Ishizaka H. Diffusion weighted EPI of cystic ovarian lesions: evaluation of cystic contents using apparent diffusion coefficients. *J Magn Reson Imag* 2000; **12**:1014–19.

35. Thomassin-Naggara I, Bazot M, Darai E, *et al.* Epithelial ovarian tumors: value of dynamic contrast-enhanced MR imaging and correlation with tumor angiogenesis. *Radiology* 2008;**248** (1):148–59.

36. Frei KA, Kinkel K, Bonél HM, *et al.* Prediction of deep myometrial invasion in patients with endometrial cancer: clinical utility of contrast-enhanced MR imaging: a meta-analysis and Bayesian analysis. *Radiology* 2000;**216**(2):444–9.

37. Shen SH, Chiou YY, Wang JH, *et al.* Diffusion-weighted single-shot echo-planar imaging with parallel technique in assessment of endometrial cancer. *Am J Roentgenol* 2008;**190**(2):481–8.

38. Lin G, Ng K, Chang C, *et al.* Myometrial invasion in endometrial cancer: diagnostic accuracy of diffusion-weighted 3.0-T MR imaging: initial experience. *Radiology* 2009;**250**:784–92.

39. Tempancy CM, Zou KH, Silverman SG, *et al.* Staging of advanced ovarian cancer: comparison of imaging modalities: report from the Radiological Diagnostic Oncology Group. *Radiology* 2000; **215**:761–7.

40. Ricke J, Sehouli J, Hach C, *et al.* Prospective evaluation of contrast enhanced MRI in the depiction of peritoneal spread in primary or recurrent ovarian cancer. *Eur Radiol* 2003;**13**:943–9.

41. Tangjitgamol S, Manusirivithaya S, Jesadapatarakul S, Leelahakorn S, Thawaramara T. Lymph node size in uterine cancer: a revisit. *Int J Gynecol Cancer* 2006;**16** (5):1880–4.

42. Yu KK, Hricak H, Subak LL, Zaloudek CJ, Powell CB. Preoperative staging of cervical carcinoma: phased array coil fast spin-echo versus body coil spin-echo T2-weighted MR imaging. *Am J Roentgenol* 1998;**171**:707–11.

43. Reinhardt MJ, Ehritt-Braun C, Vogelgesang D, *et al.* Metastatic lymph nodes in patients with cervical cancer: detection with MR imaging and FDG PET. *Radiology* 2001; **218**:776–82.

44. Rockall AG, Sohaib SA, Harisinghani MG, *et al.* Diagnostic performance of nanoparticle-enhanced magnetic resonance imaging in the diagnosis of lymph node metastases in patients with endometrial and cervical cancer. *J Clin Oncol* 2005;**23** (12):2813–21.

45. Choi HJ, Kim SH, Seo SS, *et al.* MRI for pretreatment lymph node staging in uterine cervical cancer. *Am J Roentgenol* 2006;**187**: 538–43.

46. Sironi S, Buda A, Picchio M, *et al.* Lymph node metastasis in patients with clinical early-stage cervical cancer: detection with integrated FDG PET/CT. *Radiology* 2006;**238**:272–9.

47. Chou HH, Chang TC, Yen TC, *et al.* Low value of [^{18}F]-fluoro-2-deoxy-D-glucose positron emission tomography in primary staging of early-stage cervical cancer before radical hysterectomy. *J Clin Oncol* 2006;**24**:123–8.

48. Kim J, Kim K, Park B, Kim M, Cho K. Feasibility of diffusion-weighted imaging in the differentiation of metastatic from non-metastatic lymph nodes: early experience. *J Magn Reson Imag* 2008; **28**:714–19.

49. Thoeny HC, Triantafyllou M, Birkhaeuser FD, *et al.* Combined ultrasmall superparamagnetic particles of iron oxide-enhanced and diffusion-weighted magnetic resonance imaging reliably detect pelvic lymph node metastases in normal-sized nodes of bladder and prostate cancer patients. *Eur Urol* 2009;**55** (4):770–2.

50. Schepkin VD, Chenevert TL, Kuszpit K, *et al.* Sodium and proton diffusion MRI as biomarkers for early therapeutic response in subcutaneous tumors. *Magn Reson Imag* 2006;**24**:273–8.

51. Chenevert TL, McKeever PE, Ross BD. Monitoring early response of experimental brain tumors to therapy

using diffusion magnetic resonance imaging. *Clin Cancer Res* 1997;**3**:1457–66.

52. Einarsdottir H, Karlsson M, Wejde J, Bauer HC. Diffusion-weighted MRI of soft tissue tumors. *Eur Radiol* 2004;**14**:959–63.

53. Jacobs MA, Herskovits EH, Kim HS. Uterine fibroids: diffusion weighted MR imaging for monitoring

therapy with focused ultrasound surgery-preliminary study. *Radiology* 2005; **236**:196–203.

54. Liapi E, Kamel IR, Bluemke DA, Jacobs MA, Kim HS. Assessment of response of uterine fibroids and myometrium to embolisation using diffusion-weighted echoplanar MR imaging. *J Comput Assist Tomogr* 2005; **29**:82–6.

Chapter 10

Diffusion-weighted MRI of the bone marrow and the spine

Olaf Dietrich and Andrea Baur-Melnyk

Introduction

Diffusion-weighted magnetic resonance imaging (DWI) is a well-established magnetic resonance imaging (MRI) technique, in which the MR signal intensity is influenced by the self-diffusion, i.e., the microscopic stochastic Brownian motion, of water molecules caused by the molecular thermal energy[1–7]. An overview of the physical principles of diffusion and DWI is given in a separate chapter, and elsewhere[8]. DWI can provide information about the microscopic structure and organization of biological tissues and, thus, can depict various pathological changes of organs or tissues. It has been thoroughly evaluated for a multitude of neurological pathologies[9] such as brain tumors[10], abscesses[11], or white-matter diseases[12], and in particular for the early detection of cerebral ischemia[13,14], which is generally considered the most important application of clinical DWI.

Significantly fewer studies have been published about diffusion MRI outside the brain, mainly because of the relatively low robustness of conventional DWI methods in non-neurological applications and, consequently, the rather limited image quality in such applications. This situation, however, improved significantly in recent years due to better MRI hardware as well as newly developed pulse sequences; as a consequence, several new applications of DWI have been described. Examples such as DWI studies of the liver[15,16], the kidneys[17,18], or of soft-tissue tumors[19,20] are described in detail elsewhere in this book. Recently, whole-body DWI was proposed to improve the detection of malignancies and pathological lymph nodes[21,22]. Most of these applications are based on variants of the diffusion-weighting echo-planar imaging (EPI) pulse sequence.

Since the late 1990s, DWI has also been successfully used for the detection and characterization of bone-marrow alterations – predominantly in the spine. The most important clinical application of DWI in bone marrow is the differentiation of benign (e.g., osteoporotic or traumatic) and malignant (metastatic or neoplastic) vertebral compression fractures[23–25]. Unfortunately, DWI of the bone marrow is considerably complicated by the fact that significant variations of susceptibility occur in the close anatomical neighborhood of bone structures. These susceptibility variations result in severe distortion artifacts when standard echo-planar DWI techniques are applied. Hence, several alternative diffusion-weighting pulse sequences were proposed and evaluated for DWI of the bone marrow[26] as described below in the section "Techniques for DWI of bone marrow."

In this chapter, we will discuss several specific MRI techniques, which have been used for DWI of bone marrow in general and in particular for the spine. Subsequently, we will give an extensive overview about diffusion studies of the bone marrow and particularly of vertebral compression fractures as well as of the intervertebral disks.

Techniques for DWI of bone marrow

Many different types of pulse sequences can be modified for DWI by inserting additional diffusion-sensitizing gradients. Typically, a pair of diffusion gradients is used in these sequences as proposed by Stejskal and Tanner[27]. The effect of these diffusion gradients is to attenuate the transversal magnetization, i.e., the received MR signal intensity, depending on the strength and duration of the gradients, which are summarized as the diffusion weighting or b-value of the sequence, and the extent of molecular motion described by the (apparent) diffusion coefficient[8] (see also Chapter 1).

Extra-Cranial Applications of Diffusion-Weighted MRI, ed. Bachir Taouli. Published by Cambridge University Press.
© Cambridge University Press 2011.

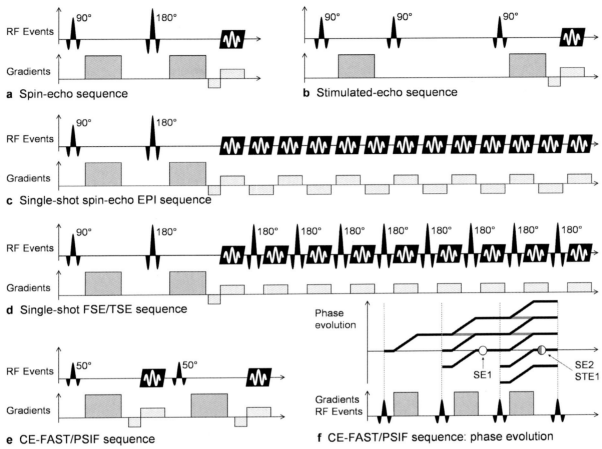

Figure 10.1 Pulse sequences used for DWI. Sequences are simplified by displaying only the diffusion gradients (dark gray boxes) and the imaging gradients in readout direction (light gray boxes). (a, b) A single repetition of a spin-echo and stimulated-echo sequence; (c, d): echo trains of single-shot spin-echo echo-planar and fast-spin-echo sequences; (e) two subsequent repetitions of a diffusion-weighted SSFP sequence; (f) evolution of phase in a diffusion-weighted SSFP sequence (phase angles are increased by diffusion gradients and partially inverted by the RF pulses).

Since the diffusion gradients are inserted in order to depict stochastic molecular motions in the range of typically some 10 μm, DWI becomes very sensitive to any macroscopic patient motion as well[28–30]. The most important sources of such motion are pulsatile blood flow, cerebrospinal fluid pulsation, cardiac and respiratory motion, as well as peristaltic bowel motion. Depending on the pulse sequence, different strategies can be chosen to reduce the influence of motion as described in the following sections.

Spin-echo and stimulated-echo sequences

Historically, DWI was first performed with stimulated-echo and spin-echo pulse sequences (Fig. 10.1a and 1b)[5–7].

These pulse sequences, however, require very long acquisition times of several minutes to acquire a single multislice dataset, since they fill the required raw data space (k-space) line-by-line with echoes (Fig. 10.2a), whose acquisition is separated by the relatively long repetition time(TR) of 2 to 5 s. These sequences are very prone to motion artifacts, which result from different states of involuntary patient motion in subsequently acquired k-space lines.

Different strategies were proposed to reduce the motion sensitivity and increase the robustness of stimulated-echo and spin-echo sequences such as navigator echo motion correction[31–33] or radial k-space sampling[34,35]. A navigator echo is an additionally acquired echo immediately following (or preceding) the conventional imaging echo that is, however,

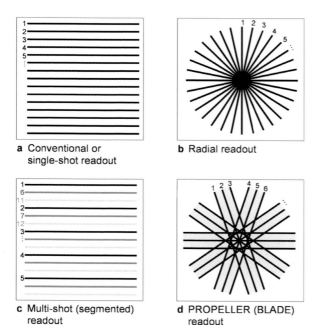

a Conventional or single-shot readout

b Radial readout

c Multi-shot (segmented) readout

d PROPELLER (BLADE) readout

Figure 10.2 Different *k*-space acquisition schemes used for DWI. (a) Conventional line-by-line readout of, e.g., a spin-echo sequence; the same *k*-space scheme is used for single-shot sequences, but with much shorter intervals (fractions of milliseconds instead of seconds) between the readout of the lines. (b) Radial readout; the central point of *k*-space is covered in each readout and can be used for motion correction. (c) Segmented or multi-shot readout; the *k*-space is covered by multiple (in this case three) echo trains (differentiated by different gray levels). (d) PROPELLER or BLADE readout; the *k*-space is covered by rotated rectangular strips that correspond to a single multi-echo readout; the center of *k*-space is acquired by all strips and can thus be used for motion correction.

acquired without phase encoding. Thus, all navigator echoes of a dataset should ideally be completely identical in the absence of motion; and any translational as well as some forms of rotational bulk motion can be deduced and subsequently corrected by comparing the navigator echoes of different acquisition steps.

In radial *k*-space sampling, all *k*-space trajectories run through the center of *k*-space (Fig. 10.2b). These sequences are called self-navigated since the central point of *k*-space contained in each echo can be used similarly to the navigator echo described above to correct motion effects or to discard echoes with severe influences of motion. In addition, less motion-sensitive reconstruction techniques such as radial projection reconstruction of magnitude data are available after radial *k*-space acquisition. However, in spite of these technical developments, these sequences are generally not applied in clinical routine applications

today because of their prohibitively long acquisition times. Only few diffusion studies of bone marrow were performed with these techniques such as a study by Ward *et al.* on DWI of tibial bone marrow[36] and two studies by Dietrich *et al.* and Spuentrup *et al.* on DWI of vertebral bone marrow[35,37].

A more advanced modification of the conventional spin-echo sequence is the diffusion-weighted line-scan imaging techniques proposed by Gudbjartsson *et al.*[38]. In line-scan imaging, 1D lines of the imaged volume are excited instead of complete 2D slices. Thus, the repetition time can be considerably reduced and images can be reconstructed from 1D magnitude data that are much less sensitive to motion than the conventional 2D complex raw datasets. As a disadvantage, the signal-to-noise ratio (SNR) of this technique is reduced in comparison with conventional acquisitions due to the smaller excited volume. A second disadvantage is that line-scan imaging techniques are not available for all MRI systems. Line-scan imaging has been applied, e.g., for DWI of the spine by Maeda *et al.*, Bammer *et al.*, Newitt and Majumdar, and Carballido-Gamio *et al.*[39–42]

Echo-planar imaging (EPI) sequences

The most important and most frequently used pulse sequence for DWI in general is the single-shot spin-echo echo-planar imaging sequence (Fig. 10.1c)[43]. This sequence is relatively insensitive to influences from macroscopic patient motion because of the very fast readout of the complete image data within about 100 ms. The fast and – with respect to motion sensitivity – relatively robust acquisition was the most important reasons that the single-shot EPI sequence became the standard technique for DWI and diffusion tensor imaging (DTI) of the brain.

In the presence of susceptibility variations, however, echo-planar images frequently suffer from gross geometrical image distortions due to the relatively long gradient-echo train. Susceptibility variations translate to variations of the Larmor frequencies of spins and, thus, to phase errors in the *k*-space data that accumulate over the duration of the echo train[26]. In brain MRI, the distortion artifacts arise mainly at a few well-known locations such as the frontobasal area and in the vicinity of the brainstem; most other brain areas are depicted in acceptable image quality due to the relatively homogeneous distribution of susceptibility within the brain. However, this property of EPI is a severe limitation for the application outside the brain and particularly in the musculoskeletal system where structures or organs of interest are frequently found in the direct neighborhood of air-filled spaces or bone/soft tissue interfaces with substantially different susceptibilities. Thus, the image quality of echo-planar acquisitions of the spine is typically extremely low and often does not provide sufficient anatomical details. A second disadvantage of single-shot EPI is the relatively low spatial resolution that can be realized with this approach. The single-shot readout used to limit the spatial resolution to matrix sizes of 128×128 due to the rapid $T2^*$ decay of the signal during the gradient-echo train.

Only relatively recently have innovations in hardware and in acquisition techniques substantially improved the suitability of EPI for non-neuroradiological DWI. Improved gradient systems with reduced eddy-current effects can reduce geometric distortions. Even more important became the application of parallel imaging techniques[44] such as sensitivity-encoded (SENSE) MRI[45] or the generalized autocalibrated partially parallel acquisition (GRAPPA) technique[46]. These techniques were originally developed to accelerate the MRI acquisition by employing multiple receiver coil elements and reducing thus the number of required k-space lines. As an additional advantage, parallel MRI can be used to reduce geometric distortions in EPI and, at the same time, to increase the spatial resolution of EPI to matrix sizes of 192×192 or even 256×256[47].

A second approach to reduce artifacts and to increase the spatial resolution of EPI acquisitions is a segmented (or multishot) echo-planar readout: the echo train of a single image can be divided into several parts that are shorter than the original single-shot readout (Fig. 10.2c). Since the acquisition of these segments must be separated by a repetition time of typically a few seconds, the total acquisition time of a slice is considerably increased. On the one hand, by shortening the echo train length, the segmented EPI sequence becomes less sensitive to susceptibility variations, shows reduced distortion artifacts, and its spatial resolution can be easily increased. On the other hand, its robustness against motion artifacts is substantially reduced as different states of patient motion may now occur for each acquired segment. Navigator echo correction schemes similar to those described above for the spin-echo approach have been applied for segmented EPI to correct for the influences of motion[48].

In spite of the limited image quality of single-shot EPI for DWI of bone marrow or the spine, this sequence type has been used rather frequently for these applications as discussed below.

Fast-spin-echo or turbo-spin-echo sequences

An alternative to diffusion-weighted EPI acquisitions are diffusion-weighted single-shot sequences based on the acquisition of spin-echo trains, i.e., single-shot fast-spin-echo (FSE) or turbo-spin-echo (TSE) pulse sequences, which are also known as rapid acquisition with relaxation enhancement (RARE) or half-Fourier acquisition single-shot turbo-spin-echo (HASTE) sequences (Fig. 10.1d)[49,50]. Similarly to echo-planar sequences, these approaches are very fast (with acquisition times in the order of 200–400 ms per image) and relatively insensitive to motion, but also limited in their spatial resolution due to the T2 decay of the signal during the spin-echo train.

In comparison to EPI, an important advantage particularly for non-neurological applications such as DWI of the bone marrow is the insensitivity of these techniques to susceptibility variations: any variations of the Larmor frequencies are inherently compensated by the refocusing RF pulses. Unfortunately, inserting diffusion-sensitizing gradients into the spin-echo train destroys the originally equal spacing of refocusing RF pulses (known as Carr–Purcell–Meiboom–Gill [CPMG] condition) and, thus, can induce new image artifacts. Several approaches have been suggested to overcome this disadvantage, but most solutions also reduce the SNR of the acquired images[49,51,52]; thus, single-shot fast-spin-echo DWI frequently requires the acquisition of multiple averages in order to obtain a sufficient SNR. More recently proposed solutions can recover (at least almost) the full SNR[53,54], but are not yet generally available on most MRI systems. As for EPI, parallel imaging can be employed to increase the spatial resolution that can be acquired with a single echo train and to reduce some image artifacts such as image blurring in phase-encoding direction, which is caused by the T2 decay of signal during the echo train.

Some remaining disadvantages of single-shot fast-spin-echo techniques can be overcome by segmenting the readout as in segmented EPI acquisitions; at the cost, however, of increased acquisition times and motion sensitivity. A related and particularly promising

147

approach is the recently proposed diffusion-weighted periodically rotated overlapping parallel lines with enhanced reconstruction (PROPELLER) MRI sequence[55] or BLADE sequence[56]. With these non-Cartesian techniques, the k-space is covered by rotated rectangular strips, each consisting of a spin-echo train (Fig. 10.2d). The sequence is self-navigated since all these strips (or blades) include an area around the center of the k-space. This allows for a motion correction, as in purely radial spin-echo techniques but with higher robustness due to the larger oversampled central k-space area.

These techniques, in particular the single-shot variant, have been applied in DWI studies of the vertebral bone marrow by Zhou *et al.*, Byun *et al.*, Park *et al.*, Oner *et al.*, and Raya *et al.*[57–62] as well as in DWI studies of the intervertebral disks[42,63].

Steady-state free-precession sequences

A very different approach for DWI (in particular of the spinal column) is the application of steady-state free-precession (SSFP) sequences (Fig. 10.1e). The SSFP sequence type used for DWI is the diffusion-weighted contrast enhanced Fourier-acquired steady-state technique (CE-FAST; here, "contrast-enhanced" does not refer to any administered contrast agent, but to the inherent image contrast) or PSIF sequence[64,65]. The PSIF sequence is the reversed version (with respect to the timing of the pulse sequence events) of the "fast imaging with steady precession" (FISP) sequence; hence, the acronym PSIF was chosen as the reversed (backwards spelling) version of FISP. In contrast to the other approaches described above, only a single (monopolar) diffusion gradient is typically inserted into each TR of the PSIF sequence (Fig. 10.1e shows two subsequent TRs)[66,67]. Thus, the SSFP approach differs considerably from almost all other diffusion-weighting pulse sequences, which employ variants of the conventional Stejskal–Tanner diffusion gradient scheme.

Spins dephased by the diffusion sensitizing gradients are rephased by a second diffusion gradient later in the sequence scheme (i.e., in one of the following repetitions); however, not necessarily by the immediately subsequent one, since the dephased spins can be partially stored for several TRs in the longitudinal direction. This is illustrated in the phase-evolution diagram in Fig. 10.1f: The first diffusion gradient (gray box) adds an extra phase to the spins (indicated by the first ramp in the upper part of the diagram). The next RF pulse partially reverts the phase, leaves other spins in their current state, and rotates a third fraction of the spins into the longitudinal direction (indicated by the gray line; these spins cannot be dephased by the following diffusion gradient). Only the reverted spins form the first spin echo (SE1) after the second diffusion gradient and have then experienced a diffusion-sensitizing duration of about $1 \times TR$; the other spins remain dephased and evolve further until the next RF pulse acts on them. Again, some spins are flipped by 180°, some are left unchanged, and some are moved from the longitudinal direction back into the transversal plane. The last group forms the first stimulated echo (STE1) in the following cycle and has experienced a diffusion-sensitizing duration of about $2 \times TR$. Other spins are rephased even later. Thus, the duration of the diffusion-sensitizing preparation can be very different for the spins that contribute to the observed signal and, hence, the diffusion-weighting, b, of the PSIF sequence cannot easily be determined, but depends on the relaxation times of tissue, T1 and T2, as well as on the sequence parameters, echo time (TE), TR, and the flip angle[68,69]. Although this makes the exact quantification of the apparent diffusion coefficient (ADC) very difficult, diffusion-weighted images acquired by the PSIF sequence have been shown to be extremely valuable for the differential diagnosis of vertebral compression fractures based on the visual (non-quantitatively evaluated) image contrast between lesions and surrounding vertebral bodies[23–25].

The diffusion-weighted PSIF approach is relatively fast due to the short repetition times in the order of typically 20 to 30 ms. Consequently, the PSIF sequence is also relatively insensitive to the influence of bulk motion. Newer developments of SSFP DWI include the implementation of diffusion-weighted 3D sequences, which have been applied, e.g., for DWI of the cartilage[70].

The optimal diffusion weighting for DWI of the bone marrow

An important parameter for all DWI studies is the diffusion weighting or the b-value of the applied pulse sequence. On the one hand, the contrast between tissues with different ADCs increases with higher b-values. On the other hand, this process is limited by the available SNR, since the signal intensity decreases with increasing diffusion weightings and, thus, the tissue signal approximates the noise level of the image, which can bias the determined ADCs if too high b-values are applied[71]. As a consequence, an optimal diffusion weighting should balance between sufficient diffusion contrast and sufficient SNR. A frequently found rule of thumb is that the b-value should be about the inverse of the expected ADC; e.g., for ADCs of 1.0×10^{-3} mm^2/s, the b-value should be chosen around 1000 s/mm^2.

However, in DWI of normal and pathological bone marrow the range of observed ADCs is relatively large (varying between about 0.2 and 2.0×10^{-3} mm^2/s) and, therefore, is not very helpful in order to define an optimal b-value. The SNR of bone marrow is generally very low in DWI, and, thus, the optimal diffusion weighting for DWI of bone marrow is somewhat lower than the value of about 1000 s/mm^2 typically used for DWI of the brain. From our own experience and in agreement with several other publications, the optimal b-value for DWI of the bone marrow is in the range of 500 to 600 s/mm^2 for both EPI-based or TSE-based measurements. To obtain a more acceptable image quality with EPI sequences, even lower optimal b-values of about 300 s/mm^2 have been proposed[72], although this may reduce the precision of the determined ADCs.

If diffusion-weighting SSFP techniques are applied, the signal attenuation cannot be easily described by a single b-value; instead, different attenuations are observed depending not only on the ADC but also on the relaxation times, in particular on the longitudinal relaxation time, T1, of the imaged object or organ. Thus, the diffusion weighting can only be specified by the area (i.e., the zeroth moment) of the diffusion gradient and by other sequence parameters such as flip angle and TR. Typical values used for DWI studies are gradient moments between 69 and 138 mT/m·ms (e.g., gradients with an amplitude of 23 mT/m and durations between 3 and 6 ms) in SSFP sequences with a TR of 25 ms, and a flip angle of 50°. In pure water, this sequence results in a signal attenuation by about 50% and 75%, which would correspond to "hypothetical b-values" of about 350 s/mm^2 and 700 s/mm^2. However, it is important to note that these values would be valid only in pure water, while tissue (with typically shorter T1 relaxation times) will show smaller signal attenuations corresponding to lower b-values even if the same ADC is assumed. This means that no unique b-value can be defined for these SSFP sequences, and that the concept of "b-values" cannot be applied in this context.

Sequence recommendations for DWI of the bone marrow and the spine

In contrast to DWI of the brain, for which EPI sequences are the established and generally accepted acquisition technique, there is no such general agreement on the optimal method for DWI of the bone marrow and the spine. Based on our own experience, the image quality and the reliability of the quantitative parameters is frequently very low when applying EPI sequences for DWI of the bone marrow and in particular of the spine due to severe image distortions. Thus, we prefer single-shot turbo-spin-echo techniques for quantitative DWI of structures affected by substantial susceptibility variations. Typical parameters include three to four b-values between 50 and 600 s/mm^2, a minimized echo time, between four and ten signal averages, and low to moderate matrix sizes of, e.g., 128×128. However, as mentioned above and described in detail below, special applications such as the assessment of vertebral compression fractures can be effectively based on non-quantitative DWI using SSFP sequences with a diffusion gradient amplitude of 23 mT/m and durations between 3 and 6 ms, a TR of 25 ms, and a flip angle of 50°.

DWI studies of bone marrow and the spinal column

Non-quantitative DWI of vertebral bone marrow and fractures

As mentioned above, one of the most successful applications of diffusion-weighted imaging of the bone marrow is the differentiation of benign osteoporotic and malignant vertebral compression fractures, which was first demonstrated by Baur *et al.* in 1998[23]. In this study, the pathological differentiation was based on the relative signal intensity of the affected vertebra in non-quantitative DWI with a diffusion-weighted SSFP sequence, i.e., on purely non-quantitative DWI without any determination of the corresponding apparent diffusion coefficient. Baur and co-workers demonstrated that benign osteoporotic fractures appear hypointense or isointense in SSFP-based DWI, while malignant fractures caused by bone marrow tumors and metastases appear hyperintense.

Table 10.1 Non-quantitative DWI of vertebral bone marrow

Study	Pulse sequence type[a]	Diffusion weighting (gradient moment or *b*-values)	Number of patients	Signal relative to normal vertebral bone marrow[b]		
				Benign (osteoporotic/ traumatic) fracture	Malignant fracture or metastasis	Differentiability benign vs. malignant fracture
Baur *et al.* 1998[23]	SSFP	46 ms·mT/m	30	↓ (↔)	↑	yes
Castillo *et al.* 2000[73]	SSFP	48 ms·mT/m	15	–	↓ ↔ ↑	no
Baur *et al.* 2001[75]	SSFP	138 ms·mT/m	29	↓ (↔)	↑	yes
Spuentrup *et al.* 2001[37]	SE, STE	0, 360/598 s/mm²	34	↓	↔	yes
Yasumoto *et al.* 2002[91]	SS-EPI	30, 300, 900 s/mm²	53	↓ (↔) (↑)[c]	↑ (↔) (↓)[c]	yes
Byun *et al.* 2002[58]	SSFP	48 ms·mT/m	24	–	↑[d]	n/a
Baur *et al.* 2002[76]	SSFP	69 ms·mT/m	85	↓ (↔) (↑)	↑	yes
Abanoz *et al.* 2003[92]	SSFP	115 ms·mT/m	49	↓ ↔	↑[e]	yes
Park *et al.* 2004[60]	SS-FSE	500 s/mm²	46	↓ (↔)	↓ ↔ (↑)	low
Hackländer *et al.* 2006[74]	SSFP	25 ms·mT/m	38	–	↑ (↔)[f]	no[f]
Byun *et al.* 2007[59]	SSFP	120 ms·mT/m	22	↓	↑	yes

Notes: [a]Sequence types: SSFP, diffusion-weighted steady-state free-precession (or PSIF) sequence; SS-FSE, diffusion-weighted single-shot fast-spin-echo sequence; SS-EPI: diffusion-weighted single-shot spin-echo echo-planar imaging sequence with fat saturation; SE, STE, diffusion-weighted spin-echo or stimulated-echo sequence.
[b]↓, lesion hypointense; ↔, lesion isointense; ↑, lesion hyperintense; parentheses, sporadic observations; –, no data.
[c]Results for iliac bone marrow without (left) or with (right) infiltration of malignant lymphoma.
[d]Results from metastatic disease before therapy; all lesions became hypointense after successful radiation therapy.
[e]Three lesions in inflammatory diseases also hyperintense.
[f]Results for non-prostate carcinoma metastases; 18 metastatic lesions from prostate carcinoma showed mixed contrasts (hypo-, iso-, or hyperintense).

Several similar studies of non-quantitative DWI of vertebral compression fractures (frequently performed with diffusion-weighting SSFP techniques rendering quantitative measurements extremely difficult) are summarized in Table 10.1. The results of most of these studies are compatible with a general tendency to hypointensity in benign vertebral fractures and to hyperintensity in malignant fractures with good to excellent differentiability of both groups; image examples are shown in Figs. 10.3 and 10.4. Typically, this signal behavior showed up more clearly with the diffusion-weighted SSFP approach than with alternative pulse sequences such as single-shot EPI, single-shot FSE, or conventional spin-echo or stimulated echo sequences (cf. Table 10.1). A recently published statistical meta-analysis of several of these publications by Karchevsky *et al.*[25] concluded as well that hypointense signal in a fractured vertebra on DWI is strongly suggestive of benign etiology.

Contradictory results were reported by Castillo *et al.*[73], who found a number of hypointense vertebral metastases in diffusion-weighted SSFP acquisitions. These results may be explained by the fact that some patients with hypointense metastases were treated with radiotherapy before imaging (resulting in hypointense signal as described by Byun *et al.*[58]) and some other patients had sclerotic metastases that

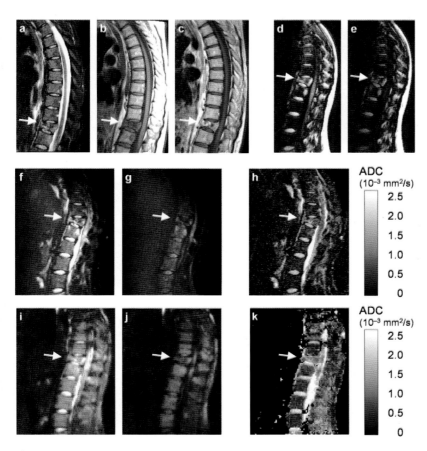

Figure 10.3 Example of a neoplastic vertebral compression fracture of the 11th thoracic vertebra (arrows) in a 50-year-old woman with breast carcinoma; a second metastatic lesion (without fracture) is present in the 12th thoracic vertebra caudal of the compression fracture. (a) Sagittal STIR image shows a slightly hyperintense lesion, (b) sagittal non-enhanced T1-weighted image shows a hypointense lesion, (c) sagittal contrast-enhanced T1-weighted image demonstrates inhomogeneous signal enhancement. (d, e) Diffusion-weighted SSFP acquisitions with diffusion gradient moments of 69 and 138 ms·mT/m; the lesion appears hyperintense, indicating a malignant fracture. (f, g) Diffusion-weighted single-shot EPI acquisitions with b-values of 50 and 600 s/mm^2, (h) corresponding ADC map with a diffusion coefficient in the lesion of 1.10×10^{-3} mm^2/s. (i, j) Diffusion-weighted single-shot FSE acquisitions (with fat saturation) with b-values of 100 and 600 s/mm^2, (k) corresponding ADC map with a diffusion coefficient in the lesion of 1.28×10^{-3} mm^2/s; the ADC of normal appearing bone marrow is about $0.6\ 10^{-3}$ mm^2/s. Note the low image quality of the EPI acquisitions (f, g) with severe distortions and signal loss cranial of the lesion; better image quality (and, thus, more reliable ADC quantification) is obtained by the single-shot FSE acquisitions (i, j). The best image quality of all diffusion-weighted acquisition is obtained with the SSFP acquisitions (d, e), which, however, cannot be used for ADC quantification.

appear hypointense due to their very low water content. Recently, Hackländer *et al.* noted that particularly vertebral metastases of prostate cancer show lower signal than metastases of other tumors[74]. This result may also explain some of the hypointense signals observed by Castillo and co-workers.

An important factor in diffusion-weighted SSFP imaging is the influence of in- and opposed-phase effects of the fat and water components. Depending on the interval between signal excitation and readout, fat and water signals may superimpose constructively ("in phase" acquisition) or destructively ("opposed phase" acquisition). This effect is particularly relevant for bone marrow, since it contains a mixture of fat and water components, whereas most other tissues consist of a single predominant component. Thus, slight modifications of the pulse sequence timing in the order of 1 ms can result in very different signal intensities of the vertebral bone marrow relative to its surroundings. This effect is demonstrated in Fig. 10.5; in acquisitions close to in-phase conditions, the signal intensity of the bone marrow is much higher than

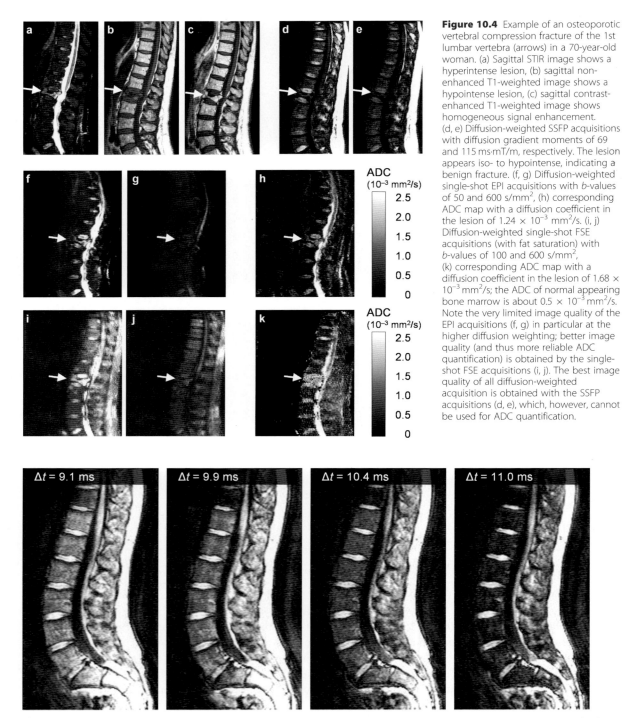

Figure 10.4 Example of an osteoporotic vertebral compression fracture of the 1st lumbar vertebra (arrows) in a 70-year-old woman. (a) Sagittal STIR image shows a hyperintense lesion, (b) sagittal non-enhanced T1-weighted image shows a hypointense lesion, (c) sagittal contrast-enhanced T1-weighted image shows homogeneous signal enhancement. (d, e) Diffusion-weighted SSFP acquisitions with diffusion gradient moments of 69 and 115 ms·mT/m, respectively. The lesion appears iso- to hypointense, indicating a benign fracture. (f, g) Diffusion-weighted single-shot EPI acquisitions with b-values of 50 and 600 s/mm², (h) corresponding ADC map with a diffusion coefficient in the lesion of 1.24×10^{-3} mm²/s. (i, j) Diffusion-weighted single-shot FSE acquisitions (with fat saturation) with b-values of 100 and 600 s/mm², (k) corresponding ADC map with a diffusion coefficient in the lesion of 1.68×10^{-3} mm²/s; the ADC of normal appearing bone marrow is about 0.5×10^{-3} mm²/s. Note the very limited image quality of the EPI acquisitions (f, g) in particular at the higher diffusion weighting; better image quality (and thus more reliable ADC quantification) is obtained by the single-shot FSE acquisitions (i, j). The best image quality of all diffusion-weighted acquisition is obtained with the SSFP acquisitions (d, e), which, however, cannot be used for ADC quantification.

Figure 10.5 Sagittal diffusion-weighted SSFP images of a healthy volunteer acquired with identical sequence parameters except for the interval, Δt, between the center of the data readout and the center of the following RF pulse. The first acquisition ($\Delta t = 9.1$ ms) is acquired approximately under in-phase conditions, the last one ($\Delta t = 11.0$ ms) under opposed-phase conditions. Note the strongly varying signal intensity of the vertebral bone marrow in contrast to the almost constant signal intensity of other tissues such as the spinal cord or muscles. Clinical applications such as the differentiation of vertebral compression fractures require a relatively low signal intensity in normal appearing bone marrow, i.e., should be acquired in approximate opposed-phase condition.

under opposed-phase conditions. It is therefore important to note that the original studies by Baur *et al.* were based on a diffusion-weighting PSIF sequence with approximately opposed-phase read-out[23,75,76]. The time interval between the center of the echo readout and the center of the following RF excitation pulse was about 7.2 ms, i.e., close to the opposed-phase state on a 1.5-T MRI scanner. Diffusion-weighting SSFP sequences with in-phase acquisition might result in substantially different signal properties (and potentially reduced differentiability) of vertebral compression fractures. Further studies are still required to understand the details of signal alterations and the influences of in- and opposed-phase effects in DWI of vertebral lesions.

Quantitative DWI of vertebral bone marrow and fractures

An alternative to non-quantitative diffusion-weighted SSFP imaging is the acquisition of diffusion-weighted images at two or more *b*-values in order to calculate the apparent diffusion coefficient as a quantitative measure of diffusion. Several studies have applied quantitative DWI to normal and pathological vertebral bone marrow as summarized in Tables 10.2 and 10.3. Although the displayed results exhibit a certain variability, there appear to be typical ADC ranges associated with normal and pathological vertebral bone marrow in the majority of these studies. Typical ADCs of normal vertebral bone marrow (but also of osteopenic or osteoporotic bone marrow) are relatively low between 0.2 and 0.6×10^{-3} mm^2/s (Fig. 10.6). Pathological bone marrow exhibits much higher diffusivities, ranging from about 0.7 to 1.0×10^{-3} mm^2/s in metastases as well as malignant fractures, and from about 1.0 to 2.0×10^{-3} mm^2/s in osteoporotic or traumatic fractures. Vertebrae affected by inflammatory disease such as spondylitis or tuberculosis have been reported with ADCs in an intermediate range from about 1.0 to 1.5×10^{-3} mm^2/s. Although a certain overlap of ADC ranges can be seen in Table 10.2, several authors concluded that ADC measurements can be useful for the differentiation of benign vertebral fractures and metastatic lesions[57,77,78]. The overlap of ADC ranges in particular with respect to infectious diseases is typically not a problem for the differential diagnosis of vertebral lesions since infectious alterations can in general be well distinguished independently of diffusion measurements based on the image morphology alone.

The general variability of the reported ADCs can be explained by the different pulse sequences and different diffusion weightings used in these studies. The most important difference with respect to the applied pulse sequences is the use of fat saturation, which is required for single-shot EPI (due to the large chemical-shift-related displacement of fat relative to other tissue) but is optional in combination with spin-echo or fast-spin-echo techniques. Since the ADC of vertebral fat is very close to zero, the calculated diffusion coefficients of normal bone marrow are systematically decreased when fat saturation is not applied[79]. Typical values are in the range of 0.2 to 0.4×10^{-3} mm^2/s without fat saturation, in contrast to 0.3 to 0.6×10^{-3} mm^2/s with fat saturation (Fig. 10.6). Smaller differences are seen in lesions, since the relative fat content is much lower there than in normal bone marrow.

The chosen range of *b*-values can also systematically influence the measured ADCs: at very low *b*-values, the diffusion effect is known to be overestimated due to the contribution of perfusion to the signal attenuation[80,81], while the choice of relatively high *b*-values greater than about 600 s/mm^2 may result in an underestimation due to signal intensities comparable to the noise level as discussed above.

The pathophysiological background of the described diffusion properties in vertebral bone marrow is not yet fully understood. Currently, the most probable hypothesis is that the molecular diffusion of water is substantially increased in osteoporotic fractures because of bone marrow edema and the disruption of the trabecular structure. In contrast, the diffusion is restricted in malignant vertebral compression fractures due to the high cellularity of tumor tissue[23]. In addition, if DWI without fat suppression is applied, the ratio of the fat and water contributions to the signal, i.e., the presence of red and yellow bone marrow or of tumor tissue, plays an important role as well. In general, the lower the fat contribution to the signal, the higher becomes the diffusivity of the composite tissue signal.

DWI of bone marrow outside the spine

Only very few studies examined DWI of the bone marrow outside of the vertebrae as listed in Table 10.4. The number of these studies is too small (and the results are too inhomogeneous) to establish typical ADC ranges for normal or pathological bone marrow

Table 10.2 Quantitative DWI of vertebral bone marrow (v.b.m.) with fractures, metastases, or inflammatory disease

Study	Pulse sequence type[a]	b-values (s/mm²)	Number of subjects	Apparent diffusion coefficient (10⁻³ mm²/s)			
				Benign (osteoporotic/traumatic) fracture	Malignant fracture (#) or metastasis (M)	Inflammatory disease[b]	Normal v.b.m.
Herneth et al. 2000[77]	MS-EPI	0, 440, 880	5	0.86	0.39 ± 0.11 (M)	–	1.13 ± 0.23
Zhou et al. 2002[57]	SS-FSE	0, 150, 250	27	0.32 ± 0.05	0.19 ± 0.03 (M)	–	0.27 – 0.35
Chan et al. 2002[78]	SS-EPI	200...1000	32	1.94 ± 0.35	0.82 ± 0.20 (#)	0.98 ± 0.21 (S)	0.23 ± 0.05
Byun et al. 2002[58]	SS-STE	0, 650	3	–	0.78 ± 0.03 (M)	–	0.33 ± 0.03
Herneth et al. 2002[93]	MS-EPI	440, 880	22	1.61 ± 0.37	0.71 ± 0.27 (#)[c]	–	1.66 ± 0.38
Bammer et al. 2003[40]	LSDI	5, 650	15	1.02 – 1.97	–	–	0.23 ± 0.08
Maeda et al. 2003[39]	LSDI	5, 1000	64	1.21 ± 0.17	0.92 ± 0.20 (#)[d]	–	–
Ballon et al. 2004[94]	SS-EPI	0, 1000	1	–	0.70 ± 0.21 (M)	–	–
Pui et al. 2005[95]	SS-EPI	0 ... 1000	51	–	1.02 ± 0.36 (M)	1.15 ± 0.42 (TB)	0.30 ± 0.21
Oner et al. 2007[61]	SS-FSE	0, 600	24	1.54 ± 0.36	0.69 ± 0.30 (M)	1.21 ± 0.24 (SD)	0.35 ± 0.15
Oner et al. 2007[61]	SS-EPI	0, 600	24	1.61 ± 0.46	0.72 ± 0.31 (M)	1.51 ± 0.25 (SD)	0.53 ± 0.15
Raya et al. 2007[62]	SS-FSE	0 ...750	32	1.25 ± 0.26	0.97 ± 0.14 (M)	1.48 ± 0.033 (SD)	0.21 ± 0.06
Tang et al. 2007[72]	SS-EPI	0, 300	34	2.23 ± 0.21	1.04 ± 0.03 (#)	–	–
Byun et al. 2007[59]	SS-STE	0, 650	7	0.88 ± 0.07	0.78 ± 0.03 (#)	–	0.21 ± 0.06
Gašperšič et al. 2008[96]	SS-EPI	0, 400	30	–	–	≈1.3 (AS)	–
Bozgeyik et al. 2008[97]	SS-EPI	100...1000	42	–	–	≈1.1 (S, AS)[e]	0.65 – 0.83[e]
Balliu et al. 2009[98]	MS-EPI	0, 500	45	1.90 ± 0.39	0.92 ± 0.13 (M)	0.96 ± 0.49 (S)	–
Typical values				1.0 – 2.0	0.7 – 1.0	1.0 – 1.5	0.2 – 0.6

Notes: [a]Sequences: MS-EPI, diffusion-weighted multi-shot (segmented) spin-echo echo-planar imaging sequence with fat saturation; SS-EPI, diffusion-weighted single-shot spin-echo echo-planar imaging sequence with fat saturation; SS-STE, diffusion-weighted single-shot stimulated-echo sequence; SS-FSE, diffusion-weighted single-shot fast-spin-echo sequence; LSDI, line-scan diffusion-weighted-imaging sequence; rad-SE, diffusion-weighted spin-echo sequence with radial readout.
[b]S, spondylitis; AS, ankylosing spondylitis; SD, spondylodiskitis; TB, tuberculosis.
[c]Non-collapsed metatstatic lesions: (0.69 ± 0.24) × 10⁻³ mm²/s.
[d]Non-collapsed metatstatic lesions: (0.83 ± 0.17) × 10⁻³ mm²/s.
[e]ADCs determined with b = 600 s/mm².

Table 10.3 Quantitative DWI of normal and osteoporotic vertebral bone marrow (v.b.m.)

Study	Pulse sequence type[a]	b-values (s/mm²)	Number of subjects	Apparent diffusion coefficient (10^{-3} mm²/s) Osteoporotic v.b.m.	Osteopenic v.b.m.	Normal v.b.m.
Dietrich et al. 2001[35]	rad-SE	50 … 350	6	–	–	0.33 ± 0.06
Yeung et al. 2004[81]	SS-EPI	0 … 500	44	0.42 ± 0.11	0.42 ± 0.14	0.44 ± 0.11[b]
Griffith et al. 2006[99]	SS-EPI	0 … 500	103	0.43 ± 0.12	0.41 ± 0.12	0.46 ± 0.08
Hatipoglu et al. 2007[100]	SS-EPI	0, 600	51	0.38 ± 0.02	0.42 ± 0.03	0.46 ± 0.03
Sugimoto et al. 2008[101]	SS-EPI	0, 1000	25	–	–	≈0.2[c]

Notes: [a]Sequences: SS-EPI, diffusion-weighted single-shot spin-echo echo-planar imaging sequence with fat saturation; rad-SE, diffusion-weighted spin-echo sequence with radial readout.
[b]normal v.b.m. in young healthy subjects: $(0.50 ± 0.09) × 10^{-3}$ mm²/s.
[c]ADCs of vertebrae that showed fracture in follow-up examination: $≈0.6 × 10^{-3}$ mm²/s.

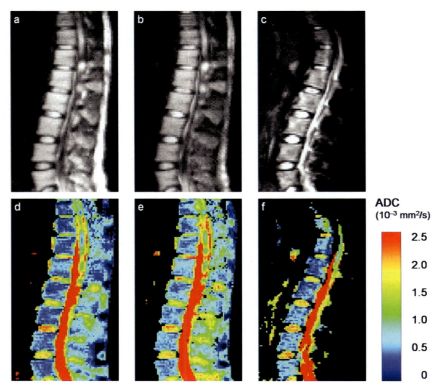

Figure 10.6 DWI of the spine of a 35-year-old female healthy volunteer: (a–c) Sagittal diffusion-weighted images with an intermediate b-value of 300 s/mm²; (d–f) corresponding ADC maps calculated from seven b-values (10, 100, 200, 300, 400, 500, 600 s/mm²). (a, d) Single-shot FSE acquisition © fat suppression; (b, e) single-shot FSE acquisition © fat suppression; (c, f) single-shot EPI acquisition © fat suppression. Note the lower ADCs of bone marrow measured without fat suppression (d; ADC ≈ $0.56 × 10^{-3}$ mm²/s) than with fat suppression (e; ADC ≈ $0.67 × 10^{-3}$ mm²/s), while the large intervertebral disks have almost identical ADCs without fat suppression (ADC ≈ $1.80 × 10^{-3}$ mm²/s) as with fat suppression (ADC ≈ $1.81 × 10^{-3}$ mm²/s). Note also the limited image quality and the considerable distortion artifacts of the echo-planar images (c, f), which were acquired with identical slice positioning and field of view as the FSE images.

Table 10.4 Quantitative DWI of non-vertebral bone marrow (b.m.)

Study	Pulse sequence[a]	b-values (s/mm²)	Number of subjects	Region/pathology	Apparent diffusion coefficient (10^{-3} mm²/s)	
					Pathology	Normal b.m.
Ward et al. 2000[36]	nav-SE	0, 980	50	Tibial b.m./bone bruise	0.40 – 1.30	0.10 – 0.25
Ballon et al. 2000[102]	SS-EPI	0, 1000	21	Iliac b.m./leukemia	0.48 ± 0.13	0.53 ± 0.07
Nonomura et al. 2001[103]	SS-EPI	30, 300	37	Iliac b.m./malignant lymphoma	1.31 ± 033[b]	0.83 ± 0.71
Ragin et al. 2006[104]	SSEPI	0, 1000	20	Cranial b.m./HIV patients	0.77 – 0.86	1.01 – 1.11
Moon et al. 2007[105]	SS-EPI	0, 1000	13	Cranial b.m. metastases	0.90 ± 0.25	–

Notes: [a]Sequences: SS-EPI: diffusion-weighted single-shot spin-echo echo-planar imaging sequence with fat saturation; nav-SE, diffusion-weighted spin-echo sequence with navigator-echo correction.
[b]Normal hypocellular iliac b.m.: $(0.36 \pm 0.31) \times 10^{-3}$ mm²/s.

in the examined regions. Only recently, these studies were complemented by whole-body applications of DWI based on a technique called diffusion-weighted whole-body imaging with background body signal suppression (DWIBS) as suggested by Takahara et al.[21] The primary focus of these studies is the sensitive depiction of lesions rather than the quantification of their ADC. Although no ADCs were determined, it was demonstrated in several studies that whole-body DWI is very sensitive to bone marrow lesions as well[22,82,83].

DWI of intervertebral disks

Another structure that has frequently been examined in diffusion-weighted musculoskeletal MRI is the intervertebral disk as summarized in Table 10.5. As in other spinal structures, a variety of different pulse sequence types has been employed for DWI of the intervertebral disks including single-shot EPI, line-scan imaging, or single-shot FSE techniques. The ADCs reported for normal intervertebral disks (see also Fig. 10.6) vary to a certain degree: while several former studies found consistent values between about 1.4 and 1.6×10^{-3} mm²/s, more recent results showed both lower values of about 1.2×10^{-3} mm²/s[42] and higher values between 1.9 and 2.3×10^{-3} mm²/s[84–86]. The lower values may be explained by the relatively high maximal b-value of almost 1000 s/mm² used in this study, which may lead to artificially increased signal

intensities at high b-values due to the influence of noise. A second source of the observed variations could be the relatively small size of the disks which results in very small regions of interest and thus in larger statistical deviations of single measurements. Finally it should be noted that the ADCs differ for different substructures found in the intervertebral disks such as the nuclei pulposi with higher and the annuli fibrosi with lower ADCs[40]. Consequently, the results will depend to a certain degree on the exact size and location of the evaluated regions. Some authors also described a dependence of the ADC on the location (higher ADCs in lumbar and lower ADCs in thoracic disks were found by Kerttula et al.[87]), on the time of the day[85], or on the extent of examination-preceding joint mobilization[86].

Several groups compared the ADCs of normal and abnormal or degenerated intervertebral disks. Generally, a lower diffusivity (by roughly 10% to 20%) has been observed in pathologically changed intervertebral disks[63,84,86,88–90]. However, it should be noted that no clear advantage of these ADC measurements in comparison to, e.g., T2 measurements could be demonstrated yet with respect to abnormal or degenerated intervertebral disks[88].

Limitations, recommendations, and future directions

DWI of the bone marrow and of spinal structures is still limited by the relatively low image quality of EPI

Table 10.5 Quantitative DWI of intervertebral disks

Study	Pulse sequence type[a]	b-values (s/mm^2)	Number of subjects	Apparent diffusion coefficient (10^{-3} mm^2/s)	
				Normal disks	Degenerated disks
Kerttula et al. 2000[87]	SS-EPI	0, 250, 500	18	1.5 ± 0.3	–
Dietrich et al. 2001[35]	Rad-SE	50 . . . 350	6	1.53 – 1.59	–
Kerttula et al 2001[88]	SS-EPI	0, 250, 500	37	1.38 – 1.60	1.09 – 1.48
Kurunlahti et al. 2001[89]	SS-EPI	0, 250, 500	37	1.38 – 1.56	1.06 – 1.21
Bammer et al. 2003[40]	LSDI	5, 650	15	1.65 ± 0.21	–
Newitt and Majumdar 2005[41]	LSDI	5, 255, 505, 755	11	1.33/1.87 (fs)[b]	–
Kealey et al. 2005[84]	SS-EPI	0, 400	44	2.27 ± 0.58	2.06 ± 0.47
Tokuda et al. 2007[63]	SS-FSE	0, 900	75	1.14 – 2.35	0.30 – 2.31
Carballido-Gamio et al. 2007[42]	LSDI	0 – 995	6	1.19 ± 0.16	–
Carballido-Gamio et al. 2007[42]	SS-FSE	0 – 995	6	1.27 ± 0.23	–
Ludescher et al. 2008[85]	SS-STE-EPI	0, 600	6	2.08 – 2.11	–
Beattie et al. 2008[90]	SS-EPI	0, 400	30	1.89 – 1.99	1.45 – 1.68
Beattie et al. 2009[86]	SS-EPI	0, 400	24	1.90 – 2.03	1.53 – 1.85
Niinimäki et al. 2009[106]	SS-EPI	0, 500	20	–	1.62 ± 0.28
Niinimäki et al. 2009[107]	SS-EPI	0, 500	228	–	2.01 ± 0.29

Notes: [a]Sequences: SS-EPI, diffusion-weighted single-shot spin-echo echo-planar imaging sequence with fat saturation; rad-SE, diffusion-weighted spin-echo sequence with radial readout; LSDI, line-scan diffusion-weighted-imaging sequence; SS-FSE, diffusion-weighted single-shot fast-spin-echo sequence; SS-STE-EPI: diffusion-weighted single-shot stimulated-echo echo-planar imaging sequence.
[b]fs: LSDI with fat saturation.

acquisitions and by the large variability of results obtained with several available alternative methods. However, ongoing optimizations of these acquisition techniques beyond EPI promise increased robustness and new perspectives for future clinical applications. Currently, the most important and most widely evaluated clinical application of DWI in bone marrow is the differentiation of benign osteoporotic and malignant neoplastic vertebral compression fractures, which is often difficult based on conventional (T1-weighted, T2-weighted, or STIR) images alone. Here, DWI presents an important additional image contrast that increases the differentiability with high sensitivities. Based on our own experience, best results are obtained with non-quantitative diffusion-weighting SSFP acquisitions; however, it should be noted that this sequence type is very sensitive to fat–water in-phase and opposed-phase effects and has to be carefully optimized to yield an appropriate signal intensity in healthy appearing bone marrow.

Future developments can be expected to include more studies on the characterization of bone marrow lesions and the staging of bone tumors or metastases. In combination with other functional imaging techniques such as dynamic contrast-enhanced perfusion MRI, DWI is a promising tool for the monitoring of therapy response and, thus, can be anticipated to play an important role in the evaluation and application of new, e.g., antiangiogenic tumor therapies in the near future.

Conclusions

Diffusion-weighted imaging of the bone marrow and the spinal column requires considerably more robust imaging techniques than typical neurological DWI applications. Several different techniques apart from EPI and also different protocol parameters have been used for diffusion studies of the spine resulting in a relatively large variability of results. Although the optimization of the DWI technique is still an active subject of research, the application of diffusion-weighted MRI in bone marrow is today an established examination technique that provides a unique contrast and that can help in the detection of bone marrow pathologies and the differentiation of benign and malignant bone marrow lesions. It has been applied particularly successfully in DWI studies of vertebral lesions and of vertebral compression fractures.

References

1. Brown R. A brief account of microscopical observations made in the months of June, July, and August 1827, on the particles contained in the pollen of plants; and on the general existence of active molecules in organic and inorganic bodies. *The Edinburgh New Philosophical Journal* 1828; July–September: 358–71.

2. Brown R. Additional remarks on active molecules. *The Edinburgh New Philosophical Journal* 1830; January–April: 41–6.

3. Einstein A. Über die von der molekularkinetischen Theorie der Wärme geforderte Bewegung von in ruhenden Flüssigkeiten suspendierten Teilchen. *Ann Phys-Berlin* 1905;**17**:549–60.

4. Hahn EL. Spin echoes. *Phys Rev* 1950;**80**:580–94.

5. Merboldt KD, Hänicke W, Frahm J. Self-diffusion NMR imaging using stimulated echoes. *J Magn Reson* 1985;**64**:479–86.

6. Taylor DG, Bushell MC. The spatial mapping of translational diffusion coefficients by the NMR imaging technique. *Phys Med Biol* 1985;**30**:345–9.

7. Le Bihan D, Breton E, Lallemand D, *et al.* MR imaging of intravoxel incoherent motions: application to diffusion and perfusion in neurologic disorders. *Radiology* 1986;**161**:401–7.

8. Dietrich O. Diffusion-weighted imaging and diffusion tensor imaging. In: Reiser MF, Semmler W, Hricak H, eds. *Magnetic Resonance Tomography*. New York: Springer; 2008, 130–52.

9. Karaarslan E, Arslan A. Diffusion weighted MR imaging in non-infarct lesions of the brain. *Eur J Radiol* 2008;**65**:402–16.

10. Provenzale JM, Mukundan S, Barboriak DP. Diffusion-weighted and perfusion MR imaging for brain tumor characterization and assessment of treatment response. *Radiology* 2006;**239**:632–49.

11. Cartes-Zumelzu FW, Stavrou I, Castillo M, *et al.* Diffusion-weighted imaging in the assessment of brain abscesses therapy. *Am J Neuroradiol* 2004;**25**:1310–17.

12. Horsfield MA, Jones DK. Applications of diffusion-weighted and diffusion tensor MRI to white matter diseases: a review. *NMR Biomed* 2002;**15**:570–7.

13. Schaefer PW, Copen WA, Lev MH, *et al.* Diffusion-weighted imaging in acute stroke. *Magn Reson Imag Clin N Am* 2006;**14**:141–68.

14. Davis DP, Robertson T, Imbesi SG. Diffusion-weighted magnetic resonance imaging versus computed tomography in the diagnosis of acute ischemic stroke. *J Emerg Med* 2006;**31**:269–77.

15. Parikh T, Drew SJ, Lee VS, *et al.* Focal liver lesion detection and characterization with diffusion-weighted MR imaging: comparison with standard breath-hold T2-weighted imaging. *Radiology* 2008;**246**:812–22.

16. Zech CJ, Herrmann KA, Dietrich O, *et al.* Black-blood diffusion-weighted EPI acquisition of the liver with parallel imaging: comparison with a standard T2-weighted sequence for detection of focal liver lesions. *Investig Radiol* 2008;**43**:261–6.

17. Zhang J, Tehrani YM, Wang L, *et al.* Renal masses: characterization with diffusion-weighted MR imaging – a preliminary experience. *Radiology* 2008;**247**:458–64.

18. Cova M, Squillaci E, Stacul F, *et al.* Diffusion-weighted MRI in the evaluation of renal lesions: preliminary results. *Br J Radiol* 2004;**77**:851–7.

19. Nagata S, Nishimura H, Uchida M, *et al.* Diffusion-weighted imaging of soft tissue tumors: usefulness of the apparent diffusion coefficient for differential diagnosis. *Radiat Med* 2008;**26**:287–95.

20. Dietrich O, Raya JG, Sommer J, *et al.* A comparative evaluation of a RARE-based single-shot pulse sequence for diffusion-weighted MRI of musculoskeletal soft-tissue tumors. *Eur Radiol* 2005;**15**:772–83.

21. Takahara T, Imai Y, Yamashita T, *et al.* Diffusion weighted whole body imaging with background body signal suppression (DWIBS): technical improvement using free breathing, STIR and high resolution 3D display. *Radiat Med* 2004;**22**:275–82.

22. Kwee TC, Takahara T, Ochiai R, *et al.* Diffusion-weighted whole-body imaging with background body signal suppression (DWIBS): features and potential applications in oncology. *Eur Radiol* 2008;**18**:1937–52.

23. Baur A, Stäbler A, Brüning R, *et al.* Diffusion-weighted MR imaging of bone marrow: differentiation of benign versus pathologic compression fractures. *Radiology* 1998;**207**:349–56.

24. Raya JG, Dietrich O, Reiser MF, *et al.* Methods and applications of diffusion imaging of vertebral bone marrow. *J Magn Reson Imag* 2006;**24**:1207–20.

25. Karchevsky M, Babb JS, Schweitzer ME. Can diffusion-weighted imaging be used to differentiate benign from pathologic fractures? A meta-analysis. *Skeletal Radiol* 2008;**37**:791–5.

26. Raya JG, Dietrich O, Reiser MF, *et al.* Techniques for diffusion-weighted imaging of bone marrow. *Eur J Radiol* 2005;**55**:64–73.

27. Stejskal EO, Tanner JE. Spin diffusion measurements: spin echoes in the presence of a time-dependent field gradient. *J Chem Phys* 1965;**42**:288–92.

28. Norris DG. Implications of bulk motion for diffusion-weighted imaging experiments: effects, mechanisms, and solutions. *J Magn Reson Imag* 2001;**13**:486–95.

29. Bammer R. Basic principles of diffusion-weighted imaging. *Eur J Radiol* 2003;**45**:169–84.

30. Le Bihan D, Poupon C, Amadon A, *et al.* Artifacts and pitfalls in diffusion MRI. *J Magn Reson Imag* 2006;**24**:478–88.

31. Ordidge RJ, Helpern JA, Qing ZX, *et al.* Correction of motional artifacts in diffusion-weighted MR images using navigator echoes. *Magn Reson Imag* 1994;**12**:455–60.

32. Anderson AW, Gore JC. Analysis and correction of motion artifacts in diffusion weighted imaging. *Magn Reson Med* 1994;**32**:379–87.

33. Dietrich O, Heiland S, Benner T, *et al.* Reducing motion artefacts in diffusion-weighted MRI of the brain: efficacy of navigator echo correction and pulse triggering. *Neuroradiology* 2000;**42**:85–91.

34. Gmitro AF, Alexander AL. Use of a projection reconstruction method to decrease motion sensitivity in diffusion-weighted MRI. *Magn Reson Med* 1993;**29**:835–8.

35. Dietrich O, Herlihy A, Dannels WR, *et al.* Diffusion-weighted imaging of the spine using radial k-space trajectories. *MAGMA Magn Reson Mater Phys* 2001;**12**:23–31.

36. Ward R, Caruthers S, Yablon C, *et al.* Analysis of diffusion changes in posttraumatic bone marrow using navigator-corrected diffusion gradients. *Am J Roentgenol* 2000;**174**:731–4.

37. Spuentrup E, Buecker A, Adam G, *et al.* Diffusion-weighted MR imaging for differentiation of benign fracture edema and tumor infiltration of the vertebral body. *Am J Roentgenol* 2001;**176**:351–8.

38. Gudbjartsson H, Maier SE, Mulkern RV, *et al.* Line scan diffusion imaging. *Magn Reson Med* 1996;**36**:509–19.

39. Maeda M, Sakuma H, Maier SE, *et al.* Quantitative assessment of diffusion abnormalities in benign and malignant vertebral compression fractures by line scan diffusion-weighted imaging. *Am J Roentgenol* 2003;**181**:1203–9.

40. Bammer R, Herneth AM, Maier SE, *et al.* Line scan diffusion imaging of the spine. *Am J Neuroradiol* 2003;**24**:5–12.

41. Newitt DC, Majumdar S. Reproducibility and dependence on diffusion weighting of line scan diffusion in the lumbar intervertebral discs. *J Magn Reson Imag* 2005;**21**:482–8.

42. Carballido-Gamio J, Xu D, Newitt D, *et al.* Single-shot fast spin-echo diffusion tensor imaging of the lumbar spine at 1.5 and 3 T. *Magn Reson Imag* 2007;**25**:665–70.

43. Turner R, Le Bihan D, Maier J, *et al.* Echo-planar imaging of intravoxel incoherent motion. *Radiology* 1990;**177**:407–14.

44. Schoenberg SO, Dietrich O, Reiser MF. *Parallel Imaging in Clinical MR Applications.* New York: Springer; 2007.

45. Pruessmann KP, Weiger M, Scheidegger MB, *et al.* SENSE: sensitivity encoding for fast MRI. *Magn Reson Med* 1999;**42**:952–62.

46. Griswold MA, Jakob PM, Heidemann RM, *et al.* Generalized autocalibrating partially parallel acquisitions (GRAPPA). *Magn Reson Med* 2002;**47**:1202–10.

47. Jaermann T, Pruessmann KP, Valavanis A, *et al.* Influence of SENSE on image properties in high-resolution single-shot echo-planar DTI. *Magn Reson Med* 2006;**55**:335–42.

48. Brockstedt S, Moore JR, Thomsen C, *et al.* High-resolution diffusion imaging using phase-corrected segmented echo-planar imaging. *Magn Reson Imaging* 2000;**18**:649–57.

49. Norris DG, Börnert P, Reese T, *et al.* On the application of ultra-fast RARE experiments. *Magn Reson Med* 1992;**27**:142–64.

50. Lövblad KO, Jakob PM, Chen Q, *et al.* Turbo spin-echo diffusion-weighted MR of ischemic stroke. *Am J Neuroradiol* 1998;**19**:201–8.

51. Schick F. SPLICE: sub-second diffusion-sensitive MR imaging using a modified fast spin-echo acquisition mode. *Magn Reson Med* 1997;**38**:638–44.

52. Alsop DC. Phase insensitive preparation of single-shot RARE: application to diffusion imaging in humans. *Magn Reson Med* 1997;**38**:527–33.

53. Le Roux P. Non-CPMG fast spin echo with full signal. *J Magn Reson* 2002;**155**:278–92.

54. Norris DG. Selective parity RARE imaging. *Magn Reson Med* 2007;**58**:643–9. (Erratum: *Magn Reson Med* 2008;**59**:440.)

159

55. Pipe JG, Farthing VG, Forbes KP. Multishot diffusion-weighted FSE using PROPELLER MRI. *Magn Reson Med* 2002;**47**:42–52. (Erratum: *Magn Reson Med* 2002;**47**:621.)

56. Deng J, Miller FH, Salem R, *et al*. Multishot diffusion-weighted PROPELLER magnetic resonance imaging of the abdomen. *Investig Radiol* 2006; **41**:769–75.

57. Zhou XJ, Leeds NE, McKinnon GC, *et al*. Characterization of benign and metastatic vertebral compression fractures with quantitative diffusion MR imaging. *Am J Neuroradiol* 2002;**23**:165–70.

58. Byun WM, Shin SO, Chang Y, *et al*. Diffusion-weighted MR imaging of metastatic disease of the spine: assessment of response to therapy. *Am J Neuroradiol* 2002;**23**:906–12.

59. Byun WM, Jang HW, Kim SW, *et al*. Diffusion-weighted magnetic resonance imaging of sacral insufficiency fractures: comparison with metastases of the sacrum. *Spine* 2007;**32**:E820–4.

60. Park SW, Lee JH, Ehara S, *et al*. Single shot fast spin echo diffusion-weighted MR imaging of the spine: is it useful in differentiating malignant metastatic tumor infiltration from benign fracture edema? *Clin Imag* 2004;**28**:102–8.

61. Oner AY, Tali T, Celikyay F, *et al*. Diffusion-weighted imaging of the spine with a non-Carr–Purcell–Meiboom–Gill single-shot fast spin-echo sequence: initial experience. *Am J Neuroradiol* 2007;**28**:575–80.

62. Raya JG, Dietrich O, Birkenmaier C, *et al*. Feasibility of a RARE-based sequence for quantitative diffusion-weighted MRI of the spine. *Eur Radiol* 2007;**17**:2872–9.

63. Tokuda O, Okada M, Fujita T, *et al*. Correlation between diffusion in lumbar intervertebral disks and lumbar artery status: evaluation with fresh blood imaging technique. *J Magn Reson Imag* 2007; **25**:185–91.

64. Gyngell ML. The application of steady-state free precession in rapid 2DFT NMR imaging: FAST and CE-FAST sequences. *Magn Reson Imag* 1988;**6**:415–19.

65. Bruder H, Fischer H, Graumann R, *et al*. A new steady-state imaging sequence for simultaneous acquisition of two MR images with clearly different contrasts. *Magn Reson Med* 1988;**7**:35–42.

66. Le Bihan D. Intravoxel incoherent motion imaging using steady-state free precession. *Magn Reson Med* 1988;**7**:346–51.

67. Merboldt KD, Bruhn H, Frahm J, *et al*. MRI of "diffusion" in the human brain: new results using a modified CE-FAST sequence. *Magn Reson Med* 1989;**9**:423–9.

68. Kaiser R, Bartholdi E, Ernst RR. Diffusion and field-gradient effects in NMR Fourier spectroscopy. *J Chem Phys* 1974;**60**:2966–79.

69. Wu EX, Buxton RB. Effect of diffusion on the steady-state magnetization with pulsed field gradients. *J Magn Reson* 1990;**90**:243–53.

70. Miller KL, Hargreaves BA, Gold GE, *et al*. Steady-state diffusion-weighted imaging of in vivo knee cartilage. *Magn Reson Med* 2004;**51**:394–8.

71. Dietrich O, Heiland S, Sartor K. Noise correction for the exact determination of apparent diffusion coefficients at low SNR. *Magn Reson Med* 2001;**45**:448–53.

72. Tang G, Liu Y, Li W, *et al*. Optimization of b value in diffusion-weighted MRI for the differential diagnosis of benign and malignant vertebral fractures. *Skeletal Radiol* 2007;**36**:1035–41.

73. Castillo M, Arbelaez A, Smith JK, *et al*. Diffusion-weighted MR imaging offers no advantage over routine noncontrast MR imaging in the detection of vertebral metastases. *Am J Neuroradiol* 2000;**21**:948–53.

74. Hackländer T, Scharwächter C, Golz R, *et al*. Value of diffusion-weighted imaging for diagnosing vertebral metastases due to prostate cancer in comparison to other primary tumors. *Rofo Fortschr Röntgenstr* 2006;**178**:416–24.

75. Baur A, Huber A, Ertl-Wagner B, *et al*. Diagnostic value of increased diffusion weighting of a steady-state free precession sequence for differentiating acute benign osteoporotic fractures from pathologic vertebral compression fractures. *Am J Neuroradiol* 2001;**22**:366–72.

76. Baur A, Huber A, Dürr HR, *et al*. Differentiation of benign osteoporotic and neoplastic vertebral compression fractures with a diffusion-weighted, steady-state free precession sequence. *Rofo Fortschr Röntgenstr* 2002;**174**:70–5.

77. Herneth AM, Naude J, Philipp M, *et al*. The value of diffusion-weighted MRT in assessing the bone marrow changes in vertebral metastases. *Radiologe* 2000;**40**:731–6.

78. Chan JH, Peh WC, Tsui EY, *et al*. Acute vertebral body compression fractures: discrimination between benign and malignnant causes using apparent diffusion coefficients. *Br J Radiol* 2002;**75**:207–14.

79. Mulkern RV, Schwartz RB. In re: characterization of benign and metastatic vertebral compression fractures with quantitative diffusion MR imaging. *Am J Neuroradiol* 2003;**24**:1489–90.

80. Le Bihan D, Breton E, Lallemand D, *et al*. Separation of diffusion and perfusion in intravoxel incoherent motion MR imaging. *Radiology* 1988;**168**:497–505.

81. Yeung DK, Wong SY, Griffith JF, *et al.* Bone marrow diffusion in osteoporosis: evaluation with quantitative MR diffusion imaging. *J Magn Reson Imag* 2004;**19**:222–8.

82. Mürtz P, Krautmacher C, Träber F, *et al.* Diffusion-weighted whole-body MR imaging with background body signal suppression: a feasibility study at 3.0 Tesla. *Eur Radiol* 2007;**17**:3031–7.

83. Koh DM, Takahara T, Imai Y, *et al.* Practical aspects of assessing tumors using clinical diffusion-weighted imaging in the body. *Magn Reson Med Sci* 2007;**6**:211–24.

84. Kealey SM, Aho T, Delong D, *et al.* Assessment of apparent diffusion coefficient in normal and degenerated intervertebral lumbar disks: initial experience. *Radiology* 2005;**235**:569–74.

85. Ludescher B, Effelsberg J, Martirosian P, *et al.* T2- and diffusion-maps reveal diurnal changes of intervertebral disc composition: an in vivo MRI study at 1.5 Tesla. *J Magn Reson Imag* 2008;**28**:252–7.

86. Beattie PF, Donley JW, Arnot CF, *et al.* The change in the diffusion of water in normal and degenerative lumbar intervertebral discs following joint mobilization compared to prone lying. *J Orthop Sports Phys Ther* 2009;**39**: 4–11.

87. Kerttula LI, Jauhiainen JP, Tervonen O, *et al.* Apparent diffusion coefficient in thoracolumbar intervertebral discs of healthy young volunteers. *J Magn Reson Imag* 2000;**12**:255–60.

88. Kerttula L, Kurunlahti M, Jauhiainen J, *et al.* Apparent diffusion coefficients and T2 relaxation time measurements to evaluate disc degeneration: a quantitative MR study of young patients with previous vertebral fracture. *Acta Radiol* 2001;**42**:585–91.

89. Kurunlahti M, Kerttula L, Jauhiainen J, *et al.* Correlation of diffusion in lumbar intervertebral disks with occlusion of lumbar arteries: a study in adult volunteers. *Radiology* 2001;**221**:779–86.

90. Beattie PF, Morgan PS, Peters D. Diffusion-weighted magnetic resonance imaging of normal and degenerative lumbar intervertebral discs: a new method to potentially quantify the physiologic effect of physical therapy intervention. *J Orthop Sports Phys Ther* 2008;**38**:42–9.

91. Yasumoto M, Nonomura Y, Yoshimura R, *et al.* MR detection of iliac bone marrow involvement by malignant lymphoma with various MR sequences including diffusion-weighted echo-planar imaging. *Skeletal Radiol* 2002;**31**:263–9.

92. Abanoz R, Hakyemez B, Parlak M. Diffusion-weighted imaging of acute vertebral compression: differential diagnosis of benign versus malignant pathologic fractures. *Tani Girisim Radyol* 2003;**9**:176–83.

93. Herneth AM, Philipp MO, Naude J, *et al.* Vertebral metastases: assessment with apparent diffusion coefficient. *Radiology* 2002;**225**:889–94.

94. Ballon D, Watts R, Dyke JP, *et al.* Imaging therapeutic response in human bone marrow using rapid whole-body MRI. *Magn Reson Med* 2004;**52**:1234–8.

95. Pui MH, Mitha A, Rae WI, *et al.* Diffusion-weighted magnetic resonance imaging of spinal infection and malignancy. *J Neuroimaging* 2005;**15**:164–70.

96. Gašperšič N, Sersa I, Jevtic V, *et al.* Monitoring ankylosing spondylitis therapy by dynamic contrast-enhanced and diffusion-weighted magnetic resonance imaging. *Skeletal Radiol* 2008;**37**:123–31.

97. Bozgeyik Z, Ozgocmen S, Kocakoc E. Role of diffusion-weighted MRI in the detection of early active sacroiliitis. *Am J Roentgenol* 2008;**191**:980–6.

98. Balliu E, Vilanova JC, Peláez I, *et al.* Diagnostic value of apparent diffusion coefficients to differentiate benign from malignant vertebral bone marrow lesions. *Eur J Radiol* 2009;**69**:560–6.

99. Griffith JF, Yeung DK, Antonio GE, *et al.* Vertebral marrow fat content and diffusion and perfusion indexes in women with varying bone density: MR evaluation. *Radiology* 2006;**241**:831–8.

100. Hatipoglu HG, Selvi A, Ciliz D, *et al.* Quantitative and diffusion MR imaging as a new method to assess osteoporosis. *Am J Neuroradiol* 2007;**28**:1934–7.

101. Sugimoto T, Tanigawa N, Ikeda K, *et al.* Diffusion-weighted imaging for predicting new compression fractures following percutaneous vertebroplasty. *Acta Radiol* 2008;**49**:419–26.

102. Ballon D, Dyke J, Schwartz LH, *et al.* Bone marrow segmentation in leukemia using diffusion and T (2) weighted echo planar magnetic resonance imaging. *NMR Biomed* 2000;**13**:321–8.

103. Nonomura Y, Yasumoto M, Yoshimura R, *et al.* Relationship between bone marrow cellularity and apparent diffusion coefficient. *J Magn Reson Imag* 2001;**13**:757–60.

104. Ragin AB, Wu Y, Storey P, *et al.* Bone marrow diffusion measures correlate with dementia severity in HIV patients. *Am J Neuroradiol* 2006;**27**: 89–92.

105. Moon WJ, Lee MH, Chung EC. Diffusion-weighted imaging with sensitivity encoding (SENSE) for detecting cranial bone marrow metastases: comparison with T1-weighted images. *Korean J Radiol* 2007;**8**:185–91.

106. Niinimäki J, Korkiakoski A, Parviainen O, *et al.* Association of lumbar artery narrowing, degenerative changes in disc and endplate and apparent diffusion in disc on postcontrast enhancement of lumbar intervertebral disc. *MAGMA Magn Reson Mater Phys* 2009;**22**:101–9.

107. Niinimäki J, Korkiakoski A, Ojala O, *et al.* Association between visual degeneration of intervertebral discs and the apparent diffusion coefficient. *Magn Reson Imag* 2009;**27**:641–7.

Diffusion-weighted MRI of soft tissue tumors

Masayuki Maeda

Introduction

Magnetic resonance imaging (MRI) has evolved as an important diagnostic tool for assessing soft tissue tumors due to its excellent soft tissue contrast and multiplanar reconstruction capabilities. The imaging characteristics of common benign lesions, such as lipoma and hemangioma, are often specific enough to allow a conclusive diagnosis. However, conventional MRI is limited in providing clinically satisfactory information about soft tissue tumor characterization and the presence and extent of viable tumor tissue and/or tumor necrosis.

Diffusion-weighted imaging (DWI) has been used in the assessment of tumors, particularly those of the central nervous system[1–4]. Results of studies correlating apparent diffusion coefficient (ADC) values and histopathological findings have suggested that higher cellularity is associated with more restricted diffusion (i.e., lower ADC)[1,3,4]. Recently, DWI has been utilized to characterize soft tissue tumors[5–9], and is expected to provide additional useful information such as lesion characterization and the presence and extent of viable tumor tissue and/or tumor necrosis that is not available with conventional MRI. In this chapter, DWI is reviewed with regard to soft tissue tumors.

Diffusion acquisition and processing for assessment of soft tissue tumors

Several diffusion acquisition techniques have been used to investigate the diffusivity of soft tissue tumors, including spin-echo (SE), multi-shot echo-planar imaging (MS-EPI), SE single-shot echo-planar imaging (SS-EPI), and SE and line-scan sequences [5–9]. Scanning times for these techniques vary from 25 s (SS-EPI) to 12 min (SE). The maximum b-values (such as 600 and 701 s/mm^2) used in early reports appeared too low to enable full evaluation of tumor diffusivity[5,6]. For brain tumors, DWI has been performed using maximum b-values of 1000 s/mm^2 or higher[1–4]; therefore, such high values may be more appropriate for quantitative evaluation of diffusivity in soft tissue tumors.

Trace ADC maps are generated using the equation described by Stejskal and Tanner[10], $S = S_0 e^{-b\mathrm{ADC}}$, where b is the diffusion weighting factor, S is the signal intensity of the diffusion trace for b = maximum, and S_0 is the signal intensity for b = minimum. The ADC value measurements are obtained from the trace ADC maps using regions of interest (ROIs) placed over the tumors. When multiple tumor components (solid vs. cystic, necrotic) are present, ROI measurements are taken to include the solid-appearing portions of the tumors and to exclude obviously necrotic or cystic regions, as demonstrated in the corresponding T2-weighted and contrast enhanced MR images.

Echo-planar imaging sequences have the advantage of short scanning times compared with SE or line-scan sequences, but are intrinsically sensitive to magnetic heterogeneity, with possibility of susceptibility artifacts due to air and metal. In addition, EPI techniques employ fat suppression and are thus unsuitable for the evaluation of fatty components within tumors. In MS-EPI, phase navigation and pulse triggering were applied to minimize phase errors induced by motion[6]. Peripheral pulse triggering was used and body parts containing the tumors were immobilized to prevent motion artifacts for SE-DWI[5]. Line-scan DWI provides diagnostic images for assessment of soft tissue tumors in the body and extremities without the need for specialized hardware, cardiac gating, or respiratory

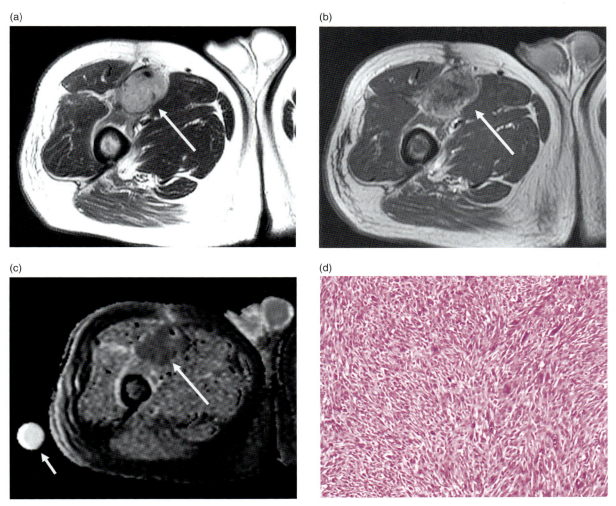

Figure 11.1 Undifferentiated high-grade pleomorphic sarcoma of the right thigh in a 76-year-old man. (a) Axial FSE T2-weighted image reveals high signal intensity mass in the right thigh (arrow). (b) Axial contrast-enhanced T1-weighted image shows moderate and heterogeneous enhancement of the mass (arrow). (c) Axial ADC map of the mass obtained using line-scan DWI ($b = 5$, 1000 s/mm^2) shows reduced diffusivity (long arrow), with ADC value of 0.66×10^{-3} mm^2/s, compared to high ADC of the water phantom (2.52×10^{-3} mm^2/s; short arrow). (d) Photomicrograph shows tumor hypercellularity (hematoxylin and eosin $\times$ 100).

compensation. With this technique, multiple diffusion-weighted SE column excitations are used to obtain a 2D image[11]. This method is relatively insensitive to motion artifacts because the images are constructed column by column and the acquisition time for an individual column is approximately equal to the echo time (TE). Importantly, in areas near large bone structures or air, the sensitivity of SS-EPI to susceptibility variations can distort images or cause complete signal loss, whereas images obtained with line-scan and SE-DWI display no such artifacts[5,7,11,12].

Results and pitfalls of DWI in soft tissue tumors

Tumor characterization

Diffusivity and cellularity of tumors

The results of experimental studies reveal that tumor cellularity strongly influences the diffusivity of tumors[13]. Clinical data of brain tumors present a clear inverse relationship between ADC values and the cellularity of tumors[1,3,4], suggesting that greater cellularity is associated with more restricted diffusivity. Similarly, it appears that this relationship might be applicable to soft tissue tumors[7,14]. Densely packed tissue structures with a high nucleus-to-cytoplasm ratio might be reflected by lower ADC values for these lesions (Fig. 11.1).

Diffusivity and bulk tumor necrosis/cystic degeneration of soft tissue tumors

Bulk necrosis and cystic degeneration of tumors generally result in increased diffusivity (Fig. 11.2)[13,15]. This finding might be explained by the free movement of water molecules that occurs when these histological changes are present. The massive necrotic region of the tumor contains material that is less viscous, resembling serous fluid. These changes are commonly observed, particularly in malignant tumors. Therefore, in measuring ADC for tumor characterization, special care should be taken to include solid-appearing regions of tumors and to exclude obviously necrotic or cystic regions demonstrated in the corresponding T2-weighted and contrast-enhanced MR images.

Diagnostic pitfall: epidermal cysts do not show increased diffusivity

Fluid-containing cysts show increased diffusivity, as mentioned above (Fig. 11.2). In contrast, epidermal cysts (or sebaceous cysts) do not (Fig. 11.3). The latter is a common, benign, soft tissue mass lined with

keratin-producing squamous epithelium filled with keratin debris and cholesterol crystals. Such lesions are commonly encountered in the hair-bearing parts of the body such as the scalp, face, and trunk[16]. The tumor is usually diagnosed clinically without imaging because it is a small tumor that is typically located in subcutaneous regions; rarely, however, this tumor grows sufficiently large to require a radiological examination. Subcutaneous epidermal cysts show a fluid-like signal and central non-enhancement with or without peripheral rim enhancement on contrast enhanced T1-weighted images[17], in addition to subcutaneous tumor location and a well-circumscribed margin. The differential diagnoses of subcutaneous epidermal cysts include other subcutaneous fluid-containing masses such as ganglion cyst or bursitis, some solid tumors, and vascular lesions that exhibit fluid-like signals on conventional MR sequences[17]. ADC appears to be useful in differential diagnosis because this value is much lower for epidermal cysts than for other masses that contain fluid[18].

Influence of myxoid matrix of soft tissue tumors on diffusivity

Although the diffusivity of a tumor is significantly influenced by its cellularity, the tumor matrix is also of importance[19]. The various tumor matrices include collagen fiber, myxoid, hyalinization, and

(a)

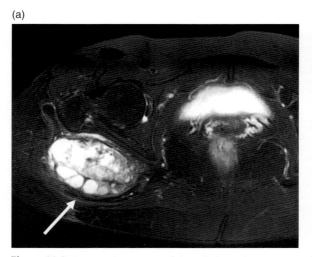

(b)

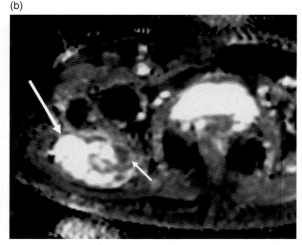

Figure 11.2 Benign schwannoma of the right buttock in a 70-year-old woman. (a) Axial FSE T2-weighted image with fat suppression reveals heterogeneous high T2 signal intensity mass in the right buttock (arrow). (b) Axial ADC map obtained with SS-EPI DWI ($b = 0$, 1000 s/mm^2) shows that diffusivity of the cystic component is very high (ADC = 3.0×10^{-3} mm^2/s; long arrow), while diffusivity of the solid component is low (ADC = 1.2×10^{-3} mm^2/s; short arrow).

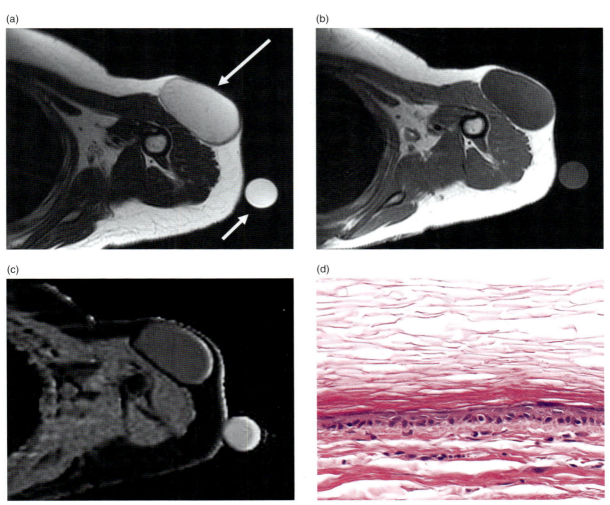

Figure 11.3 Epidermal cyst (sebaceous cyst) of the left arm in a 37-year-old woman. (a) Axial fast-spin-echo (FSE) T2-weighted image shows hyperintense mass (long arrow), but lower in intensity than the water phantom (short arrow). (b) Axial contrast-enhanced T1-weighted image shows no internal tumor enhancement. (c) Line-scan DWI, $b = 5$, 1000 s/mm^2. Axial ADC map shows that diffusivity is much lower in the tumor than in the water phantom. The ADC of the tumor is 0.94×10^{-3} mm^2/s, whereas that of the water phantom is 2.47×10^{-3} mm^2/s. (d) Photomicrograph shows keratin debris and a wall of stratified squamous epithelium (hematoxylin and eosin $\times$ 200).

lymphoid tissue. The pathological composition of interstitial spaces, in particular, is peculiar to soft tissue tumors, as distinct to that of brain tumors. For example, myxoid matrix, which is rarely seen in brain tumors, is found occasionally in several soft tissue tumors, whether benign or malignant[20].

Several reports describe that myxoid-containing soft tissue tumors have significantly higher ADC values than those recorded for non-myxoid soft tissue tumors (Fig. 11.4)[7,8]. Our data showed that the ADC (mean $\pm$ SD) in myxoid-containing tumors was $1.92 \pm 0.41 \times 10^{-3}$ mm^2/s, whereas that in non-myxoid tumors was $0.97 \pm 0.33 \times 10^{-3}$ mm^2/s ($p < 0.01$)[7]. Another study supported our data, reporting significantly higher ADC values in myxoid tumors ($2.08 \pm 0.51 \times 10^{-3}$ mm^2/s) than in non-myxoid tumors ($1.13 \pm 0.40 \times 10^{-3}$ mm^2/s)[8]. The most likely cause of increased diffusivity in myxoid-containing tumors is the abundance of free water in the myxoid matrix. Among myxoid soft tissue tumors, intramuscular myxoma shows the highest ADC values, a direct reflection of the high mucin and low collagen content of this lesion, which contains a large amount of water as seen histologically (Fig. 11.5).

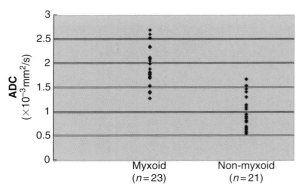

Figure 11.4 Scatterplot of ADC values of myxoid ($n = 23$) and non-myxoid ($n = 21$) soft tissue tumors. A significant difference in ADC values exists between myxoid and non-myxoid tumors ($p < 0.01$). The ADC (mean ± SD) is $1.92 ± 0.41 × 10^{-3}$ mm^2/sec in myxoid-type tumors, whereas the ADC is $0.97 ± 0.33 × 10^{-3}$ mm^2/sec in non-myxoid-type. [Reused with permission from Maeda et al. 2007[7].]

Differentiation between benign and malignant tumors using ADC

An initial report showed that the ADCs of malignant soft tissue tumors were significantly lower than those of benign tumors[5]. More recent reports state that benign soft tissue tumors and malignant soft tissue tumors cannot be differentiated based on ADC values[6–8] due to significant overlap of ADC values between benign and malignant soft tissue tumors (Fig. 11.6). It should be kept in mind that ADC values of soft tissue tumors are influenced by many factors, including tumor cellularity, tumor matrix, and necrosis/cystic degeneration. ADC values are relatively low in several non-myxoid malignant tumors such as lymphoma, Ewing sarcoma, malignant peripheral nerve sheath tumor, and undifferentiated high-grade pleomorphic sarcoma (Fig. 11.1). The pathologic findings of such tumors reveal hypercellularity (Fig. 11.1). In contrast, myxoid-containing tumors, either benign or malignant, show significantly higher ADC values than non-myxoid tumors (Fig. 11.7). Another factor influencing ADC is the fat component within the tumor. A large amount of fatty tissue greatly reduces the ADC of a soft tissue tumor (Fig. 11.8), although ADC is not usually necessary to identify the tumor characteristics of a typical lipoma. A small or moderate amount of fatty tissue can exist in either benign or malignant soft tissue tumors, such as spindle cell lipoma or well-differentiated liposarcoma, which may have an influence on the ADC of tumors. Thus, the ADC values of soft tissue tumors are so complicated that they alone may not be useful in differentiating between benign and malignant tumors.

Treatment response

Results of MRI have been used in the evaluation of therapeutic effects on soft tissue tumors; however, assessment is commonly achieved by comparing tumor size and contrast enhancement before and following completion of therapeutic interventions. It would be advantageous to evaluate early response to a particular treatment at the early stage of therapeutic intervention, thus enabling unnecessary treatment to be avoided and optimizing individual management.

Detection of early changes within the tumor during treatment is of great clinical value because intratumoral changes such as vascular shutdown and consequent increase in the necrotic tumor fraction can precede morphologic changes. Previous experimental studies report the use of DWI to monitor reductions in both perfusion and diffusion changes in the extent of rhabdomyosarcoma necrosis following therapy with vascular targeting agents[15,21]. DWI has several potential advantages over other methods: it is non-invasive, does not use ionizing radiation, and requires no administration of contrast medium. It also has a shorter examination time than other techniques, with an easily reproducible technique that enables close follow-up of cancer treatment. The use of low b-values ($b = 0$–100 mm^2/s) enables perfusion changes to be detected at the very early stages after treatment with vascular targeting agents[15]. The use of higher b-values (for example, 1000 mm^2/s) enables good differentiation of viable tumor tissue and necrotic tissue: viable tumor tissues with high cellular density show low ADC because the mobility of water protons is impeded by the higher amounts of cell membranes, whereas necrotic tissues show high ADC due to rapid diffusivity of water protons as a consequence of lost membrane integrity[15]. The results of animal studies have confirmed that after the initiation of novel therapy, an increase in the ADC value may be observed in those responding to treatment[15]. Furthermore, treatment effects can be observed within the first 24 h after initiating treatment due to cell swelling, which results in a transient decrease in the ADC[15].

(a)

(b)

(c)

(d)

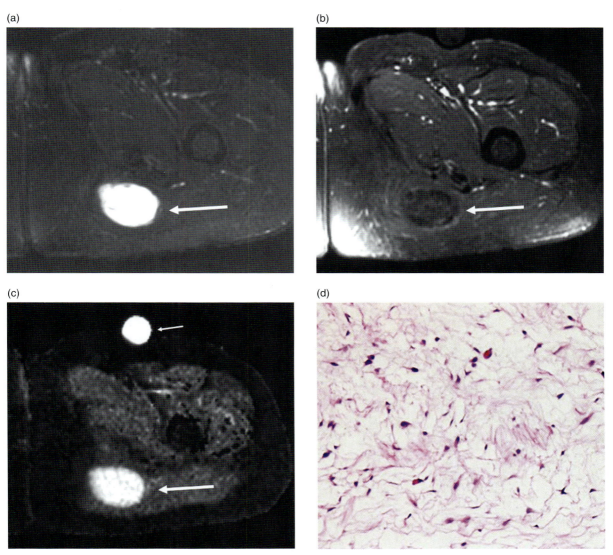

Figure 11.5 Intramuscular myxoma of the left buttock in a 54-year-old woman. (a) Axial FSE T2-weighted image with fat suppression reveals a homogeneous high signal mass in the left buttock (arrow). (b) Axial contrast enhanced T1-weighted image with fat suppression shows faint tumor enhancement (arrow). (c) Line-scan DWI, $b = 5$, 1000 s/mm². Axial ADC map of the mass shows remarkably high signal intensity (long arrow), almost equal to that of the water phantom (small arrow). The ADC values of the mass and the water phantom are 2.53×10^{-3} mm²/s and 2.70×10^{-3} mm²/s, respectively. (d) Photomicrograph shows abundant myxoid matrix of the tumor (hematoxylin and eosin × 200).

A recent report found that DWI could be used as a supplement to morphologic imaging in evaluating tumor response to anticancer therapy in patients with soft tissue sarcomas[9]; an increase in ADC value could be associated with a reduction of tumor size (Fig. 11.9). Likewise, a decrease in ADC could be associated with an increase in tumor volume. Thus, DWI is a promising tool for monitoring the effects of treatment.

Limitations of DWI for assessment of soft tissue tumors

A major limitation is that there have been only a few reports on soft tissue tumors using DWI[5–9,13–15,21]. Particularly, clinical evidence is not sufficient to determine the usefulness of DWI in comparison to conventional MRI or to other MR techniques such as dynamic enhanced MRI. This may be due to a lack of

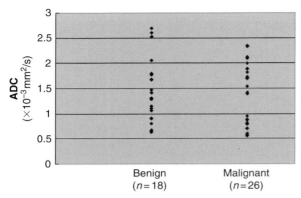

Figure 11.6 Scatterplot of ADC values for benign ($n = 18$) and malignant ($n = 26$) soft tissue tumors. No significant difference in ADC values is apparent between the two types of soft tissue tumors. The ADC (mean ± SD) is $1.45 ± 0.59 × 10^{-3}$ mm^2/s in malignant tumors, whereas the ADC is $1.50 ± 0.64 × 10^{-3}$ mm^2/s in benign tumors. [Reused with permission from Maeda *et al.* 2007[7].]

recognition by radiologists of DWI as a tool that provides unique information that can help in tumor evaluation at extra-cranial sites. Active engagement in applying DWI would facilitate its adoption to clinical practice. Another limitation is that the lack of standardization hinders the widespread use of DWI for soft tissue tumors. The DWI techniques and the choice of *b*-values vary considerably. Consequently, considerable differences in the ADC values of similar diseases have been reported using different techniques. Standardization of protocols (e.g., type of sequence, *b*-values) for both image acquisition and data analysis is important.

Future directions

According to the advance and wide spread of DWI techniques, DWI will be more widely used for soft tissue tumors in future, as for other tumors of extra-cranial

(a)

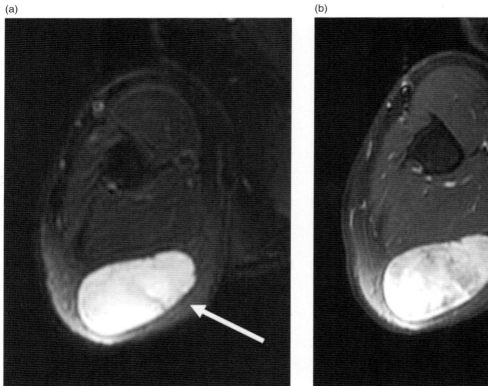

(b)

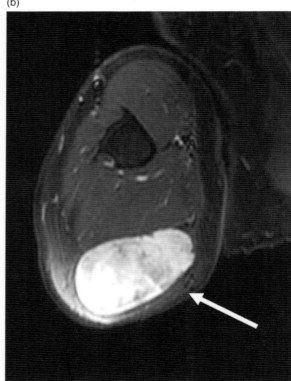

Figure 11.7 Myxoid liposarcoma of the right arm in a 57-year-old man. (a) Axial FSE T2-weighted image with fat suppression reveals a homogeneous high signal mass in the right arm (arrow). (b) Axial contrast enhanced T1-weighted image with fat suppression shows intense enhancement of the mass (arrow). (c) Line-scan DWI, $b = 5$, 1000 s/mm^2. Axial ADC map shows increased diffusivity of the mass (arrow). The ADC value of the mass is $2.0 × 10^{-3}$ mm^2/s. (d) Photomicrograph shows abundant myxoid matrix (hematoxylin and eosin × 200).

(c)

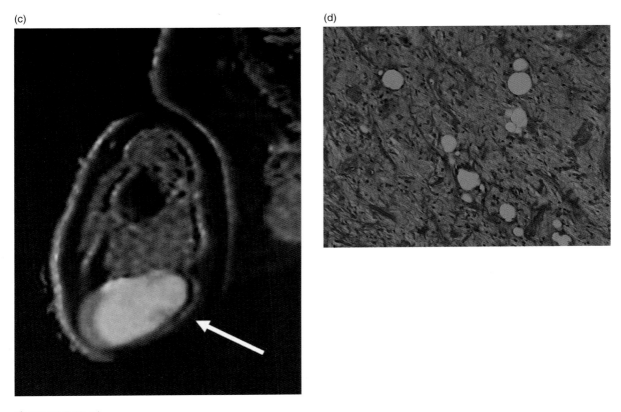

Figure 11.7 (*Cont.*)

(a)

(b)

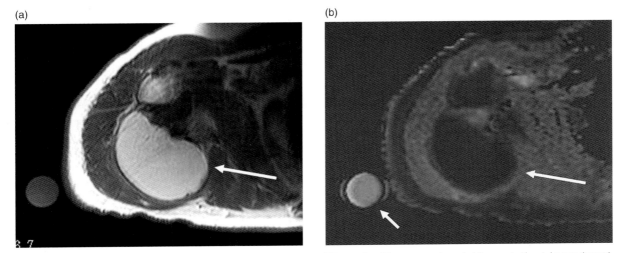

Figure 11.8 Lipoma of the right arm in an 80-year-old woman. (a) Axial T1-weighted image reveals typical lipoma in the right arm (arrow). (b) Line-scan DWI, $b = 5$, 1000 s/mm^2. Axial ADC map shows decreased diffusivity of the lipoma. The respective ADC values of the lipoma (long arrow) and water phantom (short arrow) are 0.43×10^{-3} mm^2/s and 2.70×10^{-3} mm^2/s.

(a)

(b)

(c)

(d)

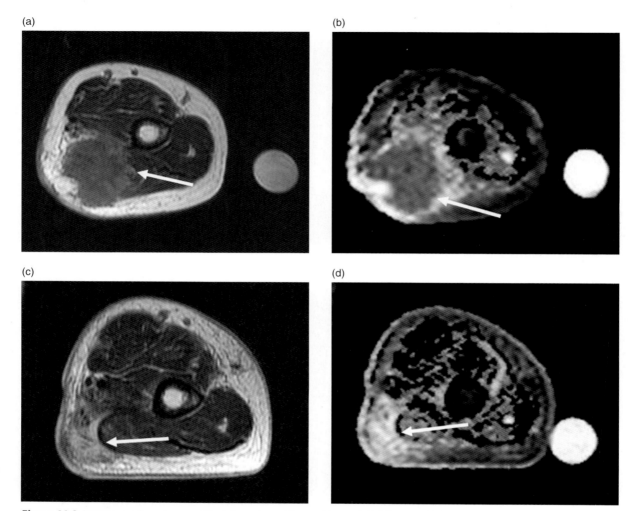

Figure 11.9 Squamous cell carcinoma of the left arm in an 87-year-old man. (a,b) MR images before treatment. (c,d) MR images after radiation therapy. (a) Axial T2-weighted image shows a mass of moderate signal intensity (arrow). (b) Line-scan DWI, $b = 5$, 1000 s/mm^2. The ADC of the mass (arrow) is 0.86×10^{-3} mm^2/s before treatment. (c) Axial T2-weighted image shows that the mass has decreased in size following radiation therapy (arrow). (d) Line-scan DWI, $b = 5$, 1000 s/mm^2. The ADC of the mass (arrow) is 2.0×10^{-3} mm^2/s post radiation therapy. The diffusivity of the tumor is increased after radiation therapy.

sites. Since DWI has a great potential to monitor the early response to treatment for soft tissue sarcoma, this method will be particularly used in the assessment of treatment efficacy.

Conclusion

Although the clinical usefulness of DWI for soft tissue tumors has yet to be sufficiently investigated, DWI techniques have come to be used in the clinical setting for a wide variety of soft tissue tumors. However, there are major challenges to the widespread use of DWI and the standardization of DWI sequence and

data analysis. Importantly, DWI could be a promising tool for monitoring the effects of treatment in malignant soft tissue tumors.

References

1. Sugahara T, Korogi Y, Kochi M, *et al.* Usefulness of diffusion-weighted MRI with echo-planar technique in the evaluation of cellularity in gliomas. *J Magn Reson Imag* 1999;**9**:53–60.

2. Filippi CG, Edgar MA, Ulug AM, *et al.* Appearance of meningiomas on diffusion-weighted images: correlating diffusion constants with histopathologic findings. *Am J Neuroradiol* 2001;**22**:65–72.

3. Kono K, Inoue Y, Nakayama K, *et al.* The role of diffusion-weighted imaging in patients with brain tumors. *Am J Neuroradiol* 2001;**22**:1081–88.

4. Guo AC, Cummings TJ, Dash RC, *et al.* Lymphomas and high-grade astrocytomas: comparison of water diffusibility and histologic characteristics. *Radiology* 2002;**224**:177–83.

5. van Rijswijk CSP, Kunz P, Hogendoorn PCW, *et al.* Diffusion-weighted MRI in the characterization of soft-tissue tumors. *J Magn Reson Imag* 2002;**15**:302–7.

6. Einarsdottir H, Karlsson M, Wejde J, *et al.* Diffusion-weighted MRI of soft tissue tumours. *Eur Radiol* 2004;**14**:959–63.

7. Maeda M, Matsumine A, Kato H, *et al.* Soft-tissue tumors evaluated by line-scan diffusion-weighted imaging: influence of myxoid matrix on the apparent diffusion coefficient. *J Magn Reson Imag* 2007;**25**:1199–204.

8. Nagata S, Nishimura H, Uchida M, *et al.* Diffusion-weighted imaging of soft tissue tumors: usefulness of the apparent diffusion coefficient for differential diagnosis. *Radiat Med* 2008;**26**:287–95.

9. Dudeck O, Zeile M, Pink D, *et al.* Diffusion-weighted magnetic resonance imaging allows monitoring of anticancer treatment effects in patients with soft-tissue sarcomas. *J Magn Reson Imag* 2008;**27**:1109–13.

10. Stejskal EO, Tanner JE. Spin diffusion measurements: spin echoes in the presence of a time-dependent field gradient. *J Chem Phys* 1965;**42**:288–92.

11. Gudbjartsson H, Maier SE, Mulkern RV, *et al.* Line scan diffusion imaging. *Magn Reson Med* 1996;**36**:509–19.

12. Maeda M, Sakuma H, Maier SE, *et al.* Quantitative assessment of diffusion abnormalities in benign and malignant vertebral compression fractures by line scan diffusion-weighted imaging. *Am J Roentgenol* 2003;**181**:1203–9.

13. Lyng H, Haraldseth O, Rofstad EK. Measurement of cell density and necrotic fraction in human melanoma xenografts by diffusion weighted magnetic resonance imaging. *Magn Reson Med* 2000;**43**:828–36.

14. Niwa T, Aida N, Fujita K, *et al.* Diffusion-weighted imaging of retroperitoneal malignant peripheral nerve sheath tumor in a patient with neurofibromatosis type 1. *Magn Reson Med Sci* 2008;**7**:49–53.

15. Thoeny HC, De Keyzer F, Chen F, *et al.* Diffusion-weighted MR imaging in monitoring the effect of a vascular targeting agent on rhabdomyosarcoma in rats. *Radiology* 2005;**234**:756–64.

16. Fisher BK, Macpherson M. Epidermoid cyst of the sole. *J Am Acad Dermatol* 1986;**15**:1127–9.

17. Hong SH, Chung HW, Choi JY, *et al.* MRI findings of subcutaneous epidermal cysts: emphasis on the presence of rupture. *Am J Roentgenol* 2006;**186**:961–6.

18. Suzuki C, Maeda M, Matsumine A, *et al.* Apparent diffusion coefficient of subcutaneous epidermal cysts in the head and neck comparison with intracranial epidermoid cysts. *Acad Radiol* 2007;**14**:1020–8.

19. Matsushima N, Maeda M, Takamura M, *et al.* Apparent diffusion coefficients of benign and malignant salivary gland tumors. Comparison to histopathological findings. *J Neuroradiol* 2007;**34**:183–9.

20. Peterson KK, Renfrew DL, Feddersen RM, *et al.* Magnetic resonance imaging of myxoid-containing tumors. *Skeletal Radiol* 1991;**20**:245–50.

21. Thoeny HC, De Keyzer F, Chen F, *et al.* Diffusion-weighted magnetic resonance imaging allows noninvasive in vivo monitoring of the effects of combretastatin a-4 phosphate after repeated administration. *Neoplasia* 2005;**7**:779–87.

Chapter 12

Evaluation of tumor treatment response with diffusion-weighted MRI

Andriy M. Babsky, Shenghong Ju, and Navin Bansal

Abbreviations

5FU	5-fluorouracil
ADC	apparent diffusion coefficient
BCNU	1,3-bis(2-chloroethyl)-1-nitrosourea
DCE	dynamic contrast enhancement
Cp	cyclophosphamide
CT	computed tomography
DWI	diffusion-weighted imaging
rECS	(relative) extracellular space
FDG-6-P	2-[^{19}F]luoro-2-deoxyglucose-6-phosphate
HCC	hepatocellular carcinoma
ICS	intracellular space
IH	intrahepatic
MRI	magnetic resonance imaging
[Na$^+$]$_e$	extracellular Na$^+$
[Na$^+$]$_i$	intracellular Na$^+$
[Na$^+$]$_t$	total tissue Na$^+$
NACT	neoadjuvant chemotherapy
PET	positron emission tomography
RIF-1	radiation-induced fibrosarcoma-1
sc	subcutaneous
SI	signal intensity
SPECT	single-photon emission computerized tomography
SQ	single-quantum
SR	shift reagent
TACE	transarterial chemoembolization
TQF	triple-quantum-filtered
TRAIL	tumor necrosis factor-related apoptosis-inducing ligand
UFE	uterine fibroid embolization

Introduction

Prediction and detection of therapeutic response, as well as characterization of residual disease, are very important for effective cancer therapy. Current assessment of tumor treatment response relies on evaluating changes in the maximal cross-sectional area or the diameter of the tumor, weeks to months after the conclusion of a therapeutic protocol. Several non-invasive imaging methods, such as computed tomography (CT), positron-emission tomography (PET), single-photon emission computerized tomography (SPECT), magnetic resonance spectroscopy (MRS), contrast-enhanced MRI and perfusion, and diffusion-weighted magnetic resonance imaging (DWI) are being evaluated for assessing early therapeutic responses that are independent of late changes in tumor volume.

DWI is a well-known diagnostic tool to evaluate central nervous system pathologies. The primary metric used in DWI is the apparent diffusion coefficient (ADC). The first reported evaluation of mean tumor ADC following chemotherapy of an animal model was performed by Ross *et al.* in 1994[1], who studied the effect of 1,3-bis(2-chloroethyl)-1-nitrosourea (BCNU) treatment on orthotopic 9L glioma in a rat model. For many years, the use of DWI was limited to the brain.

Extra-Cranial Applications of Diffusion-Weighted MRI, ed. Bachir Taouli. Published by Cambridge University Press.
© Cambridge University Press 2011.

Physiologic motion and the challenging magnetic environment outside the brain made it difficult to obtain accurate ADC measurements within a reasonable acquisition time. Recently, however, advances in MRI hardware and software have improved image quality considerably, resulting in several reports describing the potential of DWI in the evaluation of extracranial diseases.

DW-MRI has a number of advantages over other imaging techniques (e.g., CT and PET). DW-MRI is non-invasive, and does not require the use of ionizing radiation or the administration of contrast medium. The short examination time, especially when using parallel imaging, is an additional advantage, as is the ability to assess the tumor completely. In addition, parallel imaging may reduce magnetic susceptibility and motion artifacts, which are the major limitation to the use of DW-MRI. In cancer imaging, the early detection of non-responders or the prediction of response to treatment may allow changes of therapy in order to minimize treatment-related toxicity. Furthermore, both conventional morphologic and physiologic assessments can be made during the same examination[2]. DWI provides also both quantitative and qualitative information that can be useful for tumor treatment. The challenges and recommendations concerning the application of DWI as a cancer biomarker are widely discussed in a recent review by Padhani et al.[3]

In pre-clinical models, there is abundant evidence that the ADC in tumors increases early in response to successful treatment. This has been shown in sarcoma, glioma, and breast carcinoma xenografts treated with cytotoxic chemotherapies, cytostatic chemotherapies, radiation therapy, and gene therapies[4–5]. Treatments that caused cells to shrink led to early increases in ADC that were predictive of the ultimate tumor response. Changes detected in mean tumor ADC values after treatment in rodent tumor models have revealed that DWI has merit for pre-clinical drug development studies as a sensitive and early predictor of therapeutic efficacy[5–15]. Prediction of tumor response is critical for DWI to become a validated clinical biomarker of early treatment response. However, because of tumor heterogeneity and suboptimal methods of digital image analysis[11,16–18], determining the clinical utility of this approach is more complicated and therefore its application to humans has been more difficult than initially thought. Many of the clinical studies

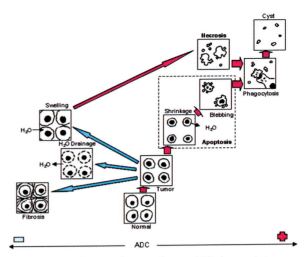

Figure 12.1 Schematic diagram of water ADC changes in tumor. [Adapted from Moffat et al. 2005[20] and Koh and Collins 2007[19].]

evaluating DWI for assessing treatment response have been performed in relatively small numbers of patients. Nevertheless, there is clear evidence that ADC measurement is a potentially useful tool that provides unique prognostic information and should be more widely investigated in large clinical studies.[19]

The common points of view on mechanisms of ADC changes in tumor tissue are summarized in Figure 12.1. Neoplastic transformation can lead to an increase in water ADC due to less efficient cell packing in tumors compared to the healthy tissue. Ross et al. hypothesized that the changes in tumor ADC that occur after effective therapy can be related to changes in cell density[1] as a result of necrotic and/or apoptotic processes. Both of these processes should lead to an increase in relative extracellular space (rECS) and an increase in water ADC. On the other hand, the loss of tumor membrane integrity can cause water inflow, cell swelling, and thus can lead to a decrease in both rECS and water ADC, especially in the beginning of the post-treatment period. Heterogeneous tumor tissues usually contain regions of intratumoral edema, necrosis, and cyst with high extracellular water content. Post-treatment dynamic reorganization of these regions involving tissue water drainage can also decrease water ADC. Furthermore, intensive fibrosis in tumor tissue can also contribute to restriction of water diffusion. Moffat et al. stated that "the changes in cell density due to cell killing along with tissue reorganization may lead to heterogeneous changes in the underlying tissue morphology (e.g., ratio of intra- to extracellular water), resulting in spatially varying changes in tumor ADC values"[20]. Koh and Collins consider that the explanation of ADC changes has to include not only the rECS changes but also the contribution of intra-vascular perfusion to the diffusion measurement, especially when DWI must be performed using low b-values, which are sensitive to vascular perfusion effects[19]. The simplified model in Figure 12.1 also does not include the possibility of changes in ADC of intracellular compartment and its contribution to the total tissue ADC value. The direct measurements of ADC of small molecules like sodium, gadolinium, mannitol, glucose, and others show that intra- and extracellular ADCs are rather more similar than different and ischemic tissue injury can cause changes in the ADC values of both the compartments[21–22].

Monitoring of the treatment response using ADC measurements in animal tumors

The use of ADC to estimate chemotherapy efficiency has been assessed in a number of animal studies and summarized in Table 12.1. The following section discusses the variabilities in the MRI techniques and animal models used in evaluating the application of DW-MRI for monitoring therapy response. Then the applications of the technique in the study of different animal body tumor models, such as a tumor of connective tissue, muscle, colon, breast, liver, prostate, and other tissues will be discussed.

Variabilities in MRI techniques and animal models in water ADC studies

The extensive application of water ADC as a marker of animal body tumor chemotherapy efficiency began about 10 years ago, using mainly rats (Fisher, Wistar, Ludwig, etc.) and mice (C3H, BALB nude, SCID, GBNIH nude, etc.). For that purpose, both clinical (1.5–4.7 T) and small animal (4.7–14 T) MRI systems have been used. Different type of MR coils, such as birdcage[23–24], loop gap[25–27], wrist,[28] and surface coils[29] have been used according to the tumor location and volume. Most of these experiments were performed using subcutaneous (sc-) implanted tumors. Sc-implanted tumor models may provide high-quality

MR images because they avoid the motion effects present in the abdominal area and allow close location of the MR coil to the tumor tissue. The values of water ADC before treatment for many sarcomas[25,30–32] and human breast cancer xenografts[33–34] were reported to be 0.4–0.7 × 10^{-3} mm^2/s. However, Thoeny et al.[14,28] found a higher water ADC value for rhabdomyosarcoma (1.26 × 10^{-3} mm^2/s). Water ADC in sc-implanted gliomas (gliosarcomas)[23–24,26] and mammary tumor xenografts[29] were found before treatment to be 0.9–1.1 × 10^{-3} mm^2/s. Pre-treated sc-implanted tumor volumes used for the water ADC estimation varied from 0.1–0.6 cm^3 (mostly for carcinomas) to 1–2 cm^3 (mostly for gliomas). Absolute ADC values, however, depend on the b-values applied for DW-MRI. Unfortunately, the number of b-values used in the different post-treatment studies of ADC greatly varied, from two (0 and 300 s/mm^2)[23–24, 35] to fourteen (15–2741 s/mm^2)[36]. In some studies, b-values higher than 1000 s/mm^2 been used[23–27,36]. Some investigators use a b-value = 0 s/mm$^{2[25–28,32,34]}$, and others do not[24,29–30,33,37]. These variations in b-values make the comparison of the ADC data complicated. As a quantitative parameter of DWI, ADC reflects not only diffusion but also perfusion in microvessels[38]. Previous studies show that for low b-values (<100 s/mm^2), perfusion dominates diffusion by a factor of 10[38–39]. However, when high b-values (>500 s/mm^2) are used, the influence of perfusion is largely attenuated. Thoeny et al.[28] divided b-values into low (0, 50, and 100 s/mm^2) and high (500, 750, and 1000 s/mm^2) groups. They propose to use the difference between ADC_{low} and ADC_{high} as a perfusion component of the tissue ADC. However, Zhao et al.[30] has assumed that the vascular contribution to tumor tissue water diffusion is minimal despite the greater water ADC in blood. This conclusion is based on the Braunschweiger study[40] showing that blood occupied less than 5% of sc-implanted fibrosarcoma-1 (RIF-1) volume. In addition, the effect of perfusion is diminished when wide ranges of b-values are used in a study.

Fibrosarcomas and myosarcomas

The first report on the application of water ADC measurements for monitoring response to body cancer therapy was published by Zhao et al. in 1996[37]. This study was performed using a diffusion-weighted spectroscopy pulse sequence. The effects of cyclophospha-mide (Cp), an alkylating agent, on sc-implanted

Table 12.1 Assessment of treatment response of body tumors using ADC measurements in animal studies

Tumor	Treatment	*b*-values	Post-treatment ADC changes	References
RIF-1, sc, mice	Cyclophosphamide	100–2500	Increase in the fraction of interstitial water at day 4	Zhao *et al.* 1996 [30]
RIF-1, sc, mice	Cyclophosphamide	0–1679	Increase after days 2 and 3 correlated with tumor shrinkage, increase in [Na$^+$]$_t$ relative decrease in [Na$^+$]$_i$	Babsky *et al.* 2005 [25]
RIF-1, sc, mice	5-Fluorouracil	0–1679	Increase after days 2 and 3 correlated with tumor shrinkage and with increase in [Na$^+$]$_t$	Babsky *et al.* 2007 [27]
Rhabdomyosarcoma, sc, rats	Combretastatin	0- 1000	Decrease at 1 and 6 h; increase in ADC by days 2 and 9 correlated with necrosis and tumor regrowth	Thoeny 2005 [28]
Human colon tumor xenografts, sc, mice	Inhibition of HIF-1α by PX-478	25- 950	Increase after 24 and 36 h correlated with reduction of cellularity	Jordan *et al.* 2005 [37]
C26 colon cancer, sc, mice	Doxorubicin or aminolevulinic acid-based photodynamic therapy	15–2,741	Low pre-ADC predicted response to chemotherapy; ADC rise at 48 hr predicted response to both chemo- and photo-therapies	Roth *et al.* 2004 [36]
Human colon adenocarcinoma HT29, sc, mice	Fractional irradiation	0, 300	Decrease after day 3 (correlated with fibrosis) and increase at days 1, 7, and 11 (correlated with necrosis)	Seierstad *et al.* 2007 [35]
Breast tumor xenografts, sc, mice	TRIAL and fractional radiation	Delta of two *b*-values = 1,148	Increase at day 7 correlated with loss of cellularity & apoptosis	Chinnaiyan *et al.* 2000 [15]
Breast tumor xenografts MCF-7, mice	Palitaxel	27–472	Early increase in drug nonresistant tumors indicated drug activity prior to tumor shrinkage	Galons *et al.* 1999 [7]
N-methyl-*N*-nitrosourea-induced mammary tumor, rat	5-Fluorouracil	15–1000	Tumors with low ADC (but not with high) showed an increase in ADC at day 7 correlated with necrosis	Lemaire *et al.* 1999 [29]
DU-145 human prostate cancer, sc, mice	Anti-vascular agent ZD6126	0–800	ADC values $>0.9 \times 10^{-3}$ mm^2/sec correlated with necrosis in tumors pre-treatment and at 48–72 h post-treatment	Vogel-Claussen *et al.* 2007 [51]
Prostate cancer xenografts, sc, rats	Docetaxel	200–800	Increase at days 2 and 3 correlated with prostate-specific antigen (PSA) and tumor volume	Jennings *et al.* 2002 [50]
VX2 liver tumor, rabbit	Chemoembolization with iodized oil and pharmorubicin	100, 300	Decrease in the tumor periphery 6 and 16 h post-treatment while at 32 and 48 h it started to increase	Yuan *et al.* 2007, 2008 [46,48]
VX2 liver tumor, rabbits	Chemoembolization	?	Increase correlated with a greater necrotic area	Geschwind *et al.* 2000 [4]

Table 12.1 (cont.)

Tumor	Treatment	b-values	Post-treatment ADC changes	References
Orthotopically implanted pancreatic tumor model	Anti-death receptor 5 antibody (TRA-8) combined with gemcitabine		Increase at days 1–3 correlated with increase in apoptotic cells and density of tumors	Kim et al. 2008 [49]
Glioma, sc, rats	BCNU	117, 1082	Increase after days 3–12 correlated with tumor growth delay and increase in $[Na^+]_t$	Schepkin et al. 2006 [23]
Glioma, sc, rats	BCNU	0–1679	Decrease in BCNU-non-resistant tumors compared to the increased in the growing tumors; changes correlated with $[Na^+]_t$	Babsky et al. 2006 [26]

radiation-induced RIF-1 in C3H mice were investigated using a 4.7-T MR system. Cyclophosphamide itself is a pro-drug, which is oxidized in the liver to 4-hydroxycyclophosphamide and subsequently converted to nitrogen mustard and other metabolites. In tumors, Cp metabolites do not directly disrupt cell metabolism, but rather these metabolites alkylate DNA and proteins. Water ADC of RIF-1 tumors increased at days 2, 3, and 4 after Cp treatment in the absence of or before a decrease in tumor volume (Figure 12.2). The magnitude and duration of the changes in ADC were dose dependent. A 300-mg/kg Cp dose caused a larger and more sustained increase in the ADC compared to a 150-mg/kg dose. Because water ADC was increased substantially at a time when there was no change in tumor volume for a dose which produces minimal cell kill, the authors suggest that ADC measurement could provide a novel means for early detection of response to anti-cancer therapy.

More recently, the increase in water ADC in sc-implanted RIF-1 tumors after chemotherapy with Cp and 5-fluorouracil (5FU) treatment has been confirmed using DW ^{1}H MRI[25,27]. A single injection of Cp (300 mg/kg) or 5FU (25 mg/kg) significantly increased the water ADC of RIF-1 tumors 2 and 3 days post-treatment while tumor volume was significantly decreased. Unlike Cp, the action of 5FU involves its incorporation into RNA and metabolic activation to 5-fluoro-2'-deoxyuridine-5'-monophosphate, which inhibits thymidilate synthetase, a key enzyme in DNA synthesis and repair. Changes in water ADC in control (untreated) and Cp-treated tumors before and 1, 2, and 3 days after Cp injection are shown in Figure 12.3. After Cp injection, water

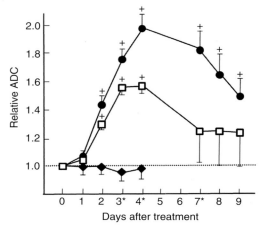

Figure 12.2 Time and dose dependence of the effect of cyclophosphamide (Cp) on RIF-1 ADC (relative to ADC on day 0 for each tumor). ◆, control (n = 6, mean tumor ADC on day 0 [ADC_0]); □, 150 mg/kg Cp (n = 6); ●, 300 mg/kg Cp. ADC_0 did not differ among groups (p = 0.8). Symbols represent mean ± s.e. (bars). Significance: +, vs. day 0 value; *, 150 mg/kg vs. 300 mg/kg Cp groups; (. . .), pre-treatment (day 0) ADC. [Reproduced with permission from Zhao et al. 1996[30].]

ADC increased progressively during the first three days post-treatment. The water ADC increase was observed not only in the tumor regions with low cell density, but throughout the tumor. In the Cp group, the average water ADC increased from 0.47×10^{-3} mm^2/s (before treatment) to 0.58×10^{-3} mm^2/s (day 2) and 0.73×10^{-3} mm^2/s (day 3). In the 5FU group, the average water ADC increased from 0.52×10^{-3} mm^2/s (before treatment) to 0.61×10^{-3} mm^2/s (day 2) and 0.65×10^{-3} mm^2/s (day 3). In the untreated control group tumor ADC remained unchanged throughout the experiment. The average water ADC

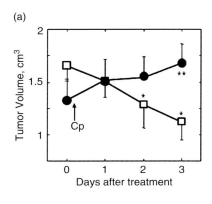
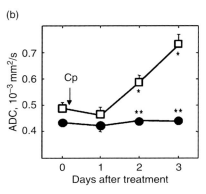

Figure 12.3 Effects of Cp therapy (300 mg/kg, ip) on tumor volume (a) and water ADC (b) in sc-implanted RIF-1 tumors. The tumor volumes were measured from ^{1}H MRI. Water ADC are the mean values from the whole tumor. Cp treatment caused a significant decrease in tumor volume and significant increases in water ADC 2 and 3 days post-therapy. Significance: $p < 0.05$ (* – vs. before treatment), $p < 0.01$ (** – Control vs. Cp-treated). Data are presented as mean $\pm$ SEM. [Reproduced with permission from Babsky et al. 2005[25].]

of treated tumors was significantly higher ($p < 0.05$) compared to both the pre-treatment ADC value and the ADC of untreated control tumors. Braunschweiger[40] has shown that Cp treatment reduces cell proliferation and increases extracellular, interstitial, and plasma water volumes during the initial 5 days after treatment. The increase in extracellular water, cell death, and/or reduction in cell volume may increase the overall mobility of water in the damaged tissue and lead to an increase in water ADC. Destructive chemical analysis and histological results of RIF-1 tumors support this hypothesis. Measurement of rECS by destructive chemical analysis shows $46 \pm 8\%$ rECS in treated tumors compared to $26 \pm 4\%$ in untreated tumors. Similarly, histologic data shows a decrease in the number of cells and an increase in extracellular space[25,27]. It has been shown previously that the increase in water ADC correlates with both the increase in tumor necrotic fraction in RIF-1 tumors[41] and with the decrease in tumor cell density in 9L glioma[11]. Similar to the Cp-treatment, treatment of RIF-1 tumors with 5FU also led to an increase in rECS. The ratio of necrotic to total tumor area in histologic sections was 52% higher than controls 3 days after the treatment. Furthermore, cellular density was 26% lower in necrotic areas of the treated tumors[27]. In necrotic areas of tumors, much evidence of apoptotic and necrotic change was found, such as dusting nuclei, pyknosis, neutrophil invasion, and/or karyorrhexis.

Thoeny et al. used a rhabdomyosarcoma tumor model to study the effects of the vascular targeting agent combretastatin A4 on water ADC using a 1.5-T MR system[14,28,42]. Combretastatin A4 produces a reversible disruption of the vascular network in tumors causing cell death without damaging the vasculature of normal organs[43]. The authors proposed

that the difference between the ADC values calculated using low b-values of 0, 50, and 100 s/mm^2 (ADC$_{low}$) and high b-values of 500, 750, and 1,000 s/mm^2 (ADC$_{high}$) provides information about the perfusion component in ADC (ADC$_{perf}$)[14]. They showed that treatment of sc-implanted rhabdomyosarcoma with a single ip dose of 25 mg/kg combretastatin A4 leads to significant decreases in ADC$_{low}$, ADC$_{high}$, and ADC$_{perf}$ 1 and 6 h post-treatment and is associated with tumor growth delay. However, at 2 and 9 days after combretastatin A4 injection when the tumor growth delay turned up to significant growth, ADC$_{low}$ and ADC$_{high}$ started to increase, overlapping the before treatment values. ADC$_{perf}$ was still lower on day 2 but increased on day 9 compared to the before treatment value. The changes in ADC$_{perf}$ were correlated with the volume transfer constant k ($R^2 = 0.46$) and the initial slope ($R^2 = 0.67$) calculated from perfusion data using dynamic contrast-enhanced MRI. The changes of mean ADC from the entire rhabdomyosarcoma showed a similar trend to the ADC$_{high}$ changes[42]. Thus, total tumor ADC showed an early decrease after combretastatin A4 injection, from 1.26×10^{-3} mm^2/s (before) to 1.18×10^{-3} mm^2/s (1 h) and 1.08×10^{-3} mm^2/s (6 h), histologically corresponding to vessel congestion and vascular shutdown in periphery but no necrosis. An increase of total tumor ADC (1.79×10^{-3} mm^2/s) 2 days after the drug injection was associated with progressive necrosis and a significant decrease in ADC 9 days after treatment (1.41×10^{-3} mm^2/s) corresponded to tumor regrowth. Repeated combretastatin A4 administration at a dose of 25 mg/kg, injected with an interval period of 9 days, retains efficacy in rat rhabdomyosarcomas, with similar effects on water ADC after each drug administration[28]. The authors concluded that both DW and dynamic contrast-enhanced MRIs provide information about intratumoral cell viability and necrosis, and allow monitoring of perfusion changes after administration of vascular targeting agents.

Colon cancer

The earliest increase in water ADC after chemotherapy was reported for the treatment of sc-implanted human colon H29 carcinoma xenografts in GBNIH nude mice with inhibition of HIF-1α by PX-478.[37] PX-478 is a novel agent that suppresses both constitutive and hypoxia-induced levels of HIF-1α in cancer cells.[44] PX-478-induced inhibition of tumor growth is associated with HIF-1α levels in different human tumor xenografts. At 24 and 36 h after the treatment with this drug water ADC increased by 94.5% and 38.4% ($p < 0.01$), respectively, before returning to the pre-treatment ADC level. However, PX-478 had no effect on the ADC of a drug-resistant tumor system.

Roth et al. treated sc-implanted C26 colon carcinomas with doxorubicin and with aminolevulenic acid-based photodynamic therapy (PDT)[36]. In malignant cells, doxorubicin-induced intercalation inhibits nucleotide replication and action of DNA and RNA polymerases. The interaction of doxorubicin with topoisomerase II to form DNA-cleavable complexes appears to be an important mechanism of doxorubicin cytocidal activity. The PDT is a regional therapy that induces early destruction of tissue, whereas the effect of doxorubicin chemotherapy is systemic and seen much later. To quantify the diffusion characteristics of the tumor tissue, the authors defined a diffusion index, R_D, which is the normalized summation over the curve

$$R_D = -\sum_{j=0}^{m} \ln(I_j/I_0),$$

where the summation is over m data points of the diffusion curve. As compared to ADC, which is the slope of b-values vs. signal intensities curve, R_D is the integral of the curve. A decrease in R_D corresponds to an increase in water ADC. In doxorubicin-treated carcinomas, a significant correlation was found between R_D measured prior to treatment, and changes in tumor volume after therapy. An average negative change in tumor R_D was observed after chemotherapy ($\Delta R_D = -3.1 \pm 0.5$) and PDT ($\Delta R_D = -4.4 \pm 1.0$) 24 or 48 h post-treatment. No substantial changes in R_D

were observed in control tumors. Tumors with high pre-treatment viability responded better to chemotherapy with doxorubicin than more necrotic tumors. In tumors treated with PDT, no such correlation was detected. Changes observed in water diffusion 24–48 h after treatment correlated with later carcinoma growth rate for both therapies.

The most persistent increase in water ADC (till 19 days post-treatment) was reported by Seierstad et al.[32] when sc-implanted human HT29 colon adenocarcinoma xenografts were treated weekly with the 5FU pro-drug capecitabine, daily oxaliplatin, and fractional irradiation. Oxaliplatin is a platinum-based chemotherapy drug in the same family as cisplatin and carboplatin. Compared to cisplatin, the two amine groups are replaced by cyclohexyldiamine for improved antitumor activity. The chlorine ligands are replaced by the oxalato bidentate derived from oxalic acid in order to improve water solubility. The authors found an increase in water ADC by ~19% with combinations of the capecitabine and oxaliplatin at 11 days after the drug applications (Figure 12.4). The combination of these drugs with fractionated irradiation showed a significant growth delay compared to the tumors that received radiation only. Histologic examination showed that both treated and control tumors had necrotic centers, ranging from 12% to 84% of total tumor volume, and that there was a much higher ADC value in the necrotic regions (Figure 12.5). However, the statistical analysis revealed no differences in necrotic fraction between the treatment groups. The same authors have studied the effect of 15 Gy irradiation alone on the same tumor model, and have found that at 24 h post-radiation the water ADC was increased by 5.0% ($p < 0.002$)[35]. This increase was followed by a significant decrease (−6.9%, $p < 0.001$) 3 days post-radiation and a renewed increase of the water ADC on days 7 (+6.2%, $p < 0.03$) and 11 (+11.1%, $p < 0.001$). The decrease in ADC 3 days post-radiation was accompanied with increased fibrosis in the treated tumors.

Breast cancer

Galons et al. monitored the chemotherapy response of human breast MCF7 cancer tumor xenografts to paclitaxel (27 mg/kg after the first MRI experiment and 18 mg/kg every other day)[33]. Paclitaxel binds to the β subunit of tubulin, interfering with normal

(a)

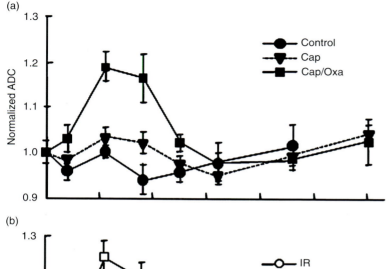

Figure 12.4 Changes in mean tumor ADC for non-irradiated (a) and irradiated (b) colon adenocarcinoma HT29 as a function of time. The ADC value of each tumor is normalized with respect to the pre-treatment ADC value. Chemoradiotherapy was given from days 1 to 13, and consisted of capecitabine (Cap, 359 mg/kg per day, 5days/week starting on day1), oxiplatin (oxa,10 mg/kg, days 2 and 9), and irradiation (IR, 2 Gy for 5 consecutive days, 5 days/week for 2 weeks starting on day2). [Reproduced with permission from Seierstad et al. 2007[32].]

(b)

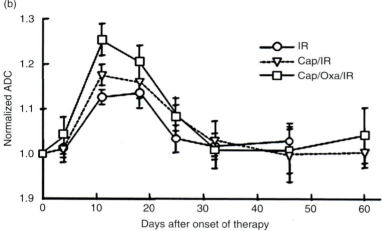

Days after onset of therapy

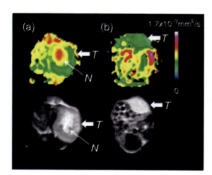

Figure 12.5 ADC maps (upper row) and T2-weighted images (bottom row) of colon adenocarcinoma HT29 illustrating the differences between a tumor with a large necrotic central area (a) and a tumor with mostly viable cells (b). Tumors (T) and their necrotic regions (N) are marked by bold and thin arrows, respectively. Histologic analysis of corresponding tumor slices revealed necrotic fractions of 80% and 20%, respectively, in these two tumors. [Reproduced with permission from Seierstad et al. 2007[32].]

microtubule breakdown during cell division. This drug is related to taxanes, which also induce apoptosis in cancer cells by binding to an apoptosis stopping protein called Bcl-2 and thus arresting its function. ADC increased from 0.5–0.7×10^{-3} mm^2/s to 0.7–1.5×10^{-3} mm^2/s 48 h after successful therapy in parental drug-sensitive MCF-7/S tumors, but there was no change in ADC in p-glycoprotein-positive tumors MCF-7/D40, which are resistant to paclitaxel. The authors concluded that the mechanism underlying these changes is consistent with apoptotic cell shrinkage and a concomitant increase in the extracellular water fraction.

Chinnaiyan et al. monitored the human breast MCF-7 cancer xenografts therapy with tumor necrosis factor-related apoptosis-inducing ligand (TRAIL)[15]. TRAIL is a ligand molecule which induces caspase-8-dependent apoptosis. It is a type II transmembrane protein homologous to other members of the tumor necrosis factor family that can bind to the death receptors, DR4 and DR5. The authors found an increase in water ADC from 0.7 to 1.7×10^{-3} mm^2/s in combined TRAIL- and radiation-treated tumors 7 days post-treatment, but not in tumors treated with these therapies separately (Figure 12.6). Histologic analysis confirmed a decrease in cellularity and activation of apoptotic activity in tumor cells after TRAIL and radiation therapy.

Morse *et al.* treated the human breast MCF-7 and MDA-mb-231 cancer xenografts with the chemotherapeutic agent docetaxel (15 and 30 mg/kg)[34]. The main mode of therapeutic action of docetaxel is the suppression of microtubule dynamic assembly and disassembly, rather than microtubule bundling leading to apoptosis, or the blocking of Bcl-2[45]. Docetaxel has greater cytotoxicity than paclitaxel, possibly due to its more rapid intracellular uptake. MCF-7 cells are partially deficient for apoptosis, and MDA-mb-231 cells are not. The authors examined whether ADC is altered in response to therapies that induce cell death via non-apoptotic mechanisms and correlated ADC changes with cell death regionally within the tumor. The increased ADC in the central regions of

the untreated tumors may correspond to spontaneous necrosis (Figure 12.7). While there was a post-treatment increase in ADC throughout the tumor, much of the increase was associated with the central region of

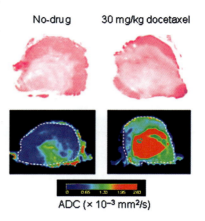

Figure 12.7 ADC maps and histology sections of sc-implanted MDA-mb-231 human breast carcinoma. ADC maps are shown from center axial slices through MDA-mb-231 tumors and surrounding tissue (bottom), after treatment with drug carrier only (left) and after treatment with 30 mg/kg docetaxel (right). Tumor boundaries are delineated by white dashed lines. H&E-stained middle sections of the same tumors, not registered (top). [Reproduced with permission from Morse *et al.* 2007[34].]

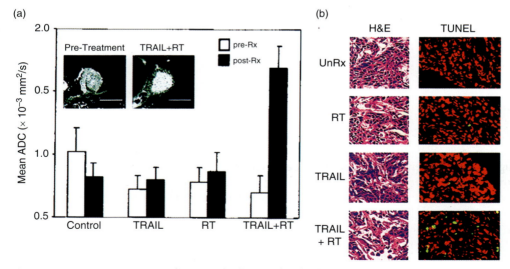

Figure 12.6 Non-invasive imaging of TRAIL- and radiation-induced (RT) apoptosis activity in breast carcinoma MCF-7 as monitored by diffusion MRI. (a) ADC changes in control and treated tumors. Mice were imaged at day 0 and 7 days after start of various treatments. The bar graphs displayed are the mean ADC value (± SD) across pixels within regions of interest defined on a representative animal from each treatment or control group. Isotropic ADC images of a representative tumor before and after TRAIL and radiation treatment are presented. Pixel intensity is directly proportional to the measured ADC. There is a noticeable increase in water mobility after radiation- and TRAIL-combined treatment. (b) Imaged tumors were then assessed for apoptosis. Tumors were sectioned and subsequently stained with hematoxylin and eosin (H&E) or TUNEL. TUNEL-positive cells stain green. Nuclei are counterstained red with propidium iodide. [Reproduced with permission from Chinnaiyan *et al.* 2000[15].]

the tumor, which had low cellularity as determined by histology. ADC decreased in the tumor periphery, which had a higher cell density. The water ADC values from multiple slices in both MCF-7 and MDA-mb-231 tumors show an increase from about 0.5×10^{-3} mm^2/s to 1.0–1.5×10^{-3} mm^2/s 2 to 4 days post-treatment. The authors observed a general trend towards increasing water ADC with increasing dose. Both tumors showed a decrease in the number of pixels after treatment relative to carrier-treated controls, implying tumor shrinkage. These results indicated that early and significant changes in ADC can be related to mitotic catastrophe and lytic necrosis in the absence of apoptosis. The authors proposed to use changes in ADC as a generalized measure of cytotoxic reaction to chemotherapy.

Lemaire et al. examined the effects of 5FU (100 mg/kg, ip) on the water ADC in a rat mammary tumor induced by N-methyl-N-nitrosurea[29]. They showed that the 5FU-treated tumors were not distinguishable in terms of tumor volume change up to day 5, whereas the ADC trend over the same period of time did distinguish the sensitive and non-sensitive groups. They found that mammary tumors with low initial ADC values responded to a single 5FU bolus therapy by a 30% increase in ADC at day 7 after treatment, whereas tumors with high initial ADC showed a 30% decrease and tumors with intermediate values showed no significant change in ADC.

Liver, prostate, and other tumors

The effect of chemotherapy in animal liver tumors has been studied using orthotopic tumors. Transcatheter hepatic arterial chemoembolization (TACE) is a classic interventional therapy for hepatocellular carcinoma (HCC) and some types of liver metastases. TACE enables a higher drug concentration to be in contact with the tumor for a longer period of time. Geschwind et al. used TACE with carboplatin to treat VX2 tumor in the rabbit liver[4]. The ADC in the rabbit VX2 liver carcinoma was evaluated after sacrificing the animals to prevent motion artifacts. DWI delineated regions of tumor cell death as zones of lower signal intensity (SI) in both control and treated groups. ADC was significantly greater in the area of tumor necrosis compared to the area of viable tumor. Histologic analysis showed a significantly lower amount of viable cells after treatment (<1%) compared to the untreated control group (55%).

Bcl-2 was expressed in the liver tumor after chemoembolization, suggesting an apoptotic pathway of cell death.

Yuan et al. used iodized oil (0.3 mL/kg) and pharmorubicin (2 mg/kg) for chemoembolization of the rabbit VX2 tumor in the liver[46]. Similar to doxorubicin, pharmorubicin is an anthracycline antibiotic that interacts with DNA by intercalation and inhibits macromolecular biosynthesis[47]. This inhibits the progression of the enzyme topoisomerase II, which unwinds DNA for transcription. The authors anesthetized rabbits with 3% soluble pentobarbitone into auriborder vein to slow and stabilize animal breathing. Using b-values of 100 s/mm^2 and 300 s/mm^2, ADC in surrounding liver tissue (2.71×10^{-3} mm^2/s, and 2.30×10^{-3} mm^2/s, respectively) was higher than in the tumor center (1.77×10^{-3} mm^2/s and 1.55×10^{-3} mm^2/s, respectively). They found that under both b-values, the water ADC decreased in the tumor periphery 6 and 16 h post-treatment while at 32 and 48 h post-treatment it started to increase. A similar trend was found for water ADC changes in normal liver parenchyma around the tumor. DWI showed potential ability on detecting and differentiating viable tumor from necrotic tumor. The authors concluded that the areas of viable VX2 cells are associated with high signal on DWI and low signal on the ADC map. In contrast, the necrotic areas in the tumors show low signals on DWI and equal or low signals on the ADC map. However, high signals on DWI and on the ADC map appear when the areas of necrotic tumor are liquefied or have become cystic[46,48].

An orthotopic pancreatic tumor model was used to study the early therapeutic efficacy of monometric monoclonal anti-death receptor 5 antibody (TRA-8) combined with gemcitabine using DWI[49]. An anti-death receptor 5 is predominantly expressed in most cancer cells but not in normal cells. TRA-8 was developed specifically to target this receptor. As with fluorouracil and other analogs of pyrimidines, gemcitabine replaces cytidine of nucleic acids during DNA replication, arresting tumor growth as new nucleosides cannot be attached to the "faulty" nucleoside resulting in apoptosis. To prevent the transfer of the respiratory motion in the chest and abdominal area, an orthogonally bent plastic board was used. At day 1 after the beginning of the combined TRA-8 and gemcitabine therapy, water ADC in tumor regions was 27% higher than in untreated controls or those treated with gemcitabine only. At that time point, no statistical difference in tumor volume was found. The mean water ADC values gradually increased over 3 days, which were concurrent with tumor volume regression. An increase in ADC was correlated with an increase in apoptotic cell density of tumors and with mean survival times of animals treated with the same drugs.

Jennings et al. studied the effect of docetaxel (10, 30, and 60 mg/kg) on water ADC in prostate cancer xenografts sc-implanted into the flanks of SCID mice, which are severely deficient in T and B cells and fail to reject allogenic grafts or produce antibodies to common antigens[50]. They showed that tumor volume and secreted prostate-specific antigen both vary inversely with docetaxel dose, and that the ADC increased significantly by day 2 and day 4 post-treatment with all drug doses. They concluded that DWI can be used for early detection of prostate carcinoma xenograft response to docetaxel chemotherapy, and ADC changes may be used to optimize timing of fractioned chemotherapy such that effective doses may be applied when the tumor shows its highest ADC related to the high tumor vulnerability.

Vogel-Claussen et al. used the vascular-targeting agent ZD6126 to treat sc-implanted DU-145 human prostate cancer xenografts in SCID mice[51]. ZD6126 is a pro-drug for N-acetycholinol (NAC), a tubulin-binding agent that inhibits tubulin polymerization and leads to microtubule destabilization selectively in the immature endothelial cells of the tumor neo-vasculature[52]. After intravenous administration, ZD6126 rapidly converts to NAC. In tumors that were not resistant to the drug, the treatment caused progressive cell necrosis in the central tumor region within 24 h post-treatment that was associated with a trend towards restricted diffusion. They explained this effect as a result of acute tumor ischemia, followed by cell swelling and a relative decrease in extracellular space. These data are consistent with the results of Thoeny et al. for angiogenic therapy in rhabdomyosarcomas presented above[42]. A significant linear correlation was observed between the area of ADC values $\geq 0.9 \times 10^{-3}$ mm^2/s and the amount of necrosis in tumors at 48 and 72 h after ZD6126 treatment. The authors mentioned that in cystic malignancies with high pre-treatment ADC values, DWI may not adequately assess early tumor response to antivascular therapy.

Dev et al. used a new type of cancer treatment that combines a pulsed electric field (PEF) with the anticancer drug bleomycin. PEF may create transient pores in the membranes which allow entry of drugs into the cells[53]. Intratumor injection of bleomycin with PEF significantly increased ADC 24 to 48 h post-treatment of sc-implanted laryngeal tumor from 0.73 to 0.82×10^{-3} mm^2/s. During this interval, spin–lattice T1 relaxation time was unchanged while spin–spin T2 relaxation time significantly increased in the treated group. The longer T2 values may reflect early apoptosis and tumor death, reflecting less density of the tumor cells, and higher ADC may indicate looser structural organization and necrosis after treatment.

The studies presented in this chapter allow one to conclude that in animal models, with a few exceptions, effective tumor therapy is associated with an increase in tumor ADC.

Tumor tissue water ADC and ^{23}Na MRI signal intensity reflects structural post-treatment changes

Because of its concentration, ubiquity, and short T1, ^{23}Na is the second most sensitive MR nucleus in tissue, with only ^{1}H being more sensitive. It has been shown that, on average, both ^{23}Na SI and water ADC increased throughout the tumor after the chemotherapy treatment[25,31]. The effects of the alkylating anticancer drug Cp (300 mg/kg, ip) on water ADC measured by DW ^{1}H MRI and [Na$^+$]$_t$ measured by ^{23}Na MRI were examined in subcutaneously implanted RIF-1 tumors[25]. Tumor volumes were significantly lower in Cp-treated animals 2 and 3 days post-treatment (Figure 12.8). At the same time points, in vivo MRI experiments showed an increase in both water ADC and ^{23}Na signal intensity in the treated tumors, while the control tumors did not show any significant changes. Water ADC increased from $0.49 \pm 0.02 \times 10^{-3}$ mm^2/s (before treatment) to $0.73 \pm 0.04 \times 10^{-3}$ mm^2/s (day 3 after treatment) ($p \leq 0.05$); [Na$^+$]$_t$ increased from 34.2 ± 1.9 mM (before treatment) to 43.5 ± 2.7 mM (day 3 after treatment) ($p \leq 0.05$). The correlation between the water ADC and [Na$^+$]$_t$ changes was dramatically increased in the Cp-treated group ($R^2 = 0.97$) compared to the untreated group ($R^2 = 0.29$), suggesting that the observed increases in both water ADC and [Na$^+$]$_t$ were caused by the same

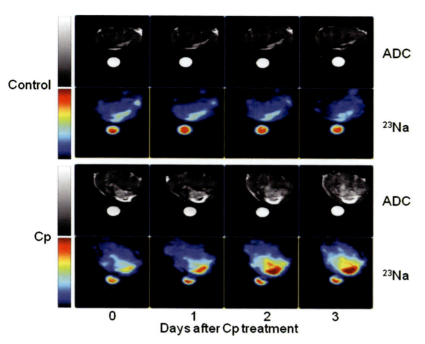

Figure 12.8 Water ADC maps and ^{23}Na MR images of representative control and Cp-treated RIF-1 tumors. Water ADC and ^{23}Na signal intensity increased with time after Cp treatment. A vial filled with a 154 mM NaCl solution was placed near the tumor as a reference. [Reproduced with permission from Babsky et al. 2005[25].]

mechanism. The increase in ^{23}Na MRI SI after Cp treatment was due to increases in $[Na^+]_t$, but not due to changes in ^{23}Na relaxation characteristics, because T1, T2$_s$, and T2$_f$ values did not change after treatment or during untreated growth. The increase in ^{23}Na SI after chemotherapy could be due to an increase in concentration of total tumor tissue sodium ($[Na^+]_t$) or a change in ^{23}Na relaxation times. The authors showed that Cp treatment or untreated growth of RIF-1 tumors did not significantly change the T1, T2$_s$, and T2$_f$ values, or the relative contributions of T2$_s$ and T2$_f$. These results suggest that the observed increase in ^{23}Na SI after Cp treatment was due to increased $[Na^+]_t$ caused by Cp treatment. The inductively coupled plasma-mass spectroscopy data confirmed that in Cp-treated tumors, $[Na^+]_t$ is significantly increased 3 days after treatment (45 ± 7 mM control, 58 ± 10 mM Cp-treated). The value of the Cp-induced increase in $[Na^+]_t$ was comparable for both MRI (36.8%) and inductively coupled plasma spectroscopy (29.4%) methods. Histological sections showed decreased cell density in the regions of increased water ADC and $[Na^+]_t$.

Similar changes in ADC and $[Na^+]_t$ that correlated with each other were shown in the same subcutaneous RIF-1 tumor model with the antimetabolic drug 5FU[31]. The chemotherapy effects were monitored using in vivo DW ^{1}H MRI and ^{23}Na MRI. Tumor volumes were significantly lower in 5FU-treated animals (150 mg/kg, ip) 2 and 3 days posttreatment. At the same time points, in vivo MRI experiments showed a significant increase in water ADC ($\times 10^{-3}$ mm^2/s) in treated tumors from 0.52 ± 0.03 (before treatment) to 0.61 ± 0.02 (day 2 after treatment) and 0.65 ± 0.03 (day 3 after treatment) (Figure 12.9). In the control group, the water ADC value was unchanged during the experimental period. Similar to ADC changes, total tissue ^{23}Na SI increased at days 2 and 3 after treatment. At those time-points, the ^{23}Na MRI SI was significantly higher compared to both before treatment value and to mostly unchanged control values. An increase in both water ADC and total tissue ^{23}Na SI was caused mostly by the increase in rECS, due to cell death and necrotic processes following effective chemotherapy. This mechanism is similar to that described above for the effect of Cp in RIF-1.

Although the extracellular space increases after therapy, $[Na^+]_e$ may remain constant. $[Na^+]_e$ can be maintained constant by transport of Na$^+$ from the vascular and/or interstitial space of the nearby tissue. Previous ^{1}H MRI studies show that tumor perfusion

183

is indeed increased after therapy[54]. Thus, transport of Na^+ from the vascular space can maintain $[Na^+]_e$, and an increase in extracellular space results in increased $[Na^+]_t$ within the tumor after therapy.

There was a good correlation between ^{23}Na SI and ADC in the Cp- and 5FU-treated tumors. One possible reason for this effect may be that $[Na^+]_t$ increases with increased extracellular space because of cells lost via apoptosis and/or necrosis. Schepkin et al.[23–24] also showed that a large increase in ^{23}Na MRI SI occurred 7–9 days following treatment with BCNU, which correlated to the period of greatest chemotherapy-induced cellular necrosis based on water ADC changes and histopathology.

Changes in $[Na^+]_t$ and water ADC are related, and ^{23}Na images may provide additional functional information. This is because therapy can also alter $[Na^+]_i$, which depends on the cellular energy status and activity of ion transport processes. Using triple-quantum-filtered (TQF) ^{23}Na MRI, Babsky et al.[27] have found that $[Na^+]_i$ changed differently than $[Na^+]_t$ after chemotherapy. Although single quantum (SQ) ^{23}Na MRI SI (which reflects total $[Na^+]_t$) increased 2 and 3 days after 5FU treatment,

TQF ^{23}Na MRI SI (which mainly reflects changes in $[Na^+]_i$) remained almost unchanged. Furthermore, in untreated tumors, TQF ^{23}Na MRI SI was increased while SQ ^{23}Na MRI SI was unchanged at the same time-points. One possible explanation for the observed increase in TQF ^{23}Na MRI SI is that tumor growth is associated with progressive hypoxic conditions, accompanied by a decrease in the bioenergetic status that could reduce cellular ability to maintain low $[Na^+]_i$ in control tumors. Conversely, the improvement of tumor bioenergetic status and increase in intracellular pH following 5FU therapy support[55] Na^+/K^+-ATPase activity and decreased Na^+/H^+ exchange across the plasma membrane. Both of these factors help in maintaining low $[Na^+]_i$ and can explain the lower TQF ^{23}Na SI in 5FU-treated tumors compared to the control tumors. In addition, chemotherapy primarily targets weak cells, while the remaining tumor cells are stronger, more viable, and better able to maintain $[Na^+]_i$. However, because $[Na^+]_i$ (10–15 mM) is much lower than $[Na^+]_e$ (145 mM), the unchanged TQF ^{23}Na SI did not interrupt the increase in SQ ^{23}Na SI following chemotherapy.

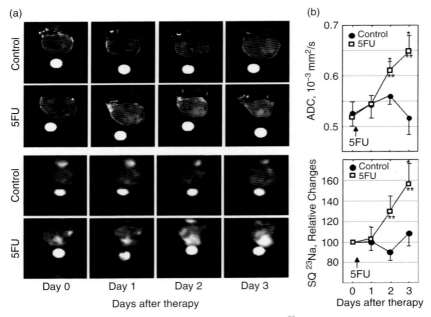

Figure 12.9 Correlation of changes in water ADC (top) and SQ ^{23}Na SI (bottom) after 5FU therapy in sc-implanted RIF-1 tumors. (a) Representative examples of water ADC map and ^{23}Na MRI for a control and a 5FU-treated tumor before (Day 0) and 1, 2, and 3 days after 5FU injection. (b) The mean water ADC and SQ ^{23}Na SI from the whole control and treated tumors. Significance: $p \leq 0.05$ (* - vs. before treatment), $p \leq 0.01$ (** - Control vs. 5FU-treated). Data are presented as mean ± SEM. [Reproduced with permission from Babsky et al. 2007[31].]

Unlike water, Na^+ signals from different tissue compartments can be effectively separated by a shift reagent (SR), such as $TmDOTP^{5-}$. It allows simultaneous monitoring of Na^+ ADCs in the intracellular space (ICS) and extracellular space (ECS). Goodman et al.[56] suggested that changes in the local environment affect water and Na^+ ADCs in a similar manner. They showed that Na^+ diffusion measurements provide a reasonable representation of water diffusion during both normal and ischemic conditions in the rat brain. The ADCs of Na^+_i and Na^+_e were found to be similar in normal resting rat skeletal muscle[21]. This is in contrast to the general belief that the ADCs of water and other small molecules are slower in the ICS compared to the ECS. The Na^+ ADC data is in agreement with the data published by Duong et al.[22], which show that the ADCs of 2FDG-6-P are similar in the ECS and ICS in the rat brain. Measurement of Na^+_i and Na^+_e ADCs in rat skeletal muscle show that the decrease in Na^+_t ADC during ischemia was largely due to a decrease in the ADC of Na^+_e[21]. The ADC of Na^+_t decreased by 25–30% after 3 h of ischemia while water ADC did not change significantly. The different postmortem changes in Na^+_t and water ADCs can be explained by the difference in their compartmental distribution. In living muscle, the concentration of Na^+ in the ECS, which composes 23% of the tissue[57], is roughly 150 mM, while Na^+ concentration in the ICS is 4.7 mM[58]. Thus, more than 80% of the tissue ^{23}Na signal comes from the ECS. This is in contrast to the water compartmental distribution, which is ~80% intracellular. Therefore, the tissue sodium signal mostly arises from the ECS and the water signal mostly arises from the ICS[56]. The SR-aided ^{23}Na ADC measurements show that Na^+_e ADC is decreased by 34% after 4 h of ischemia while Na^+_i ADC did not change significantly[21]. Thus, in the absence of a SR, the ADC of Na^+_t, which is mostly extracellular, is expected to decrease, while the ADC of water, which is mostly intracellular, is not expected to change during ischemia. In addition, the long exchange time of Na^+ allows one to measure compartmental ADCs of sodium quite accurately, unlike water, where diffusion within the ECS and ICS compartments is obscured by a very fast exchange rate.

Water ADC measurement in liver: applications and challenges

The monitoring of water ADC in the animal liver is challenging due to respiratory and cardiac motion. To avoid this problem, in animal experiments respiratory gating has been used to collect ^1H MR image only during exhalation. However, Figure 12.10 shows that even with respiratory gating DW images can be blurred, with high b-values (945 or 1679 s/mm^2) affecting the ADC calculation in both liver and tumors. In contrast, ^1H images of sc-HCC are not affected by physiological motion, and the ^1H MR images with all b-values and the water ADC

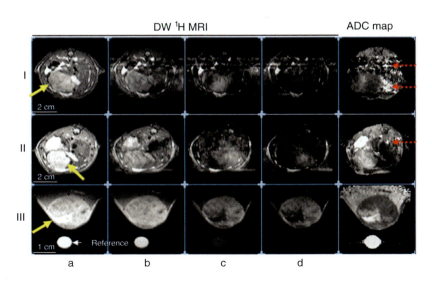

DW ^1H MRI   ADC map

Figure 12.10 Diffusion-weighted ^1H MRI and ADC maps of orthotopic (IH-) (I and II) and sc-implanted hepatocellular carcinoma (HCC) (III) at different b-values (in s/mm^2): a – 0, b – 256, c – 945, d – 1679. HCCs are marked by yellow arrows. IH tumor images could be moderately (I) or intensively (II) blurred by respiratory or cardiac motions especially at high b-values, which introduce some errors in water ADC calculation. The motion effect is marked by the dotted red arrows on the ADC map. Sc-implanted tumor image did not have a motion effect.

a   b   c   d

map were of high quality for analysis and interpretation.

Several approaches have been proposed to reduce the effects of motion on ADC measurements. Some of these include (1) avoiding undoubtedly bright spots on ADC maps when regions of interest (ROIs) are drawn, (2) using of a threshold to eliminate ADC values that are clearly higher than free water diffusion ($>3 \times 10^{-3}$ mm^2/s), and (3) comparing water ADC of intrahepatic (IH) HCC with the surrounding liver tissue, which has similar motion artifacts. A completely different approach is to monitor SQ ^{23}Na SI which, like ADC, mostly reflects rECS changes but is not sensitive to physiologic motion. These approaches have helped to achieve relatively steady ADC values for each experimental data point. It was found that ADC in IH HCC was significantly higher by 40–50% on all days of the experiment, compared to surrounding liver tissue[59]. These data correlate with other publications showing higher ADC in IH HCC compared to healthy liver tissue (see review[60]). The most reasonable explanation for this effect invokes less differentiation of tumor cells and a net increase in the tumor rECS. Histological examination of IH HCC and liver after the last MRI experiment showed that the rECS in the viable tumor cells regions is larger than in the healthy liver, mostly due to reduction in cellular cytoplasm. Furthermore, IH HCC contains areas of inflammation and necrosis with increased rECS. ADC in the ECS is generally faster compared to the ICS. Moffat et al.[20] also associated an increase in water ADC after treatment with cell lysis, apoptosis, necrosis involving cell shrinkage, and blebbing followed by phagocytosis.

The ratio of viable, necrotic, and cystic regions in growing tumor can sufficiently affect a mean of tumor ADC. Yuan et al. showed that the areas of viable and necrotic VX2 cells are associated with low ADC while high signals on the ADC map are produced when the necrosis is associated with the cystic regions[48]. In our experiments, tumor ADC remained unchanged on days 14 and 21, and even slightly decreased on day 28 using both the low (0 and 256 s/mm^2) and high (945 and 1679 s/mm^2) b-values that Koh and Collins described as flow-insensitive and flow-sensitive b-values, respectively[19]. One could explain this discrepancy by the possible contribution of the blood perfusion to the water ADC

measurement. The contribution of perfusion ADC measurement in the well-vasculated HCC needs to be considered. The possibility of an increase in density of ECS due to necrotic cell digestion and increase in macromolecular contamination in growing HCCs, leading to a decrease in water ADC, cannot be excluded. Furthermore, the decrease in bioenergetic status in growing tumor can also decrease energy-dependent ADC in intracellular space.

In our study, the ADC value in sc-implanted HCC was lower compared to IH HCC 56%, 37%, and 30% on days 14, 21, and 28, respectively. In addition, ADC in sc-implanted HCC was decreased 40–50% compared to nearby muscle tissue. Furthermore, unlike IH HCC the ADC in sc-implanted HCC increased on day 21 and 28 compared to the day 14 value. Therefore, in growing sc-implanted HCC the increase in rECS (mostly in inflamed and necrotic regions) is the key reason for the increased ADC.

Because of the contribution of motion effects to ADC measurement, the possibility of artificially higher ADC in HCC (especially in small tumors) can thus create some artifacts in the absolute values of ADC. On the other hand, neoplastic transformation in the sc-implanted tumors could differ from the same cells located in the deep tissue. Thus, data obtained with sc-implanted tumor must be translated to orthotopic tumors with caution.

Summary: Monitoring of the treatment response in animal tumors

DWI can be used widely for tumor detection and characterization, and for monitoring of response to treatment in animal tumor models. Effective tumor therapy is usually associated with an increase in ADC values, although exceptions may occur. ADC appears to have the ability to predict treatment response to chemotherapy. However, there are several challenges to wider use of DWI in cancer patients. These include a lack of accepted standards for data acquisition and analysis, variability of ADC changes depending on tumor cell type and location, motion effects on body tumor ADC measurement, incomplete theoretical understanding of DWI in ECS and ICS, and poor knowledge of multiexponential decay components which affect the calculated ADC values. Thus, DWI protocols and analyses need to be adapted to individual tumor types, anatomic locations, and therapies. We also need a better understanding of how tumor

ADC measurements can be combined with the results of other diagnostic modalities, such as ^{23}Na MRI, ^{31}P MR spectroscopy, PET, destructive chemical analysis, and histology, to improve our assessment of prognosis and monitoring of therapeutic efficiency.

Monitoring treatment response in human patients

Several studies have been published in recent years detailing changes in ADC after treatment of extracranial cancers in humans, including the liver, breast, prostate, uterus, rectum, and other tissues (Table 12.2).

Liver

The monitoring of therapy for liver tumors, including HCC and liver metastases, is the most frequently used clinical DWI application outside the brain. Kamel et al. studied 38 patients with HCC, with a mean tumor diameter of 8.0 cm, and assessed treatment response after transarterial chemoembolization (TACE) with DWI[61]. The mean reduction in tumor diameter was 8 mm after treatment, which did not fulfill response evaluation criteria in solid tumors (RECIST) for complete or partial response. Tumor ADC increased from 1.5×10^{-3} to 1.8×10^{-3} mm^2/s 4 to 6 weeks after treatment ($p = 0.026$), while the ADC values for the liver, spleen, and muscle remained unchanged. Similar results were noted in 20 HCC patients by Chen et al.[62], but in only 2 to 3 days post-TACE; the mean ADC increased from 1.56×10^{-3} to 2.09×10^{-3} mm^2/s ($p < 0.01$).

Deng et al.[63] and Kamel et al.[64] also found DWI was useful in assessing the early (30–40 days) treatment response of HCC to a single treatment with ^{90}Y-labeled microspheres. Five of six patients were determined as responders to the therapy, showing a >50% decrease in tumor size or >50% increased necrosis as determined with contrast agent-enhanced CT or MRI[63]. In this group, tumor ADC value increased significantly ~40 days after ^{90}Y Thera-Sphere administration from 1.35×10^{-3} to 2.23×10^{-3} mm^2/s ($p < 0.004$). For the non-responder, tumor ADC increased by only 0.33×10^{-3} mm^2/s, whereas tumor ADC increased by 0.84×10^{-3} mm^2/s in the five responders[63]. Kamel et al. showed an increase in HCC ADC one month after treatment with ^{90}Y microspheres even without changes in tumor size. Thirteen targeted tumors demonstrated a mean increase in ADC value

of 18%, from 1.65×10^{-3} to 1.95×10^{-3} mm^2/s ($p < 0.001$) and a decrease in arterial and venous enhancement of 22% and 25%, respectively ($p \leq 0.013$), yet the mean tumor size was unchanged ($p = 0.492$). The ADC value of the background liver and spleen also was unchanged.

The value of DW MRI has also been investigated in patients with liver metastases from different primary cancers, such as breast cancer[65], ocular melanoma[66], and leiomyosarcoma[67] for the evaluation of early (4–6 weeks) tumor response after TACE, and compared with traditional imaging response assessment based on tumor size. The treatment of breast cancer metastases in liver caused an 18% decrease in tumor size ($p = 0.002$) and a decrease in tumor enhancement in the arterial (32%) and portal venous (39%) phases. In this study, mean ADC in the tumor increased 27%, from 1.81×10^{-3} to 2.29×10^{-3} mm^2/s ($p = 0.0001$). Similar results were obtained after the treatment of liver metastases from ocular melanoma. Tumor size decreased 16% ($p = 0.003$), arterial and venous phase enhancement decreased 41% and 56%, respectively, and the mean water ADC increased 48% from 1.57×10^{-3} to 2.32×10^{-3} mm^2/s ($p = 0.00003$). TACE treatment of liver metastases from leiomyosarcoma did not cause any significant changes in tumor size, but mean water ADC increased 20% from 1.77×10^{-3} to 2.13×10^{-3} mm^2/s ($p = 0.0015$) and arterial (35%) and venous (49%) phase enhancement decreased as well. Thus, although changes in tumor size were small or absent, in liver metastases water ADC increased significantly 4–6 weeks after chemoembolization.

Breast

In patients with breast cancer receiving neoadjuvant chemotherapy (NACT) for several cycles, treatment response is traditionally assessed by physical examination and volumetric-based measurements, which are subjective and/or require macroscopic changes in tumor morphology. DWI has been explored as a reliable and quantitative measure for the early assessment of response in breast cancer.

Pickles et al.[68] examined ten patients before and after the first and second NACT cycle time-points. Treatment cycles consisted of epirubicin (90 mg/m^2) and Cp (600 mg/m^2) administered at 3-weekly intervals. A significant increase in the mean ADC was noted at the first ($1.25 \pm 0.21 \times 10^{-3}$ mm^2/s, $p = 0.005$,

187

Table 12.2 Assessing treatment response of body tumors using ADC measurements in human studies

Tumor	Treatment	b-values	Post-treatment ADC changes	Reference
HCC	TACE	500	Increase in ADC by 20% in the fraction of interstitial water at day 45	Kamel et al. 2006 [61]
HCC	TACE	500	ADC has a high correlation with the degree of necrosis at day 32	Kamel et al. 2003 [64]
HCC	TACE	0, 500	Increase in ADC at day 1–2	Chen et al. 2006 [62]
HCC	^{90}Y microspheres	0, 500	Increase in ADC at day 28–70	Deng et al. 2006 [63]
Liver metastases from ocular melanoma	TACE	500	Increase in ADC at week 4–6	Buijs et al. 2008 [66]
Liver metastatic leiomyosarcoma	TACE	500	Increase in ADC at week 4–6	Vossen et al. 2008 [67]
Liver metastatic breast cancer	TACE	500	Increase in ADC at week 4–6	Buijs et al. 2007 [65]
Liver metastatic breast cancer	Chemotherapy	0–450	ADC can predict response by 4 or 11 days after therapy	Theilmann et al. 2004 [87]
Ankylosing spondylitis	Chemotherapy	0, 400	Decrease in ADC 12 months after infliximab treatment	Gašperšič et al. 2008 [83]
Malignant primary bone tumors	Chemotherapy	0, 1000	Increase in ADC of Group B ($\geq$90% necrosis) greater than in group A (<90% necrosis)	Hayashida et al. 2006 [82]
Metastatic disease of spine	Radiation therapy	165, 650	Increase in ADC at >1 month after therapy	Byun et al. 2002 [81]
Breast cancer	Chemotherapy	0–1000	Gradual increase in ADC at 1st, 2nd, and 3rd cycle. ADC more useful for predicting early tumor response than morphological variables	Sharma et al. 2008 [69]
Breast cancer	Chemotherapy	0, 700	Increase in ADC at 1st and 2nd cycle	Pickles et al. 2006 [68]
Breast cancer	Chemotherapy	0–680	ADC can not detect early response	Manton et al. 2006 [88]
Prostate cancer	Focused ultrasonic ablation	0, 1000	DWI with T2-W MRI more specific than DCE-MRI for prediction of local tumor progression after ablation	Kim et al. 2008 [72]
Prostate cancer	Radiotherapy	0, 700	Increase in ADC at months 3–9	Takayama et al. 2008 [71]
Rectal carcinoma	Chemoradiation	30, 300, 1100	Decrease of ADC at the 2nd, 3rd, and 4th weeks due to cytotoxic edema and fibrosis	Hein et al. 2003 [16]
Rectal carcinoma	Chemoradiation	30, 300, 1100	Higher parameter levels in the non-responding group, ADC is of predictive value for therapy outcome	Devries et al. 2003 [12]
Soft tissue sarcoma	Chemotherapy	0, 500, 1000	High degree of correlation between changes in tumor volumes and ADC	Dudeck et al. 2008 [84]
Uterine fibroid	Embolization	0, 500	Decrease of ADC at day 181 due to infarction and dehydration	Liapi et al. 2005 [73]
Uterine fibroid	Ablation	0, 500, 1000	ADC was decreased just after treatment and increased at 6-month follow-up	Jacobs et al. 2005 [77]

paired t-test) and second ($1.37 \pm 0.24 \times 10^{-3}$ mm^2/s, $p = 0.004$) cycle time-points compared to the pre-treatment value ($1.08 \pm 0.19 \times 10^{-3}$ mm^2/s). However, only a borderline significant reduction ($p = 0.057$) in the mean longest diameter was noted, and not until the second cycle time-point. Their results indicate that ADC may provide a suitable biomarker capable of providing an indication of response to treatment before tumor size measurements.

Sharma et al.[69] studied 56 patients with locally advanced breast cancer to determine the value of ADC, volume, and diameter in assessing the response of NACT at four time periods (before treatment and after each of three cycles of NACT). The mean ADC before treatment of malignant breast tissue (0.95×10^{-3} mm^2/s) was significantly lower than that of controls (1.88×10^{-3} mm^2/s), contralateral tissue (1.87×10^{-3} mm^2/s) and benign lesions (1.50×10^{-3} mm^2/s), and gradually increased during the course of NACT (1.09×10^{-3}, 1.21×10^{-3}, and 1.30×10^{-3} mm^2/s at three post-treatment time-points, respectively). The change in ADC after the first cycle was statistically significant compared with volume and diameter, indicating its potential in assessing early response. A sensitivity of 84% (specificity of 60% with an accuracy of 76%) was achieved when all three variables were taken together to predict the response. The results show that ADC is more useful for predicting early tumor response to NACT than morphological variables, suggesting its potential in effective treatment management. Recently, Yankeelov et al.[70] also identified that ADC and K_{rans} from dynamic contrast enhancement (DCE) MRI data are more sensitive to longitudinal changes in breast tumor status than morphologic measurements of tumor size.

However, a study by Manton et al.[88] showed that ADC may not always be useful for evaluation of early response to treatment. Women undergoing NACT for locally advanced breast cancer underwent DWI, DCE MR and proton spectroscopy (MRS) to predict ultimate tumor response or to detect early response. Their results showed that ADC and DCE MR did not detect early response, but early changes in water to fat ratios and water T2 demonstrated substantial prognostic efficacy.

Prostate

Takayama et al. compared the ADC and diffusion tensor imaging (DTI), including fractional anisotropy (FA), before and after carbon-ion radiotherapy (CIRT) in nine patients. They reported that pre-treatment ADC values were significantly lower in prostate tumor compared to non-cancerous inner gland and peripheral zone ($p < 0.05$). The ADC values of tumor significantly increased after CIRT ($p < 0.01$), whereas that of non-cancerous inner gland and peripheral zone remained mostly unchanged. Thus, after CIRT, the pre-treatment differences between ADC in cancerous and non-cancerous tissue disappeared. Values of FA showed no significant differences in any comparisons and DTI showed changes in the direction of the main axis of the tensor in prostate cancer after CIRT. Thus, both ADC and DTI may be useful for monitoring prostatic structural changes following radiotherapy[71].

Kim et al.[72] evaluated the diagnostic performance of DCE MRI, T2-weighted imaging, and DWI for predicting local tumor progression after high-intensity focused ultrasonic ablation of localized prostate cancer in 27 patients. Qualitative analysis was performed; two readers used a five-point scale to independently assess DCE MR images, T2-weighted, and DW images. They found that for prediction of local tumor progression of prostate cancer after ablation, DCE MRI was more sensitive than T2-weighted MRI and DWI, but T2-weighted MRI and DWI were more specific than DCE MRI.

In conclusion, most studies showed that, as in most animal studies, the effectiveness of clinical therapy for liver, breast, and prostate cancers correlated with an increase in ADC. Likewise, there are some exceptions showing a decrease in ADC after treatment of human cancers. These exceptions may be related to fibrotic changes in the tumor, as discussed below.

Uterine fibroids

In 11 patients with 32 uterine fibroids, Liapi et al.[73] found that, after treatment with uterine fibroid embolization (UFE), fibroids had significantly lower ADC values at 6-month follow-up compared to untreated lesions. In assessing treatment response of uterine fibroids, the usual method is measurement of the fibroid size or T1-WI enhancing area. However, change in fibroid size or volume after treatment may not accurately predict lesion response, as embolization may be associated with hyalinizing necrosis without tissue collapse or decrease in tumor size[74].

Enhancing areas in a lesion are presumed to represent a viable component; however, residual enhancement may also result from post-embolization inflammation[75–76]. Post-UFE treatment was reported in this study to produce low ADC values, confirming infarction and dehydration of uterine fibroids after embolization[73]. Before treatment, the accumulated clusters of uniform smooth muscle cells with intervening collagen within fibroids result in a restricted pattern of water diffusion. After therapy, the low SI on T2-weighted images and the overall decrease of mean ADC values in these lesions are evidence that there is increased dehydration at a cellular level.

Jacobs et al.[77] prospectively demonstrated that DWI and ADC mapping are feasible for identification of ablated tissue after focused ultrasound treatment of uterine fibroids. The mean pre-treatment ADC value in fibroids was 1.50×10^{-3} mm^2/s (Figure 12.11). After ablation, the ADC significantly decreased within the ablated tissue (1.08×10^{-3} mm^2/s) and was increased at 6-month follow-up (1.91×10^{-3} mm^2/s) compared with baseline or non-treated fibroids. DWI SI also increased following treatment. The induction of thermal necrosis with the MR image-guided focused

ultrasound surgical treatment may present a different evolution of the ADC than is currently seen in ischemic tissue. For example, thermal coagulation can induce a range of tissue changes, including protein denaturation, cell membrane rupture or dysfunction, increased vasoconstriction, disruption of fiber networks, and cauterization of blood vessels[78–79]. These changes within the tissue can lead to a heterogeneous pattern of both restricted and non-restricted movement of water and, hence, a range of ADC values within uterine fibroids. Even though the exact mechanism for ADC changes following focused ultrasound surgery is still unknown, these changes may provide a measure by which to gauge the effectiveness of treatment.

Rectal carcinoma

Recent studies have further explored the clinical utility of DWI for monitoring response of rectal carcinoma to pre-operative chemoradiation by measuring ADC. Comparison of mean ADC and cumulative radiation dose showed a significant decrease of mean ADC after 2 weeks (0.64×10^{-3} mm^2/s), 3 weeks (0.58×10^{-3} mm^2/s), and 4 weeks (0.55×10^{-3} mm^2/s)

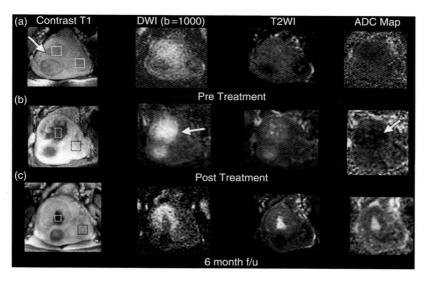

Figure 12.11 Representative coronal post-contrast T1-weighted MR images (*Contrast T₁*), DW images (*DWI*), T2-weighted MR images (*T2WI*), and ADC maps acquired in a 48-year-old woman. Arrows show location of fibroid, and squares demonstrate the region of interest selected for quantification of ADC values. Row (a), enhancing fibroids were seen on baseline T1-weighted MR image (185/1.5) with no discernible signal changes on DW image (5000/90, b = 1000 s/mm²) or T2-weighted MR image (5000/90, b = 0 s/mm²). ADC map shows no discernible signal changes. Row (b), after treatment, post-contrast T1-weighted MR image demonstrates area of hypointensity within the treated region, with increased signal intensity in the same regions on the DW image and corresponding decreased signal intensity on ADC map. Row (c), at 6-month follow-up, a persistent area of hypointensity is noted in the area of treated fibroid as shown on the T1-weighted post-contrast image. The DW image signal intensity is heterogeneous with the treated region, and the central region shows increased signal intensity on the ADC map that is co-localized with the T1-weighted MR image. [Reproduced with permission from Jacobs et al. 2005[77].]

of treatment compared to the pre-treatment value $(0.76 \times 10^{-3}$ mm^2/s)[16]. Cytotoxic edema and fibrosis were postulated as the reasons for the ADC decrease. The pathway of necrotic cell death shows cell swelling due to failure of the Na$^+$/K$^+$-ATPase pump. Cytotoxic edema arises from a shift of water from the ECS to the ICS[80]. Chemoradiation results in increased interstitial fibrosis as documented by post-surgical, histological examination. The limiting effect of fibers reduces free diffusion in the ECS. It can be hypothesized that at the end of therapy, increasing development of fibrous connective tissue will decrease ADCs.

Musculoskeletal diseases

Only a few reports are available describing the effect of tumor treatment and tissue diffusivity in human diseases involving bone marrow. Buyn et al.[81] reported 23 cases where the ADC of radiation-treated vertebral bone marrow metastatic lesions increased from 0.78×10^{-3} mm^2/s to 1.22×10^{-3} mm^2/s. Similar results were found by Hayashida et al.[82], who evaluated DWI of chemotherapy-treated malignant primary bone tumors. The change of the ADC value of tumors with at least 90% necrosis was statistically greater than those with less than 90% necrosis.

In the first report of the use of DWI to evaluate the activity of skeletal inflammation in rheumatic diseases[83], 30 patients with active ankylosing spondylitis or bilateral sacroilitis were selected, treated with three different types of drugs, and followed up for 1 year. After 12 months the mean ADC in the infliximab treatment group significantly diminished from 1.31×10^{-3} to 0.88×10^{-3} mm^2/s.

In 23 patients with soft-tissue sarcoma, an increase in the ADC value was always associated with a reduction of tumor size[84]. Likewise, a decrease in ADC was always associated with a tumor volume increase. Hence, there was high correlation between tumor volume and ADC value ($r = -0.925$, $p < 0.0001$), regardless of the effectiveness of anticancer therapy as expressed by changes of tumor volume.

Predicting treatment response

Predicting treatment response on the basis of the pre-treatment ADC value could have considerable clinical benefit as it might indicate the eventual outcome of therapy. As described above, Lemaire et al. found that mammary tumors with low initial ADC values

($<0.95 \times 10^{-3}$ mm^2/s) responded to a single 5FU bolus therapy by a 30% increase in ADC at day 7 after treatment, whereas tumors with high initial ADC ($>1.2 \times 10^{-3}$ mm^2/s) showed a 30% decrease; tumors with intermediate values showed no significant change in ADC[29]. The high and low initial ADC groups both showed a significant decrease in tumor volume after the treatment. High and low ADC values in tumors were correlated with high and low necrosis, respectively. The authors explained these results by higher absolute concentration of 5FU in tumors with low necrosis. Kamm et al.[85] previously have shown that the absolute concentration of 5FU and metabolites was lower in the necrotic regions of tumors compared to viable regions, an effect attributed to better vascularization of the viable regions. However, it is still unclear if the initial ADC values can predict the clinically relevant tumor chemosensitivity in all types of tumors. In contrast to Lemaire's data, Babsky et al. have found that the initial levels of water ADC as well as ^{23}Na SI were higher in BCNU-responsive sc-implanted 9L gliomas compared to the BCNU non-responsive group[26]. These data suggested that a higher initial ADC level ($1.1-1.7 \times 10^{-3}$ mm^2/s) was a promising sign for effective BCNU treatment, and in contrast, tumors with a lower initial ADC value ($0.6-0.9 \times 10^{-3}$ mm^2/s) were most likely to be resistant to BCNU treatment. The higher pre-treatment ADC levels in BCNU-responsive tumors may be related to an overall weakened condition of the cells making them vulnerable to toxic therapy. Tumors with high pre-treatment ADC values are likely to be more necrotic than those with low values. Necrotic tumors frequently are hypoxic, acidotic, and poorly perfused, leading to diminished sensitivity to chemotherapy and to radiation therapy. In contradiction to presented above data, Seierstad et al.[32] did not find correlations between pre-treatment ADC values and changes in colon adenocarcinoma HT29 xenograft volumes after chemoradiation, whereas early changes in mean ADC quantitatively correlated with treatment outcome. They conclude that "it is a prerequisite for comparing different chemotherapy regimens in animal models that initial xenografts be similar so that observed effects are therapy-induced effects and not effects originating from the initial composition of necrosis, fibrosis, and viable cells in tumors."

The contradictive results in predicting treatment response on the basis of the pre-treatment ADC value were also obtained with human patients. Studies in human rectal carcinoma[12–13] and colorectal hepatic metastases[86] have shown that cellular tumors with low baseline pre-treatment ADC values respond better to chemotherapy or radiation treatment than tumors that exhibit high pre-treatment ADC values. In a preliminary study in 14 patients with locally advanced rectal cancer, a strong negative correlation was found between mean pre-treatment tumor ADC and the percentage size change of tumors after chemotherapy ($r = -0.67$, $p = 0.01$) and chemoradiation ($r = -0.83$, $p = 0.001$)[13].

DeVries et al. studied 34 patients with primary rectal carcinoma undergoing pre-operative chemoradiation[12]. They compared the pre-therapeutic ADCs of those patients that responded well to therapy (0.65 ± 0.20 × 10^{-3} mm^2/s) and the non-responders (0.66 ± 0.17 × 10^{-3} mm^2/s), and did not find a significant difference between them ($p < 0.83$). However, when they investigated the distribution of any single voxel ADC value in the tumor region in a histogram-like fashion using a three-way ANOVA, they found significant effects for therapy responder/non-responder ($p < 0.001$) and ADC ($p < 0.001$). The ADC histograms showed a higher relative fraction of high ADCs in the therapy non-responder group compared with the therapy responder group. Although single ADC intervals were not significantly different, the global distributions showed a statistically significant difference ($p < 0.001$). In Koh's study[86] of 20 patients with hepatic lesions metastatic from colorectal carcinoma, 25 responding and 15 non-responding metastatic lesions were evaluated with DWI before and after chemotherapy. Non-responding lesions had a significantly higher pre-treatment mean ADC than did responding lesions ($p < 0.002$). There was a linear regression relation ($r^2 = 0.34$, $p = 0.02$) between percentage size reduction of metastatic lesions and pre-treatment mean ADC.

Theilmann et al. proposed to use early changes in water ADC for predicting treatment response[87]. Their study of metastatic breast carcinoma has shown that an early increase in the ADC after commencing treatment was predictive of better treatment outcome. In this study, 13 patients with metastatic breast cancer and 60 measurable liver lesions were monitored by DWI after initiation of new courses of chemotherapy. The data indicated that ADC can predict response by 4 to 11 days after the start of therapy. The highest concordance was observed in tumor lesions that were less than 8 cm^3 in volume.

These results suggest that ADC calculation can be useful to predict the response of liver metastases to effective chemotherapy.

Summary: Monitoring treatment response in patients

Generally, DWI may have practical usefulness for cancer patients in detection and diagnosis of cancerogenic transformation, and in evaluation of therapy efficacy. Whether ADC values can be used as a tool for distinguishing tumor from normal tissue depends on tumor type, tissue differentiation, apoptosis, and necrosis. Thus, tumors can have higher or lower ADC values compared to normal tissue. The absolute values of ADC for the different tumor types and organs need to be calculated considering data acquisition parameters. DWI may be an effective early biomarker for treatment efficacy for chemotherapy with different types of drugs that induce tumor cell apoptosis and necrosis. DWI protocols and analysis need be adapted to individual tumor types, anatomy structure, and therapies. Effective therapy is usually associated with an increase in ADC values, although exceptions may occur as well, as transient early decreases in ADC values can be observed after treatment. The significance of pre-treatment ADC values in predicting and evaluating treatment response needs to be studied further.

Limitations of DWI

Several limitations to the DWI technique as a tool for body tumor studies have to be taken to consideration. The ADC values are highly dependent on the parameters, such as b-values, that can affect the absolute values of ADC. In the tumors with a relatively well developed vascular system, such as liver tumor, the use of a variety of b-values can mix up diffusion and perfusion components of ADC. It leads to variability of post-treatment ADC data and makes reproducibility of the method quite challenging. Thus, standardization of acquisition parameters and processing methods is necessary. In abdominal organs, the monitoring of ADC is affected by physiological motion and that problem cannot be fully avoided by using respiratory gating. The traditional ADC measurement does not separate extra- and intracellular ADC values, and the latter may have a significant impact to the total tissue ADC. Another limitation is the overlapping of processes that can simultaneously decrease (e.g., fibrosis, increase in tortuosity) and increase (e.g., increase in ECS, necrosis, vessel leakage) ADC.

Future directions

ADC could be used as a biomarker for prediction and assessment of treatment efficacy in body tumors. The use of ^{23}Na and other modalities such as, PET, histology, and destructive chemical analysis will further improve our understanding of the mechanism of post-treatment changes in ADC. Another interesting application is to separate the perfusion and diffusion component of water ADC, and analyze separately "perfusion" (0–500 mm^2/s) and "diffusion" (> 500 mm^2/s) b-values. For clinical application, the image quality may require improvement, perhaps by using parallel imaging, respiratory gating, and a navigator echo acquisition.

Summary

In conclusion, non-invasive DWI shows utility for predicting and monitoring response to treatment in body tumors. DWI may be an effective early biomarker for treatment efficacy for chemotherapy with drugs that induce tumor cell apoptosis and necrosis. However, DWI protocols and analysis need to be adapted to individual tumor types, location, volume, and anatomical structure, as well as types of therapy.

Acknowledgments

The authors thank Dr. S. Gregory Jennings for valuable comments and assistance in the preparation of the manuscript.

References

1. Ross B, Chenvert T, Kim B, Ben-Yoseph O. Magnetic resonance imaging and spectroscopy: application to experimental neurooncology. *Q Magn Reson Biol Med* 1994;**1**:89–106.

2. Thoeny HC, De Keyzer F. Extracranial applications of diffusion-weighted magnetic resonance imaging. *Eur Radiol* 2007;**17**(6):1385–93.

3. Padhani A, Liu G, Koh DM, *et al.* Diffusion weighted magnetic resonance imaging as a cancer biomarker: consensus and recommendations. *Neoplasia* 2009;**11**(2):102–25.

4. Geschwind JF, Artemov D, Abraham S, *et al.* Chemoembolization of liver tumor in a rabbit model: assessment of tumor cell death with diffusion-weighted MR imaging and histologic analysis. *J Vasc Intervent Radiol* 2000;**11**(10):1245–55.

5. Stegman LD, Rehemtulla A, Hamstra DA, *et al.* Diffusion MRI detects early events in the response of a glioma model to the yeast cytosine deaminase gene therapy strategy. *Gene Ther* 2000;**7**(12):1005–10.

6. Chenevert TL, McKeever PE, Ross BD. Monitoring early response of experimental brain tumors to therapy using diffusion magnetic resonance imaging. *Clin Cancer Res* 1997;**3**(9):1457–66.

7. Galons JP, Altbach MI, Paine-Murrieta GD, Taylor CW, Gillies RJ. Early increases in breast tumor xenograft water mobility in response to paclitaxel therapy detected by non-invasive diffusion magnetic resonance imaging. *Neoplasia* 1999;**1**(2):113–17.

8. Poptani H, Puumalainen AM, Grohn OH, *et al.* Monitoring thymidine kinase and ganciclovir-induced changes in rat malignant glioma in vivo by nuclear magnetic resonance imaging. *Cancer Gene Ther* 1998;**5**(2):101–9.

9. Ross BD, Chenevert TL, Garwood M, *et al.* Evaluation of (E)-2'-deoxy-2'-(fluoromethylene)cytidine on the 9L rat brain tumor model using MRI. *NMR Biomed* 2003;**16**(2):67–76.

10. Zhao M, Pipe JG, Bonnett J, Evelhoch JL. Early detection of treatment response by diffusion-weighted ^{1}H-NMR spectroscopy in a murine tumour in vivo. *Br J Cancer* 1996;**73**(1):61–4.

11. Chenevert TL, Stegman LD, Taylor JM, *et al.* Diffusion magnetic resonance imaging: an early surrogate marker of therapeutic efficacy in brain tumors. *J Natl Cancer Inst* 2000;**92**:2029–36.

12. DeVries AF, Kremser C, Hein PA, *et al.* Tumor microcirculation and diffusion predict therapy outcome for primary rectal carcinoma. *Int J Radiat Oncol Biol Phys* 2003;**56**(4):958–65.

13. Dzik-Jurasz A, Domenig C, George M, *et al.* Diffusion MRI for prediction of response of rectal cancer to chemoradiation. *Lancet* 2002;**360**(9329):307–8.

14. Thoeny HC, De Keyzer F, Vandecaveye V, *et al.* Effect of vascular targeting agent in rat tumor model: dynamic contrast-enhanced versus diffusion-weighted MR imaging. *Radiology* 2005;**237**(2):492–9.

15. Chinnaiyan AM, Prasad U, Shankar S, *et al.* Combined effect of tumor necrosis factor-related apoptosis-inducing ligand and ionizing radiation in breast cancer therapy. *Proc Natl Acad Sci USA* 2000;**97**(4):1754–9.

16. Hein PA, Kremser C, Judmaier W, *et al.* Diffusion-weighted magnetic resonance imaging for monitoring diffusion changes in rectal carcinoma during combined, preoperative chemoradiation: preliminary

results of a prospective study. *Eur J Radiol* 2003; **45** (3):214–22.

17. Kremser C, Judmaier W, Hein P, *et al.* Preliminary results on the influence of chemoradiation on apparent diffusion coefficients of primary rectal carcinoma measured by magnetic resonance imaging. *Strahlenther Onkol* 2003;**179** (9):641–9.

18. Ross BD, Moffat BA, Lawrence TS, *et al.* Evaluation of cancer therapy using diffusion magnetic resonance imaging. *Mol Cancer Ther* 2003;**2** (6):581–7.

19. Koh DM, Collins DJ. Diffusion-weighted MRI in the body: applications and challenges in oncology. *Am J Roentgenol* 2007;**188** (6):1622–35.

20. Moffat BA, Chenevert TL, Lawrence TS, *et al.* Functional diffusion map: a noninvasive MRI biomarker for early stratification of clinical brain tumor response. *Proc Natl Acad Sci USA* 2005;**102** (15):5524–9.

21. Babsky AM, Topper S, Zhang H, *et al.* Evaluation of extra- and intracellular apparent diffusion coefficient of sodium in rat skeletal muscle: effects of prolonged ischemia. *Magn Reson Med* 2008;**59** (3):485–91.

22. Duong TQ, Ackerman JJ, Ying HS, Neil JJ. Evaluation of extra- and intracellular apparent diffusion in normal and globally ischemic rat brain via 19F NMR. *Magn Reson Med* 1998;**40** (1):1–13.

23. Schepkin V, Chenevert T, Kuszpit K, *et al.* Sodium and proton diffusion MRI as biomarkers for early therapeutic response in subcutaneous tumors. *Magn Reson Imag* 2006;**24**:273–8.

24. Schepkin VD, Lee KC, Kuszpit K, *et al.* Proton and sodium MRI assessment of emerging tumor chemotherapeutic resistance. *NMR Biomed* 2006;**19** (8):1035–42.

25. Babsky A, Hekmatyar S, Zhang H, Solomon J, Bansal N. Application of ^{23}Na MRI to monitor chemotherapeutic response in RIF-1 tumors. *Neoplasia* 2005;**7**:658–66.

26. Babsky A, Hekmatyar S, Zhang H, Solomon J, Bansal N. Predicting and monitoring response to chemotherapy by 1,3-bis(2-chloroethyl)-1-nitrosourea in subcutaneously implanted 9L glioma using the apparent diffusion coefficient of water and ^{23}Na MRI. *J Magn Reson Imag* 2006;**24** (1):132–9.

27. Babsky A, Zhang H, Hekmatyar S, Hutchins G, Bansal N. Monitoring chemotherapeutic response in RIF-1 tumors by single-quantum and triple-quantum-filtered ^{23}Na MRI, ^{1}H diffusion-weighted MRI and PET imaging. *Magn Reson Imag* 2007;**25**:739–47.

28. Thoeny HC, De Keyzer F, Chen F, *et al.* Diffusion-weighted magnetic resonance imaging allows noninvasive in vivo monitoring of the effects

of combretastatin a-4 phosphate after repeated administration. *Neoplasia* 2005;**7** (8):779–87.

29. Lemaire L, Howe FA, Rodrigues LM, Griffiths JR. Assessment of induced rat mammary tumour response to chemotherapy using the apparent diffusion coefficient of tissue water as determined by diffusion-weighted 1H-NMR spectroscopy in vivo. *MAGMA Magn Reson Mater Phys* 1999;**8** (1):20–6.

30. Zhao M, Pipe JG, Bonnett J, Evelhoch JL. Early detection of treatment response by diffusion-weighted ^{1}H-NMR spectroscopy in a murine tumour in vivo. *Br J Cancer* 1996;**73** (1):61–4.

31. Babsky AM, Zhang H, Hekmatyar SK, Hutchins GD, Bansal N. Monitoring chemotherapeutic response in RIF-1 tumors by single-quantum and triple-quantum-filtered (23)Na MRI, (1)H diffusion-weighted MRI and PET imaging. *Magn Reson Imag* 2007;**25** (7):1015–23.

32. Seierstad T, Folkvord S, Roe K, *et al.* Early changes in apparent diffusion coefficient predict the quantitative antitumoral activity of capecitabine, oxaliplatin, and irradiation in HT29 xenografts in athymic nude mice. *Neoplasia* 2007;**9** (5):392–400.

33. Galons JP, Altbach MI, Paine-Murrieta GD, Taylor CW, Gillies RJ. Early increases in breast tumor xenograft water mobility in response to paclitaxel therapy detected by non-invasive diffusion magnetic resonance imaging. *Neoplasia* 1999;**1** (2):113–17.

34. Morse DL, Galons JP, Payne CM, *et al.* MRI-measured water mobility increases in response to chemotherapy via multiple cell-death mechanisms. *NMR Biomed* 2007;**20** (6):602–14.

35. Seierstad T, Roe K, Olsen DR. Noninvasive monitoring of radiation-induced treatment response using proton magnetic resonance spectroscopy and diffusion-weighted magnetic resonance imaging in a colorectal tumor model. *Radiother Oncol* 2007;**85** (2):187–94.

36. Roth Y, Tichler T, Kostenich G, *et al.* High-b-value diffusion-weighted MR imaging for pretreatment prediction and early monitoring of tumor response to therapy in mice. *Radiology* 2004;**232** (3):685–92.

37. Jordan BF, Runquist M, Raghunand N, *et al.* Dynamic contrast-enhanced and diffusion MRI show rapid and dramatic changes in tumor microenvironment in response to inhibition of HIF-1alpha using PX-478. *Neoplasia* 2005;**7** (5):475–85.

38. Le Bihan D, Delannoy J, Levin RL. Temperature mapping with MR imaging of molecular diffusion: application to hyperthermia. *Radiology* 1989;**171** (3):853–7.

39. Morvan D, Leroy-Willig A. Simultaneous measurements of diffusion and transverse relaxation in

exercising ske etal muscle. *Magn Reson Imag* 1995;**13**:943–8.

40. Braunschweiger PG. Effect of cyclophosphamide on the pathophysiology of RIF-1 solid tumors. *Cancer Res* 1988;**48** (15):4206–10.

41. Helmer KG, Meiler MR, Sotak CH, Petruccelli JD. Comparison of the return-to-the-origin probability and the apparent diffusion coefficient of water as indicators of necrosis in RIF-1 tumors. *Magn Reson Med* 2003;**49** (3):468–78.

42. Thoeny HC, De Keyzer F, Chen F, *et al.* Diffusion-weighted MR imaging in monitoring the effect of a vascular targeting agent on rhabdomyosarcoma in rats. *Radiology* 2005;**234** (3):756–64.

43. Tozer GM, Kanthou C, Parkins CS, Hill SA. The biology of the combretastatins as tumour vascular targeting agents. *Int J Exp Pathol* 2002;**83** (1):21–38.

44. Welsh S, Williams R, Kirkpatrick L, Paine-Murrieta G, Powis G. Antitumor activity and pharmacodynamic properties of PX-478, an inhibitor of hypoxia-inducible factor-1alpha. *Mol Cancer Ther* 2004; **3** (3):233–44.

45. Lyseng-Williamson KA, Fenton C. Docetaxel: a review of its use in metastatic breast cancer. *Drugs* 2005; **65** (17):2513–31.

46. Yuan YH, Xiao EH, Liu JB, *et al.* Characteristics and pathological mechanism on magnetic resonance diffusion-weighted imaging after chemoembolization in rabbit liver VX-2 tumor model. *World J Gastroenterol* 2007;**13** (43):5699–706.

47. Momparler RL, Karon M, Siegel SE, Avila F. Effect of adriamycin on DNA, RNA, and protein synthesis in cell-free systems and intact cells. *Cancer Res* 1976; **36** (8):2891–5.

48. Yuan YH, Xiao EH, Liu JB, *et al.* Characteristics of liver on magnetic resonance diffusion-weighted imaging: dynamic and image pathological investigation in rabbit liver VX-2 tumor model. *World J Gastroenterol* 2008;**14** (25):3997–4004.

49. Kim H, Morgan DE, Buchsbaum DJ, *et al.* Early therapy evaluation of combined anti-death receptor 5 antibody and gemcitabine in orthotopic pancreatic tumor xenografts by diffusion-weighted magnetic resonance imaging. *Cancer Res* 2008;**68** (20):8369–76.

50. Jennings D, Hatton BN, Guo J, *et al.* Early response of prostate carcinoma xenografts to docetaxel chemotherapy monitored with diffusion MRI. *Neoplasia* 2002;**4** (3):255–62.

51. Vogel-Claussen J, Gimi B, Artemov D, Bhujwalla ZM. Diffusion-weighted and macromolecular contrast enhanced MRI of tumor response to antivascular therapy with ZD6126. *Cancer Biol Ther* 2007; **6** (9):1469–75.

52. Micheletti G, Poli M, Borsotti P, *et al.* Vascular-targeting activity of ZD6126, a novel tubulin-binding agent. *Cancer Res* 2003;**63** (7):1534–7.

53. Dev SB, Caban JB, Nanda GS, *et al.* Magnetic resonance studies of laryngeal tumors implanted in nude mice: effect of treatment with bleomycin and electroporation. *Magn Reson Imag* 2002;**20** (5):389–94.

54. Poptani H, Bansal N, Graham RA, *et al.* Detecting early response to cyclophosphamide treatment of RIF-1 tumors using selective multiple quantum spectroscopy (SelMQC) and dynamic contrast enhanced imaging. *NMR Biomed* 2003;**16** (2):102–11.

55. Li S, Wehrle J, Glickson J, Kumar N, Braunschweiger P. Tumor bioenergetics and blood flow in RIF-1 murine tumors treated with 5-fluorouracil. *Magn Reson Med* 1991;**22** (1):47–56.

56. Goodman JA, Kroenke CD, Bretthorst GL, Ackerman JJ, Neil JJ. Sodium ion apparent diffusion coefficient in living rat brain. *Magn Reson Med* 2005;**53**:1040–5.

57. Lindinger MI, Heigenhauser GJ. Intracellular ion content of skeletal muscle measured by instrumental neutron activation analysis. *J Appl Physiol* 1987;**63**: 426–33.

58. Balschi JA, Bittl JA, Springer CSJ, Ingwall JS. ^{31}P and ^{23}Na NMR spectroscopy of normal and ischemic rat skeletal muscle: use of a shift reagent in vivo. *NMR Biomed* 1990;**3**:47–58.

59. Babsky A, Ju S, Topper S, *et al.* Noninvasive monitoring of the hepatocellular carcinoma growth by 1H and 23Na magnetic resonance imaging. *Ukr Biokhim Zh* 2009;**80** (4):130–7.

60. Colagrande S, Carbone SF, Carusi LM, Cova M, Villari N. Magnetic resonance diffusion-weighted imaging: extraneurological applications. *Radiol Med (Torino)* 2006;**111** (3):392–419.

61. Kamel IR, Bluemke DA, Eng J, *et al.* The role of functional MR imaging in the assessment of tumor response after chemoembolization in patients with hepatocellular carcinoma. *J Vasc Intervent Radiol* 2006;**17** (3):505–12.

62. Chen CY, Li CW, Kuo YT, *et al.* Early response of hepatocellular carcinoma to transcatheter arterial chemoembolization: choline levels and MR diffusion constants–initial experience. *Radiology* 2006; **239** (2):448–56.

63. Deng J, Miller FH, Rhee TK, *et al.* Diffusion-weighted MR imaging for determination of hepatocellular carcinoma response to yttrium-90

195

radioembolization. *J Vasc Intervent Radiol* 2006;**17** (7):1195–200.

64. Kamel IR, Reyes DK, Liapi E, Bluemke DA, Geschwind JF. Functional MR imaging assessment of tumor response after ^{90}Y microsphere treatment in patients with unresectable hepatocellular carcinoma. *J Vasc Intervent Radiol* 2007;**18** (1 Pt 1): 49–56.

65. Buijs M, Kamel IR, Vossen JA, *et al*. Assessment of metastatic breast cancer response to chemoembolization with contrast agent enhanced and diffusion-weighted MR imaging. *J Vasc Intervent Radiol* 2007;**18** (8):957–63.

66. Buijs M, Vossen JA, Hong K, *et al*. Chemoembolization of hepatic metastases from ocular melanoma: assessment of response with contrast-enhanced and diffusion-weighted MRI. *Am J Roentgenol* 2008;**191** (1):285–9.

67. Vossen JA, Kamel IR, Buijs M, *et al*. Role of functional magnetic resonance imaging in assessing metastatic leiomyosarcoma response to chemoembolization. *J Comput Assist Tomogr* 2008;**32** (3):347–52.

68. Pickles MD, Gibbs P, Lowry M, Turnbull LW. Diffusion changes precede size reduction in neoadjuvant treatment of breast cancer. *Magn Reson Imag* 2006;**24** (7):843–7.

69. Sharma U, Danishad KK, Seenu V, Jagannathan NR. Longitudinal study of the assessment by MRI and diffusion-weighted imaging of tumor response in patients with locally advanced breast cancer undergoing neoadjuvant chemotherapy. *NMR Biomed* 2009;**22** (1):104–13.

70. Yankeelov TE, Lepage M, Chakravarthy A, *et al*. Integration of quantitative DCE-MRI and ADC mapping to monitor treatment response in human breast cancer: initial results. *Magn Reson Imag* 2007; **25** (1):1–13.

71. Takayama Y, Kishimoto R, Hanaoka S, *et al*. ADC value and diffusion tensor imaging of prostate cancer: changes in carbon-ion radiotherapy. *J Magn Reson Imag* 2008;**27** (6):1331–5.

72. Kim CK, Park BK, Lee HM, Kim SS, Kim E. MRI techniques for prediction of local tumor progression after high-intensity focused ultrasonic ablation of prostate cancer. *Am J Roentgenol* 2008; **190** (5):1180–6.

73. Liapi E, Kamel IR, Bluemke DA, Jacobs MA, Kim HS. Assessment of response of uterine fibroids and myometrium to embolization using diffusion-weighted echoplanar MR imaging. *J Comput Assist Tomogr* 2005;**29** (1):83–6.

74. Fogt F, Hinds N, Zimmerman RL. Histologic features of uterine leiomyomata treated with microsphere embolization. *Obstet Gynecol* 2003;**102** (3):600–2.

75. Banovac F, Ascher SM, Jones DA, *et al*. Magnetic resonance imaging outcome after uterine artery embolization for leiomyomata with use of tris-acryl gelatin microspheres. *J Vasc Intervent Radiol* 2002; **13** (7):681–8.

76. Beaujeux R, Laurent A, Wassef M, *et al*. Trisacryl gelatin microspheres for therapeutic embolization. II. Preliminary clinical evaluation in tumors and arteriovenous malformations. *Am J Neuroradiol* 1996;**17** (3):541–8.

77. Jacobs MA, Herskovits EH, Kim HS. Uterine fibroids: diffusion-weighted MR imaging for monitoring therapy with focused ultrasound surgery – preliminary study. *Radiology* 2005;**236** (1):196–203.

78. Cheng KH, Hernandez M. Magnetic resonance diffusion imaging detects structural damage in biological tissues upon hyperthermia. *Cancer Res* 1992;**52** (21):6066–73.

79. Graham SJ, Stanisz GJ, Kecojevic A, Bronskill MJ, Henkelman RM. Analysis of changes in MR properties of tissues after heat treatment. *Magn Reson Med* 1999;**42** (6):1061–71.

80. Sevick RJ, Kanda F, Mintorovitch J, *et al*. Cytotoxic brain edema: assessment with diffusion-weighted MR imaging. *Radiology* 1992;**185** (3):687–90.

81. Byun WM, Shin SO, Chang Y, *et al*. Diffusion-weighted MR imaging of metastatic disease of the spine: assessment of response to therapy. *Am J Neuroradiol* 2002;**23** (6):906–12.

82. Hayashida Y, Yakushiji T, Awai K, *et al*. Monitoring therapeutic responses of primary bone tumors by diffusion-weighted image: Initial results. *Eur Radiol* 2006;**16** (12):2637–43.

83. Gaspersic N, Sersa I, Jevtic V, Tomsic M, Praprotnik S. Monitoring ankylosing spondylitis therapy by dynamic contrast-enhanced and diffusion-weighted magnetic resonance imaging. *Skeletal Radiol* 2008; **37** (2):123–31.

84. Dudeck O, Zeile M, Pink D, *et al*. Diffusion-weighted magnetic resonance imaging allows monitoring of anticancer treatment effects in patients with soft-tissue sarcomas. *J Magn Reson Imag* 2008; **27** (5):1109–13.

85. Kamm YJ, Heerschap A, Rosenbusch G, *et al*. 5-Fluorouracil metabolite patterns in viable and necrotic tumor areas of murine colon carcinoma determined by ^{19}F NMR spectroscopy. *Magn Reson Med* 1996;**36** (3):445–50.

86. Koh DM, Scurr E, Collins D, *et al.* Predicting response of colorectal hepatic metastasis: value of pretreatment apparent diffusion coefficients. *Am J Roentgenol* 2007;**188** (4):1001–8.

87. Theilmann RJ, Borders R, Trouard TP, *et al.* Changes in water mobility measured by diffusion MRI predict response of metastatic breast cancer to chemotherapy. *Neoplasia* 2004;**6** (6):831–7.

88. Manton DJ, Chaturvedi A, Hubbard A, *et al.* Neoadjuvant chemotherapy in breast cancer: early response prediction with quantitative MR imaging and spectroscopy. *Br J Cancer* 2006;**94** (3):427–35.

Diffusion-weighted MRI: future directions

Dow-Mu Koh and David J. Collins

Introduction

In the last few years, radiology has seen an unprecedented increase in the application of diffusion-weighted magnetic resonance imaging (DWI) for disease assessment in the body. This growing interest in body DWI is reflected by both wider clinical applications and focused research activities, and can be attributed to a greater awareness of the unique imaging information that the technique provides. In many imaging departments, DWI is now integrated into routine imaging protocols, in part to gain experience in applying the technique, but also for the diagnostic information that can be gained from an imaging technique which can be performed very quickly without detrimental effects or impact on the clinical throughput.

The current applications of DWI in the body are largely oncological[1,2], and are used in combination with conventional magnetic resonance imaging (MRI) sequences for disease detection and characterization and the assessment of treatment response. Non-oncological applications are also evolving, such as MR neurography[3], the evaluation of renal function[4], and the detection of liver fibrosis and cirrhosis[5,6]. However, as with any new technique, initial enthusiasm often gives way to a more realistic outlook, as the radiological community begins to recognize both the advantages and pitfalls of DWI. Nothing can be more damaging to the widespread adoption and application of a new imaging technique than unsubstantiated claims or unrealistic hype about its potential utility.

What is consistent across centers with greater experience in applying DWI in the body, is the recognition that careful technical optimization is important to achieve the best results[7]. Hence,

a sound understanding of the theory behind the imaging technique will ensure that the radiologist is equipped with sufficient knowledge to troubleshoot issues that may arise from its implementation. The radiologists should be familiar with imaging parameters that can be altered to improve image signal-to-noise ratio (SNR) and strategies that can be used to minimize artifacts that occur with spin-echo echo-planar imaging (EPI). The relative ease in imaging optimization varies between MR imaging platforms, with some posing more challenges than others. Not surprisingly, older MR imaging systems with poorer gradient performances or those without parallel imaging capability may struggle to achieve satisfactory results in the body.

Even when DW-MR images of different diffusion weightings (b-values) can be satisfactorily acquired, the need for accurate apparent diffusion coefficient (ADC) quantification within and between imaging centers poses additional challenges. For ADC measurements to be widely used for disease characterization and the assessment of treatment response, ADC measurements have to be accurate and reproducible[8–10] across imaging centers and MR platforms. This is yet to be fully realized, largely due to a lack of consensus as to what b-values may be appropriate for different imaging studies, how ADC calculations are to be made, as well as vendor MR system differences that make it is less straightforward to equalize imaging acquisitions across platforms[11].

In this chapter, we will survey some of the unmet needs of performing DWI in the body in terms of imaging acquisition, data analysis, image interpretation, and clinical translation of the technique. The potential ways in which these challenges could be met will be discussed.

Extra-Cranial Applications of Diffusion-Weighted MRI, ed. Bachir Taouli. Published by Cambridge University Press.
© Cambridge University Press 2011.

The future of DWI in the body

Image acquisition

DWI techniques

Currently, the most widely used DWI acquisition scheme in the body is fat-suppressed single-shot echo-planar imaging (EPI). However, there are inherent disadvantages of using an EPI-based imaging sequence in the body. First, EPI readouts are associated with relatively low signal-to-noise ratio (SNR). Second, the rapid switching of the magnetic gradients induces eddy currents and other EPI-related artifacts[12]. These include image ghosting and geometric distortion which can substantially degrade image quality. Image distortion also leads to misregistration of the DWI images, leading to errors in the calculated ADC map. As such, improvements to the EPI acquisition scheme could help to improve the quality of the DW-MR images and the accuracy of the ADC maps.

One possible approach is to employ a double spin-echo technique instead of the standard Stejskal–Tanner implementation[13,14]. This compensates for eddy current build-up, thus minimizing geometric distortion. The application of gradient reversal schemes which acquire images with positive and negative gradient polarity (bipolar gradients) can also help to cancel out the effects of eddy current[15]. The published literature has many novel schemes that have been shown to improve eddy current performance, but many have yet to be translated onto commercial MR imaging platforms. Minimizing geometric distortion is particularly relevant when there is a desire to use DWI for radiation planning purposes, since display of the anatomy without significant distortion is a requisite for accurate radiation targeting. Figure 13.1 shows the advantage of using a double spin-echo acquisition scheme compared with conventional standard Stejskal–Tanner spin-echo implementation. Using the double spin-echo sequence technique resulted in reduced geometric distortion compared with the Stejskal–Tanner acquisition scheme.

As DWI is usually performed in the body using single-shot EPI for spatial encoding, the technique is sensitive to chemical shift artifacts due to the low bandwidth in the phase encoding direction. To minimize chemical shift artifacts which can substantially degrade image quality and obscure imaging details, improvements in the fat-suppression scheme would therefore be welcomed. Currently, short tau

(a)

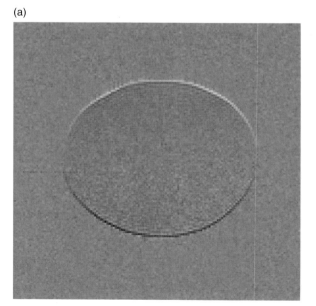

(b)

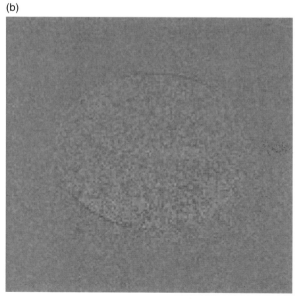

Figure 13.1 Image distortion using monopolar versus bipolar diffusion sensitizing gradients. Subtraction of $b = 1000$ s/mm^2 and $b = 0$ s/mm^2 MR images of a non-diffusing polydimethylsiloxane phantom acquired using (a) a monopolar Stejskal–Tanner diffusion sensitizing gradient and (b) a bipolar diffusion gradient. Note that in (a) the monopolar gradient scheme results in slight image distortion, resulting in the outline of the phantom being seen on the subtraction image. (b) The bipolar gradient scheme results in less eddy current-induced image distortion. Consequently, the outline of the phantom is successfully subtracted and not visible on the subtraction image.

(a) 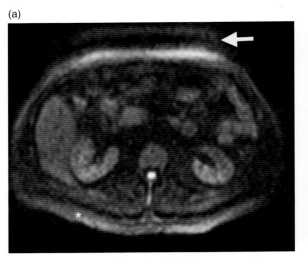 (b)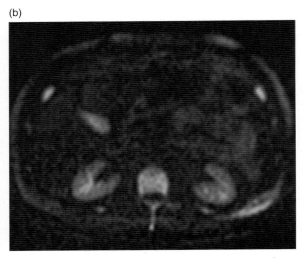

Figure 13.2 Fat suppression schemes for DWI in the body. DWI images of the abdomen acquired at 1.5 T using b-value of 750 s/mm^2 with (a) spectral attenuated inversion recovery (SPAIR) fat suppression and (b) short tau inversion recovery (STIR) fat suppression. In (a), suboptimal shimming resulted in significant chemical shift artifacts (arrow) and poor signal suppression of the fat in the posterior abdominal wall (*). By comparison, the fat signal is more effectively suppressed using the STIR fat suppression scheme. Note also that the background signal is better suppressed, including signal emanating from the contents within bowel loops.

inversion recovery (STIR) imaging is most frequently used in combination with DWI, especially over larger fields of view[16], and also at anatomical regions which are more likely to experience greater magnetic field inhomogeneity such as the breasts[17] (Figure 13.2). However, other methods are currently in development (discussed later) which aim to achieve a uniform fat suppression over a large field of view, thus improving background signal suppression and maximizing the lesion-to-background signal ratio.

Given some of the disadvantages of EPI-based imaging sequences, other DWI techniques are also currently being used or investigated. One technique that has been used with some frequency is the steady-state free precession (SSFP) DWI[18]. This technique is being used for the evaluation of the spine and has been shown to yield high-quality images, which are helpful for distinguishing between malignant and benign causes of vertebral collapse[19–21]. However, using such a gradient-echo based technique has its own inherent limitations. For example, ADC quantification using SSFP acquisitions can be challenging and requires more complex mathematical modeling[22–24]. However, as these challenges are addressed, software that will be able to process these images to obtain quantitative ADC maps may become available and could help to further widen its adoption.

Diffusion tensor imaging

DWI performed using multiple diffusion gradient encoding directions form the basis of diffusion tensor imaging (DTI) measurements. Although it is recognized that most tumors grow in a random fashion and therefore water diffusion tends to be isotropic in tumors, there is emerging evidence that the directionality of water diffusion in the body can further aid disease assessment. For example, in the normal prostate, unequal directional diffusivity has been observed due to structural organization of the glandular tissue. This is reflected by a higher fractional anisotropy (FA) measured by DTI within the normal central gland compared with the peripheral zone[25]. Interestingly, tumors in the central gland have been shown to have lower FA compared with glandular benign prostatic hypertrophy[26] (Figure 13.3).

Unequal directional diffusion has also been harnessed for image contrast. For example, in MR neurography, it has been found that applying the diffusing sensitizing gradient perpendicular to the direction of travel of the neural tracts or nerve bundles[3] resulted in improved visualization of these structures compared with trace images averaged from multi-direction image acquisition.

Diffusion tensor imaging has been used extensively in the brain to understand and delineate

(a)

(b)

(c)

(d)

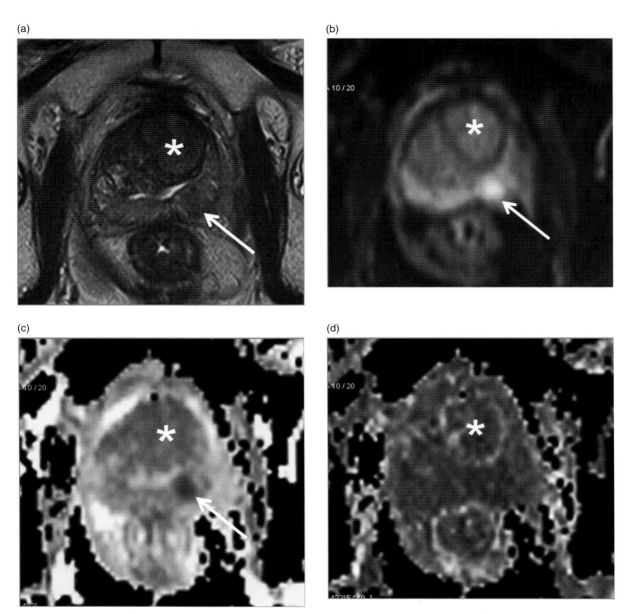

Figure 13.3 Diffusion tensor imaging (DTI) of the prostate. (a) Axial T2-weighted MR image, (b) $b= 1000$ s/mm^2 DWI image, (c) ADC map, and (d) fractional anisotropy (FA) map. There is a focus of prostate cancer in the peripheral zone of the left prostate gland (arrows). Although the cancer shows low ADC values, note that the fractional anisotropy is not significantly different from the rest of the peripheral zone. In the central gland, there is a region of glandular benign prostatic hypertrophy (*). The fibrotic capsule surrounding the prostatic hypertrophy shows low signal intensity on T2-weighted image and DWI. However, the structural organization of this fibrotic capsule also results in high fractional anisotropy observed in this area in (d). [Images courtesy of Dr. Anwar Padhani, UK.]

neurological pathways but its role in the body is not yet clearly established. Clearly, structural disruption demonstrated by DTI may prove to be a useful technique in identifying sites of disease infiltration. However, the implementation of DTI requires specialized imaging sequences, which are usually add-ons to the basic MR imaging platform, and are thus not currently universally available.

Imaging at higher magnetic fields

The experience that has been accrued so far for body DWI is largely based on studies performed at 1.5 T. Even though imaging at a higher field strength of 3 T is potentially advantageous because of higher SNR, there are many challenges to its effective implementation.

Two issues are of particular relevance when using the EPI DWI technique at 3 T: fat suppression and geometric distortion. Due to the greater inhomogeneity of the static magnetic field when a patient is placed within the scanner, achieving uniform fat suppression for body DWI can be challenging. Optimal volume shimming aids in achieving uniform fat suppression, but even this does not work consistently at 3 T over larger fields of view or where there is considerable magnetic field inhomogeneity. Poor fat suppression results in ghosting and chemical shift artifacts, which obscure disease visualization and lead to errors in ADC calculations. Hence, novel fat suppression techniques are currently being investigated and developed with the aim of achieving consistent uniform fat suppression across relatively large fields of view at 3 T. For example, on the Philips Medical 3T System (Philips Medical System, Best, The Netherlands), recent implementation of the slice selective gradient reversal (SSGR) fat suppression technique has helped to improve fat suppression at 3 T, which can be used in combination with DWI[27] (Figure 13.4). Using slice selective gradients of opposing polarity, unwanted signal arising from fat can be suppressed without affecting the water signal intensity or the image slice profile[27]. Other fat suppression techniques being investigated include the simultaneous application of STIR with chemical fat saturation techniques.

Geometric distortion arising from eddy current effects can be significant at 3 T, making it difficult to localize abnormalities observed on DWI with the corresponding morphological image. Thus, strategies to reduce eddy currents related to EPI acquisitions at 3 T should be actively pursued. Some of the possible approaches include the routine implementation of twice-refocused spin-echo sequences and the application of paired positive and negative (bipolar) gradient directions to minimize eddy current effects, as previously discussed.

Despite the improved SNR, the quality of DWI in the body can be variable at 3 T and clearly more research is needed in this area to ensure optimized imaging protocols can be consistently performed across different vendor systems. As hardware performance is enhanced by the introduction of parallel transmit technology, it is likely that the performance of DWI at 3 T will continue to improve.

Measurement reproducibility

For quantitative ADC to be widely applied for disease evaluation, knowledge of the measurement variability or reproducibility is required. The measurement

(a)

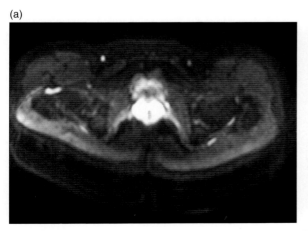

(b)

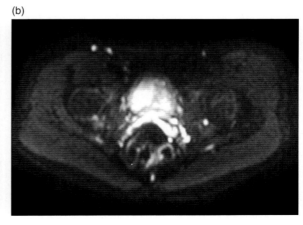

Figure 13.4 Fat suppression schemes for body DWI at 3 T. Effective fat suppression for DWI in the body can be challenging at 3 T due to the magnetic field inhomogeneity. (a) DWI acquired using STIR (TI = 240 ms) fat suppression at 3 T shows poor fat suppression posteriorly over the gluteal area with chemical shift artifacts. (b) Fat suppression can be considerably improved by applying a novel fat suppression scheme (slice selective gradient reversal, SSGR). In this example, imaging was performed slightly cranial to (a) using the combination of STIR and SSGR. Note substantial improvement in the suppression of the fat signal.

reproducibility informs us of the ADC variations that can be ascribed to measurement errors, observer errors, and biological variations. Knowledge of the reproducibility provides us with the confidence that an observed change in the measured ADC value can be ascribed to therapy rather than measurement variability.

Emerging data suggest that DWI measurements are highly reproducible in the body. Comparing techniques in the liver, free-breathing DWI was found to be more reproducible compared with breath-hold or respiratory-triggered acquisition[10]. Free-breathing DWI was also found to be reproducible across a two-center imaging study[28], with a low coefficient of reproducibility of approximately 14% (Figure 13.5). Furthermore, measurement reproducibility was found to be reasonably reproducible at

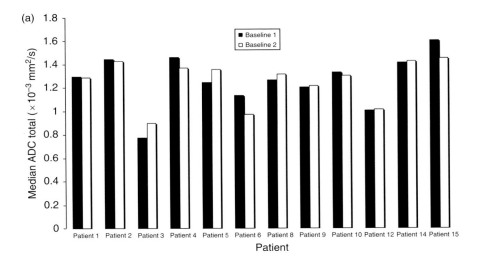

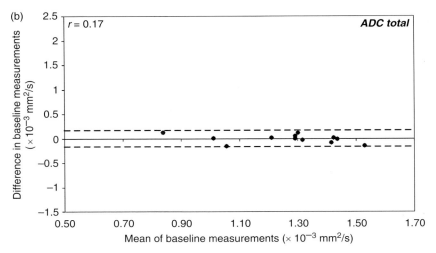

Figure 13.5 ADC measurement reproducibility. Measurement reproducibility informs us of the ADC variability that may result from measurement, observer, or biological variations. This can be estimated by a test–retest study, where ADC measurements are acquired from the same region, typically 24 h apart. In this example of a patient cohort with metastatic solid tumors in the abdomen and pelvis (a) the paired mean ADC values of a target tumor in each patient are plotted on the bar chart, which allows quick visual assessment of the variability of the paired measurements. (b) The measurement reproducibility is calculated by using Bland–Altman statistics and the Bland–Altman plot is shown here. The differences of the mean paired measurements (y-axis) are plotted against their averaged values (x-axis). The dotted lines represent the 95% confidence intervals, which also denote the coefficient of repeatability (r). [Reproduced with permission from Koh DM et al. Reproducibility and changes in the apparent diffusion coefficients of solid tumors treated with combretastatin A4 phosphate and bevacizumab in a two-centre phase I clinical trial. Eur Radiol 2009;19:2728–38.]

3 T within the abdomen, with a coefficient of repro-ducibility of approximately 27% (or coefficient of variance of 14%)[8]. In a study of ADC variability of measurements made in the brains of volunteers who were evaluated on multiple MR imaging platforms across different sites[29], it was found that ADC vari-ability was as high as 8% between imaging systems. However, this still compares favorably with the meas-urement reproducibility reported in the body.

The published findings of ADC measurement reproducibility are highly encouraging for the appli-cations of quantitative ADC values for disease char-acterization and assessment of therapy response. However, more research is needed to further under-stand the nature of measurement errors across mul-tiple sites using different vendor MR systems, so that these can be minimized to ensure confidence in the utility of quantitative DWI for disease assessment.

Imaging standardization

There is a need for standardization of acquisition techniques across imaging platforms to allow results between centers and scanner platforms to be com-pared. Review of published literature suggests that there is a wide variation in the DWI techniques applied, including the choice of b-values and other acquisition parameters when performing DWI.

The choice of b-values has a direct influence on the calculated ADC. ADC values calculated from imaging studies performed using only relatively low b-values (<100 s/mm^2) would be significantly con-taminated by perfusion effect. By contrast, ADC values calculated from higher b-values are relatively free from perfusion effects. ADC values calculated from a range of b-values, including both lower and higher b-values, may be weighted towards the higher b-values if the range of b-values used for imaging is appropriately chosen. Imaging standardization and protocol harmonization across different MR vendors would be very important to ensure consistency of ADC calculations so that results between different centers may be compared with confidence.

In 2008, a consensus meeting was held at the International Society of Magnetic Resonance in Medi-cine meeting in Toronto. This National Cancer Insti-tute (NCI)-led initiative resulted in the publication of a "white paper" which outlined the roadmap for standardization of the technique to develop DWI as a potential imaging biomarker[11]. The need for tech-nical standardization has to be championed by all involved in performing such studies to ensure that reliable results can be consistently achieved.

Quality assurance

In tandem with improvements in clinical MR acqui-sition technique for DWI, development of a well-planned quality assurance program is needed to validate hardware and MR system performance. Quality assurance checks on scanner performance are needed to ensure that ADC measurements are reliable and can be consistently reproduced.

A variety of phantoms or test objects can be used to verify the imaging performance of DWI (Figure 13.6). Of these, the iced water phantom appears to be a relatively simple and widely available solution. Imaging of a phantom containing iced water is attract-ive for a few reasons. First, the temperature of the phantom is maintained at 0–4 °C, thus controlling the temperature dependency of the ADC measure-ments. The ADC values of water at these temperatures are well known, making it easy to validate the test results. Second, iced water is widely available and is non-toxic compared with some of the phantom mater-ials. Third, the iced water phantom also allows for the evaluation of the gradient performance and eddy currents induced geometric distortion.

Other imaging phantoms that have been employed include those containing sucrose and copper sulphate solutions[30]. Another test object that can be used is made of a non-diffusing material such as polydimethylsiloxane (PDMS). As the material is non-diffusing, there should be no significant signal attenuation across the phantom with increasing b-values. Such a phantom is ideally suited to determine the degree of geometric distortion that occurs with EPI DWI, which reflects the eddy current performance of the MR system under test. Clearly, phantom con-struction for evaluating DTI performance is much more complex requiring objects with structural organ-ization[31,32]. A discussion of this is beyond the scope of the current chapter.

Data analysis

Once the DW-MR images are acquired, the images can be used for both qualitative and quantitative evaluation. DW-MR images can be viewed on stand-ard workstations of hospital picture archiving systems (PACS), although sometimes, it may be necessary to engage the help of the information system engineer to

(a)

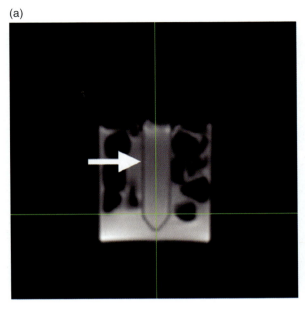

(b)

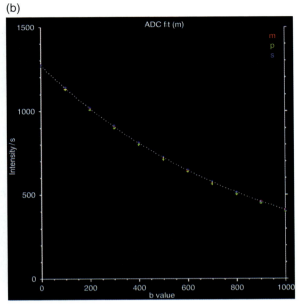

Figure 13.6 Ice water phantom for quality assurance. (a) T2-weighted MR imaging showing a simple ice water phantom, which consists of a tube of pure distilled water (arrow) submerged in a bath of ice cubes (courtesy of Prof. Thomas Chenevert, University of Michigan). (b) DWI was performed using multiple b-values (0 to 1000 s/mm^2) and diffusion gradients applied in the frequency select (m), phase select (p) and slice selection (s) directions. The signal attenuation with increasing b-value curve is as shown. The calculated ADC is compared with known published literature values.

ensure that the b-value images are appropriately displayed to facilitate viewing. The ADC map is typically generated using all the b-value images acquired. The vendor workstations usually afford greater flexibility for image display and manipulation than those available on PACS.

Workstations for image analysis

To optimize qualitative assessment, the imaging platform should allow DWI images to be displayed side-by-side with conventional imaging, and provide the ability to perform image fusion of the DWI images with conventional morphological images.

For quantitative analysis, software developments that would allow more sophisticated fitting of the ADC data would be helpful. Currently, on most vendor MR systems, the ADC is calculated across all the b-values acquired and provides limited interactivity between the user and the analysis platform. For example, the ability to check the accuracy of exponential algorithm fit to the acquired data is not possible. Furthermore, most systems will only allow output of the mean or median value of a region of interest drawn on the ADC map. It is usually not possible to obtain voxelwise ADC values within each region of interest. Voxelwise analysis has already been shown to be of value in some instances, by demonstrating heterogeneous ADC changes within the tumor voxels in response to treatment[33]. Voxelwise data would also allow for review of the data by histogram analysis (Figure 13.7). In addition, regions of interest drawn cannot be currently saved for future reference or use, making it difficult to recreate quantitative ADC data necessary for the purpose of audit trail in clinical trials. For these reasons, institutions engaged in DWI research or clinical trials are usually reliant on in-house analysis software to perform the necessary parametric calculations. Clearly, these issues need to be addressed so that robust commercial software systems would eventually become available to all to undertake ADC analysis in a clinical or research trial setting.

More sophisticated methods of modeling ADC data should also be actively explored. These include the use of a biexponential model such as by applying the principles of intravoxel incoherent motion (IVIM) (Figure 13.8)[34,35] or stretched exponentials[36]. Using voxelwise analysis will also be helpful to further understand and characterize tumor heterogeneity. For example, disease response defined by voxelwise

205

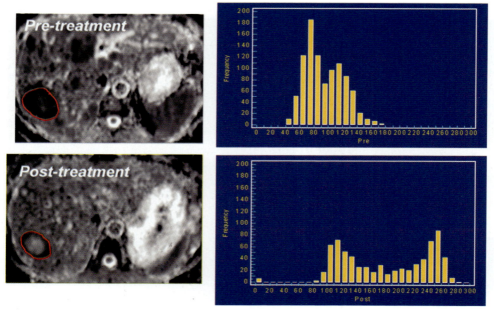

Figure 13.7 Visualizing tumor response to treatment. (a) Pre-treatment ADC map and ADC histogram of target liver metastasis (outlined in red), (b) post-treatment ADC map and ADC histogram of target liver metastasis (outlined in red) after 1 month of treatment with a novel therapeutic agent. Note slight reduction in size of the liver metastasis (<30% diameter reduction). However, there was marked increase in the median ADC values, with significant shift of tumor voxel histogram values to the right.

analysis of ADC data in patients with brain gliomas has been shown to be predictive of patient survival[37,38]. Furthermore, quantitative analysis of the entire tumor volume rather than of a single image section may also help to explore and reveal regional differences in tumors.

Data and image interpretation

As experience with DWI grows, there is no doubt that this imaging technique will increasingly be used in combination with conventional imaging, either alone or with image fusion, for clinical evaluation of diseases. As the technology continues to mature, imaging studies which are currently only performed in specialist centers could be rolled out to a wider radiological community. For example, although whole body diffusion-weighted imaging (WBDWI) has been shown in some studies to have a very high diagnostic accuracy for tumor staging[39], the technique has not been widely implemented. This is in part related to the challenges of ensuring optimal performance at all scanning stations in the body and the availability of software to display and interrogate the image dataset robustly, within the clinical workflow of the department.

Quantitative DWI has been shown to be of value for tumor response to treatment, especially for the assessment of novel therapeutics and also at sites that are deemed difficult to assess by other current imaging modalities (e.g., the bone marrow)[40]. An increase in the mean ADC value of tumors has been shown to be a consistent feature following a variety of therapeutic interventions, in keeping with cellular necrosis and cell death[1,2,41]. However, what is still unclear is the optimal timing of these measurements in relation to the therapeutic intervention, even though there is already evidence that DWI is able to detect early change within tumors as early as 3–7 days after initiating treatment[33,42,43]. Equally intriguing has been the fact that the baseline pre-treatment ADC values have been shown to be of prognostic value in various tumor types such as brain tumors[44], rectal cancer[45], head and neck tumors[46] and liver metastases[47,48]. Tumors with lower pre-treatment ADC values have been shown to respond better to chemotherapy and/or radiotherapy. Ultimately, the clinical value of quantitative ADC for the assessment of treatment response would depend on its ability to inform on patient outcome. Interestingly, recent studies have shown that the functional changes measured

(a)

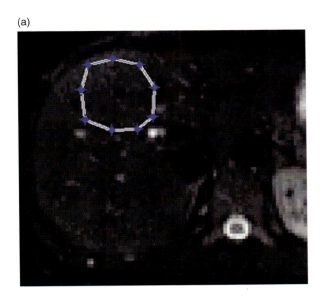

Figure 13.8 Intravoxel incoherent motion (IVIM). (a) DW-MR $b = 0$ s/mm^2 image. A region of interest is drawn over the right lobe of the liver (white circle). (b) Plot of signal intensity (y-axis) versus b-value (x-axis) averaged over the entire region of interest and fitted to the data points by applying the principles of IVIM. This shows initial higher rate of signal attenuation over the lower b-values (<100 s/mm^2) due to the effects of capillary perfusion. The signal attenuation over the higher b-values is more reflective of tissue diffusivity.

(b)

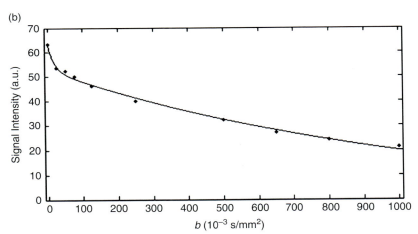

by DWI can be used to predict survival in patients with high-grade gliomas[49,50].

As the imaging technological platforms become more sophisticated, there is a huge opportunity to compare and correlate the functional information of DWI with other novel imaging techniques such as dynamic contrast-enhanced computed tomography (CT), MR spectroscopy, perfusion CT, and even positron emission tomography (PET) imaging. Recognizing that each of these functional imaging techniques provides a different biological readout of the underlying pathophysiological changes, interpreting images alongside one another is likely to further improve our understanding of the pathophysiological changes within the tumor, thus providing a better phenotypical assessment of diseases. Imaging technology has revolutionized how diseases are visualized in the body. Multidetector CT and MR imaging advancements have moved conventional imaging from a 2D to 3D perception of diseases. It is now possible to acquire information over one particular area by quick and successive measurements providing time-resolved information (4D), which has been shown to be of value for disease characterization. The next step could be seen as a "fifth-dimensional" (5D) development, by integrating spatially correlated and biologically relevant information acquired using different imaging techniques, to a provide a multifaceted assessment of disease.

As new metrics for DWI evolve, the biological basis of these observations will require further validation. Amongst the various model fitting methods being investigated for DWI, the use of IVIM[35] (Figure 13.8) and stretched exponentials have generated considerable interest. This is because of the perceived advantages of being able to quantify both tissue perfusion and tissue diffusivity using a single MR measurement without the need for intravenous contrast administration. However, for more complex data fitting, high-quality images acquired using multiple b-values would be necessary. Other DWI-derived techniques such as q-space or diffusion kurtosis imaging in the body are also currently being investigated.

Clinical translation

Understanding the biological changes that account for the appearance of DW images has been widely investigated using animal models. These experiments have provided us with better understanding of differences in the DW imaging appearances and ADC values of native tissues, as well as providing insight into tissue changes that result in ADC alterations with treatment. However, translating such knowledge from the animal model to humans can sometimes be challenging as the knowledge is not always transferable. For example, administration of the antivascular prodrug combretastatin A4 phosphate has been shown in animals to result in transient decrease in ADC values at 3 h after drug administration due to cellular edema, followed by an increase in ADC value as a result of tumor lysis or necrosis at 48 h after treatment[51]. When a similar experiment was conducted in humans[28], only an increase in ADC value could be observed at 1 week after therapy but not acutely at 3 h after drug administration. This suggests that the experiences learned in animals are not always translatable onto the human scale and there is therefore a need to constantly model and appraise our understanding of DWI by the use of appropriate back-translation studies.

Clearly, DWI is still currently not recognized as an established or a validated imaging biomarker. Validation would depend on establishing its measurement variability across multiple centers, as well as a firm understanding of the biological basis for the measurement observation. Ultimately, the aim of biomarker qualification is to provide evidence that DWI can be a reliable surrogate endpoint for a defined clinical outcome.

Currently, there is considerable interest in using DWI in early clinical trials to inform on "go"/"no-go" decision-making in drug development. However, there is a bottleneck to the clinical validation of the technology. Clinical units and radiological departments can find it challenging to perform these studies in an environment where patient throughput may be more important in defining the success of a radiological unit. Equally important, radiological education needs to embrace such new technology and provide guidance and education, to teach new functional imaging techniques to the wider radiological community so that they can be widely tested and validated. The setting up of specialist boards such as the Quantitative Imaging Biomarker Alliance (QIBA) and the various National Cancer Institute (NCI)-led quantitative imaging initiatives are vital in defining the role and standards for conducting these studies. More international collaborations will be vital to ensure that DWI becomes a useful imaging biomarker for radiological diagnosis, treatment assessment, and drug development.

References

1. Koh DM, Collins DJ. Diffusion-weighted MRI in the body: applications and challenges in oncology. *Am J Roentgenol* 2007;**188**:1622–35.

2. Patterson DM, Padhani AR, Collins DJ. Technology insight: water diffusion MRI – a potential new biomarker of response to cancer therapy. *Nat Clin Pract Oncol* 2008;**5**:220–33.

3. Takahara T, Hendrikse J, Yamashita T, *et al.* Diffusion-weighted MR neurography of the brachial plexus: feasibility study. *Radiology* 2008;**249**:653–60.

4. Thoeny HC, Zumstein D, Simon-Zoula S, *et al.* Functional evaluation of transplanted kidneys with diffusion-weighted and BOLD MR imaging: initial experience. *Radiology* 2006;**241**:812–21.

5. Annet L, Peeters F, Abarca-Quinones J, *et al.* Assessment of diffusion-weighted MR imaging in liver fibrosis. *J Magn Reson Imag* 2007;**25**:122–8.

6. Taouli B, Tolia AJ, Losada M, *et al.* Diffusion-weighted MRI for quantification of liver fibrosis: preliminary experience. *Am J Roentgenol* 2007;**189**:799–806.

7. Koh DM, Takahara T, Imai Y, Collins DJ. Practical aspects of assessing tumors using clinical diffusion-weighted imaging in the body. *Magn Reson Med Sci* 2008;**6**:211–24.

8. Braithwaite AC, Dale BM, Boll DT, Merkle EM. Short- and midterm reproducibility of apparent diffusion coefficient measurements at 3.0-T

diffusion-weighted imaging of the abdomen. *Radiology* 2009;**250**:459–65.

9. Kwee TC, Takahara T, Luijten PR, Nievelstein RA. ADC measurements of lymph nodes: inter- and intra-observer reproducibility study and an overview of the literature. *Eur J Radiol* 2009;**18**:1937–52.

10. Kwee TC, Takahara T, Koh DM, Nievelstein RA, Luijten PR. Comparison and reproducibility of ADC measurements in breathhold, respiratory triggered, and free-breathing diffusion-weighted MR imaging of the liver. *J Magn Reson Imag* 2008; **28**:1141–8.

11. Padhani AR, Liu G, Mu-Koh D, *et al.* Diffusion-weighted magnetic resonance imaging as a cancer biomarker: consensus and recommendations. *Neoplasia* 2009;**11**:102–25.

12. Le Bihan D, Poupon C, Amadon A, Lethimonnier F. Artifacts and pitfalls in diffusion MRI. *J Magn Reson Imag* 2006;**24**:478–88.

13. Finsterbusch J. Eddy-current compensated diffusion weighting with a single refocusing RF pulse. *Magn Reson Med* 2009;**61**:748–54.

14. Reese TG, Heid O, Weisskoff RM, Wedeen VJ. Reduction of eddy-current-induced distortion in diffusion MRI using a twice-refocused spin echo. *Magn Reson Med* 2003;**49**:177–82.

15. Alexander AL, Tsuruda JS, Parker DL. Elimination of eddy current artifacts in diffusion-weighted echo-planar images: the use of bipolar gradients. *Magn Reson Med* 1997;**38**:1016–21.

16. Takahara T, Imai Y, Yamashita T, *et al.* Diffusion weighted whole body imaging with background body signal suppression (DWIBS): technical improvement using free breathing, STIR and high resolution 3D display. *Radiat Med* 2004;**22**:275–82.

17. Kazama T, Nasu K, Kuroki Y, Nawano S, Ito H. Comparison of diffusion-weighted images using short inversion time inversion recovery or chemical shift selective pulse as fat suppression in patients with breast cancer. *Jap J Radiol* 2009;**27**:163–7.

18. Zur Y, Bosak E, Kaplan N. A new diffusion SSFP imaging technique. *Magn Reson Med* 1997;**37**:716–22.

19. Abanoz R, Hakyemez B, Parlak M. [Diffusion-weighted imaging of acute vertebral compression: differential diagnosis of benign versus malignant pathologic fractures.] *Tani Girisim Radyol* 2003; **9**:176–83.

20. Baur A, Huber A, Durr HR, *et al.* [Differentiation of benign osteoporotic and neoplastic vertebral compression fractures with a diffusion-weighted, steady-state free precession sequence.] *Rofo Fortschr Röntgenstr* 2002;**174**:70–5.

21. Baur A, Huber A, Ertl-Wagner B, *et al.* Diagnostic value of increased diffusion weighting of a steady-state free precession sequence for differentiating acute benign osteoporotic fractures from pathologic vertebral compression fractures. *Am J Neuroradiol* 2001;**22**:366–72.

22. Carney CE, Wong ST, Patz S. Analytical solution and verification of diffusion effect in SSFP. *Magn Reson Med* 1991;**19**:240–6.

23. Miller KL, Jezzard P. Modeling SSFP functional MRI contrast in the brain. *Magn Reson Med* 2008; **60**:661–73.

24. Petersson JS, Christoffersson JO. A multidimensional partition analysis of SSFP image pulse sequences. *Magn Reson Imag* 1997;**15**:451–67.

25. Gurses B, Kabakci N, Kovanlikaya A, *et al.* Diffusion tensor imaging of the normal prostate at 3 tesla. *Eur Radiol* 2008;**18**:716–21.

26. Xu J, Humphrey PA, Kibel AS, *et al.* Magnetic resonance diffusion characteristics of histologically defined prostate cancer in humans. *Magn Reson Med* 2009;**61**:842–50.

27. Nagy Z, Weiskopf N. Efficient fat suppression by slice-selection gradient reversal in twice-refocused diffusion encoding. *Magn Reson Med* 2008;**60**:1256–60.

28. Koh DM, Blackledge M, Collins DJ, *et al.* Reproducibility and changes in the apparent diffusion coefficients of solid tumours treated with combretastatin A4 phosphate and bevacizumab in a two-centre phase I clinical trial. *Eur Radiol* 2009;**19**:2728–38.

29. Sasaki M, Yamada K, Watanabe Y, *et al.* Variability in absolute apparent diffusion coefficient values across different platforms may be substantial: a multivendor, multi-institutional comparison study. *Radiology* 2008;**249**:624–30.

30. Delakis I, Moore EM, Leach MO, De Wilde JP. Developing a quality control protocol for diffusion imaging on a clinical MRI system. *Phys Med Biol* 2004;**49**:1409–22.

31. Latt J, Nilsson M, Rydhog A, *et al.* Effects of restricted diffusion in a biological phantom: a q-space diffusion MRI study of asparagus stems at a 3T clinical scanner. *MAGMA Magn Reson Mater Phys* 2007;**20**:213–22.

32. Yanasak N, Allison J. Use of capillaries in the construction of an MRI phantom for the assessment of diffusion tensor imaging: demonstration of performance. *Magn Reson Imag* 2006;**24**:1349–61.

33. Mardor Y, Pfeffer R, Spiegelmann R, *et al.* Early detection of response to radiation therapy in patients with brain malignancies using conventional and high

209

b-value diffusion-weighted magnetic resonance imaging. *J Clin Oncol* 2003;**21**:1094–100.

34. Le Bihan D. Intravoxel incoherent motion perfusion MR imaging: a wake-up call. *Radiology* 2008; **249**:748–52.

35. Le Bihan D, Breton E, Lallemand D, *et al.* Separation of diffusion and perfusion in intravoxel incoherent motion MR imaging. *Radiology* 1988;**168**:497–505.

36. Kwee TC, Galban CJ, Tsien C, *et al.* Intravoxel water diffusion heterogeneity imaging of human high-grade gliomas. *NMR Biomed* 2009;**23**:179–87.

37. Moffat BA, Chenevert TL, Lawrence TS, *et al.* Functional diffusion map: a noninvasive MRI biomarker for early stratification of clinical brain tumor response. *Proc Natl Acad Sci USA* 2005;**102**:5524–9.

38. Moffat BA, Chenevert TL, Meyer CR, *et al.* The functional diffusion map: an imaging biomarker for the early prediction of cancer treatment outcome. *Neoplasia* 2006;**8**:259–67.

39. Ohno Y, Koyama H, Onishi Y, *et al.* Non-small cell lung cancer: whole-body MR examination for M-stage assessment: utility for whole-body diffusion-weighted imaging compared with integrated FDG PET/CT. *Radiology* 2008;**248**:643–54.

40. Lee KC, Bradley DA, Hussain M, *et al.* A feasibility study evaluating the functional diffusion map as a predictive imaging biomarker for detection of treatment response in a patient with metastatic prostate cancer to the bone. *Neoplasia* 2007;**9**:1003–11.

41. Hamstra DA, Rehemtulla A, Ross BD. Diffusion magnetic resonance imaging: a biomarker for treatment response in oncology. *J Clin Oncol* 2007;**25**:4104–9.

42. Chen CY, Li CW, Kuo YT, *et al.* Early response of hepatocellular carcinoma to transcatheter arterial chemoembolization: choline levels and MR diffusion constants – initial experience. *Radiology* 2006; **239**:448–56.

43. Theilmann RJ, Borders R, Trouard TP, *et al.* Changes in water mobility measured by diffusion MRI predict response of metastatic breast cancer to chemotherapy. *Neoplasia* 2004;**6**:831–7.

44. Mardor Y, Roth Y, Ochershvilli A, *et al.* Pretreatment prediction of brain tumors' response to radiation therapy using high b-value diffusion-weighted MRI. *Neoplasia* 2004;**6**:136–42.

45. Dzik-Jurasz A, Domenig C, George M, *et al.* Diffusion MRI for prediction of response of rectal cancer to chemoradiation. *Lancet* 2002;**360**:307–8.

46. Kim S, Loevner L, Quon H, *et al.* Diffusion-weighted magnetic resonance imaging for predicting and detecting early response to chemoradiation therapy of squamous cell carcinomas of the head and neck. *Clin Cancer Res* 2009;**15**:986–94.

47. Koh DM, Scurr E, Collins DJ, *et al.* Predicting response of colorectal hepatic metastases: value of pre-treatment apparent diffusion coefficients. *Am J Roentgenol* 2007;**188**:1001–8.

48. Cui Y, Zhang XP, Sun YS, Tang L, Shen L. Apparent diffusion coefficient: potential imaging biomarker for prediction and early detection of response to chemotherapy in hepatic metastases. *Radiology* 2008; **248**:894–900.

49. Hamstra DA, Galban CJ, Meyer CR, *et al.* Functional diffusion map as an early imaging biomarker for high-grade glioma: correlation with conventional radiologic response and overall survival. *J Clin Oncol* 2008;**26**:3387–94.

50. Hamstra DA, Chenevert TL, Moffat BA, *et al.* Evaluation of the functional diffusion map as an early biomarker of time-to-progression and overall survival in high-grade glioma. *Proc Natl Acad Sci USA* 2005;**102**:16 759–64.

51. Thoeny HC, De Keyzer F, Vandecaveye V, *et al.* Effect of vascular targeting agent in rat tumor model: dynamic contrast-enhanced versus diffusion-weighted MR imaging. *Radiology* 2005;**237**:492–9.

Index